theclinics.com

NEUROLOGIC CLINICS

Multiple Sclerosis

GUEST EDITOR
Jerry S. Wolinsky, MD

February 2005 • Volume 23 • Number 1

SAUNDERS

An Imprint of Elsevier, Inc.
PHILADELPHIA LONDON TORONTO MONTREAL SYDNEY TOKYO

W.B. SAUNDERS COMPANY
A Division of Elsevier Inc.

The Curtis Center • Independence Square West • Philadelphia, Pennsylvania 19106

http://www.theclinics.com

NEUROLOGIC CLINICS **Volume 23, Number**
February 2005 **ISSN 0733-861**
Editor: Robert Gardler **ISBN 1-4160-2829-**

Neurologic Clinics (ISSN 0733-8619) is published quarterly by Elsevier. Corporate and editorial offices: 170 Independence Mall W 300 E, Philadelphia, PA 19106-3399. Accounting and circulation offices: 6277 Se Harbor Drive, Orlando, FL 32887-4800. Periodicals postage paid at Orlando, FL 32862, and additional mailin offices. Subscription prices are $175.00 per year for US individuals, $275.00 per year for US institutions, $88.0 per year for US students, $214.00 per year for Canadian individuals, $325.00 per year for Canadian institu tions, and $113.00 per year for Canadian students. To receive student/resident rate, orders must be accompa nied by name of affiliated institution, date of term, and the *signature* of program/residency coordinator o institution letterhead. Orders will be billed at individual rate until proof of status is received. Foreign air spee delivery is included in all *Clinics* subscription prices. All prices are subject to change without notice. POST MASTER: Send address changes to *Neurologic Clinics*, W.B. Saunders Company, Periodicals Fulfillment, Orland FL 32887-4800. **Customer Service: 1-800-654-2452 (US). From outside of the US, call 1-407-345-4000.**

Neurologic Clinics is also published in Spanish by Nueva Editorial Interamericana S.A., Mexico City, Mexic

Neurologic Clinics is covered in *Current Contents/Clinical Medicine, Index Medicus, EMBASE*/Excerpta Medic and *PsycINFO*, and *ISI/BIOMED*.

Printed in the United States of America.

GUEST EDITOR

JERRY S. WOLINSKY, MD, Bartels Family Professor of Neurology, The University of Texas, Health Sciences Center at Houston, Houston, Texas

CONTRIBUTORS

HAROLD ATKINS, MD, Assistant Professor, University of Ottawa and Ottawa Hospital Blood and Marrow Transplant Program, Ottawa, Ontario, Canada

AMIT BAR-OR, MD, FRCPC, Assistant Professor, Neurology and Neurosurgery, Montreal Neurological Institute, and Associate, Microbiology and Immunology, McGill University; and Staff Neurologist, Montreal Neurological Hospital, McGill University Hospital Center, Quebec, Montreal, Canada

WOLFGANG BRUCK, MD, Institute of Neuropathology, Göttingen, Germany

GUY J. BUCKLE, MD, Partners Multiple Sclerosis Center, Brigham and Women's Hospital; Instructor in Neurology, Harvard Medical School, Boston, Massachusetts

PATRICIA K. COYLE, MD, Professor and Acting Chair, Department of Neurology, and Director, Multiple Sclerosis Comprehensive Care Center, School of Medicine, SUNY at Stony Brook, Stony Brook, New York

MARK FREEDMAN, MD, Professor, University of Ottawa and Ottawa Hospital Multiple Sclerosis Clinic, Ottawa, Ontario, Canada

SUSAN A. GAUTHIER, DO, Partners Multiple Sclerosis Center, Brigham and Women's Hospital; Instructor in Neurology, Harvard Medical School, Boston, Massachusetts

STEPHEN L. HAUSER, MD, Professor and Chair, Department of Neurology, University of California at San Francisco, School of Medicine, San Francisco, California

ORHUN H. KANTARCI, MD, Department of Neurology, Mayo Clinic College of Medicine, Rochester, Minnesota

LUDWIG KAPPOS, MD, Professor, Department of Neurology, University Hospitals, Kantonspital, Basel, Switzerland

DAVID K.B. LI, MD, FRCPC, Professor, Department of Radiology, The University of British Columbia, Vancouver, British Columbia, Canada

FRED D. LUBLIN, MD, Saunders Family Professor of Neurology, and Director, Corinne Goldsmith Dickinson Center for Multiple Sclerosis, Mount Sinai Medical Center, New York, New York

CLAUDIA F. LUCCHINETTI, MD, Associate Professor of Neurology, Department of Neurology, Mayo Clinic, Rochester, Minnesota

AARON E. MILLER, MD, Professor of Neurology, Department of Neurology; Medical Director, Corinne Goldsmith Dickinson Center for Multiple Sclerosis, Mt. Sinai School of Medicine, New York, New York

PAUL W. O'CONNOR, MSc, MD, Associate Professor, Department of Medicine (Neurology), University of Toronto; and Director of Research, Multiple Sclerosis Clinic, and Chief, Division of Neurology, St. Michael's Hospital, Toronto, Ontario, Canada

JORGE R. OKSENBERG, PhD, Associate Professor, Department of Neurology, University of California at San Francisco, School of Medicine, San Francisco, California

JOSEPH PARISI, MD, Professor of Pathology, Department of Lab Medicine and Pathology, Mayo Clinic, Rochester, Minnesota

JOHN W. PETERSON, PhD, Department of Neurosciences, The Lerner Research Institute, The Cleveland Clinic Foundation, Cleveland, Ohio

RANDALL T. SCHAPIRO, MD, Clinical Professor, Department of Neurology, University of Minnesota, and Director, The Schapiro Center for Multiple Sclerosis, The Minneapolis Clinic of Neurology, Minneapolis, Minnesota

ANTHONY TRABOULSEE, MD, FRCPC, Clinical Assistant Professor, Division of Neurology, Department of Medicine, The University of British Columbia, Vancouver, British Columbia, Canada

BRUCE D. TRAPP, PhD, Chairman, Department of Neurosciences, The Lerner Research Institute, The Cleveland Clinic Foundation, Cleveland, Ohio

MELANIE R. URSELL, MSc, MD, Clinical Fellow, Multiple Sclerosis, University of Toronto, and Division of Neurology, St. Michael's Hospital, Toronto, Ontario, Canada

HOWARD L. WEINER, MD, Partners Multiple Sclerosis Center, Brigham and Women's Hospital; Robert L. Kroc Professor of Neurology, Harvard Medical School, Boston, Massachusetts

BRIAN G. WEINSHENKER, MD, Professor of Neurology, Department of Neurology, Mayo Clinic College of Medicine, Rochester, Minnesota

GUOJUN ZHAO, MD, Research Associate, Division of Neurology, Department of Medicine, The University of British Columbia, Vancouver, British Columbia, Canada

CONTENTS

FORTHCOMING ISSUES

May 2005

Neurotoxicology
Michael R. Dobbs, MD, and
Matthew P. Wicklund, MD, *Guest Editors*

August 2005

Otoneurology
Joseph M. Furman, MD, PhD
Guest Editor

November 2005

Sleep Disorders
Robert Fayle, MD, *Guest Editor*

RECENT ISSUES

November 2004

Neurology Illnesses and Pregnancy
Page B. Pennell, MD, *Guest Editor*

August 2004

Diagnostic Tests in Neuromuscular Diseases
Rahman Pourmand, MD, *Guest Editor*

May 2004

Perioperative Management and Preoperative Assessment of Neurologic Diseases
Néstor Gálvez-Jiménez, MD
Guest Editor

ELSEVIER
SAUNDERS

Neurol Clin 23 (2005) xi

NEUROLOGIC
CLINICS

Erratum

In the supplement to *Neurologic Clinics*, "Current Treatment Challenges and Emerging Therapies in Parkinson's Disease," a misspelling appears on the front cover, inside cover page, and the contents page. The correct spelling of the Guest Editor's name appearing second is Rajesh Pahwa, MD. We apologize for this oversight.

doi:10.1016/j.ncl.2005.01.001

ELSEVIER
SAUNDERS

NEUROLOGIC CLINICS

Neurol Clin 23 (2005) xiii–xvi

Preface

Multiple Sclerosis

This is the third issue of the *Neurologic Clinics of North America* to specifically address multiple sclerosis (MS). Each previous issue has appeared approximately a decade after its predecessor, and all have reflected substantial interval change in understanding the disease. The last issue heralded the opening of the therapeutic potential for modifying the natural history of disease as it coincided with the approval of interferon beta-1b for the prevention of MS relapses and anticipated the positive reviews of the pivotal studies of interferon beta-1a and glatiramer acetate for the same indication. This theme has been expanded greatly in this issue as we appear to be on the brink of expanding the therapeutic armamentarium to a second generation of therapeutics derived from a fundamental understanding of the molecules that are essential for central nervous system inflammation. These advances have been rather exponential, providing substantial confidence that by the time MS is revisited in the *Neurologic Clinics of North America*, control of the disease will be a reality, even if the etiology of the condition remains nearly as elusive as it was in 1983. Starting with therapy would be putting the cart before the horse; therefore, this issue begins with the critical advances over the last decade that lay the foundation for current therapy and promises for the future.

Two important consensus documents have appeared as a result of meetings held under the initiative of the National Multiple Sclerosis Society. The first addresses the usually mundane topic of nosology, attempting to derive a more universal meaning to the type of classifications used to describe various forms of MS. Consequently, clinicians, investigators and perhaps even patients now use relapsing, secondary progressive, primary progressive, and progressive relapsing designations with better precision. However, it has also raised the issue of how one reliably recognizes the differences between progression and the accumulation of disability in stepwise fashion related to relapses and that which occurs in the absence of clinically apparent attacks. The second revisits the diagnostic criteria for MS and revises them, in large part, to reflect the importance of MRI in extending our ability to image the disease process. The new diagnostic criteria and clinical classifications of MS are succinctly and ably addressed by Fred Lublin in his article "Clinical

doi:10.1016/j.ncl.2004.11.003

Features and Diagnosis of Multiple Sclerosis." The conclusions of the London panel on diagnosis will be reviewed in spring 2005 for any necessary refinements; however, they already facilitate earlier and more secure diagnosis when carefully applied. In the article "Natural History of Multiple Sclerosis," Orhun Kantarci and Brian Weinshenker provide the essentials with which every clinician should be armed for the future course of MS to provide informed answers to patients regarding prognosis and to help balance decisions on whether and when to initiate therapy. Although it is quite possible that the natural history of MS will change as we gain increasingly effective management tools, it is also likely that novel biomarkers (eg, the antibody that may differentiate neuromyelitis optica from other forms of relapsing MS) will refine our prognostic skills.

Overwhelmingly, MS is a disease of women in early life, with a shift toward men later in life. It has long been suspected that understanding these apparent differences in susceptibility might lead to better disease management. In "Gender Issues," Patricia Coyle tackles this subject with an informed review of the relevant basic and clinical literature. Many will find this article particularly helpful in providing an essential primer on unique issues raised by MS for pregnancy. Completion of the successful initiative to unravel the sequence of the human genome at the turn of this century opened the door to the age of molecular medicine. The strong genetic predisposition to MS and likely influences on presentation and course has attracted the attention of many. Jorge Oksenberg and Stephen Hauser have long been in the hunt and provide a detailed status report in "Genetics of Multiple Sclerosis." Because the majority of genetically influenced diseases of man share the extraordinary complexity of MS, a successful approach to one will likely open the door to a more rapid solution of the complex genetics of others.

With a disease that has been recognized for over 150 years, most might not expect that a fresh look at its neuropathology would add much understanding or influence our approach to its therapy. Nevertheless, an international consortium of neurologists and pathologists have not only taken a new look, but have provided a novel if controversial reclassification of the findings and acute lesions that suggest fundamental differences in the pathogenesis of the disease with potential profound clinical implications. In "The Pathology of Multiple Sclerosis," Claudia Lucchinetti, Joseph Parisi, and Wolfgang Bruck place their signal findings into the context of current concepts of the immunopathogenesis of MS with superb illustrations of these newly defined disease types. Pressing issues remain as to whether these types are patient-specific or vary within patient overtime. No doubt these will be resolved in time. No matter what emerges, these observations have reinvigorated fresh approaches. Similarly, in their article "Neuropathobiology of Multiple Sclerosis," John Peterson and Bruce Trapp review the rediscovery of axonal injury in MS and its importance in potentially understanding the dynamics of the natural history of the disease. Moreover, the application of immunochemical techniques has allowed much better recognition of the intracortical pathology associated with the disease. Their demonstration of this aspect of the pathology should stimulate those interested in imaging MS to find efficient ways of capturing these lesions in vivo. These articles on the evolving pathology of MS are appropriately followed by a practical approach to modern neuroimaging in which Anthony Traboulsee, Guojun Zhao, and David Li call on their extensive experience ("Neuroimaging in Multiple Sclerosis").

Amit Bar-Or nicely sets the stage for understanding modern immunotherapy in "Immunology of Multiple Sclerosis." Increasingly, the lessons derived from experimental allergic encephalomyelitis and other autoimmune models have pushed our perceptions of human immunology, particularly as applied to MS. This article is conceptually rich and draws heavily from human observations. This primer prepares clinicians for the articles on escalating immunotherapy that will follow. One should first stop to gather in the experience of a seasoned clinician with extensive understanding in managing the symptoms of MS. Randy Schapiro provides a structured approach in "Managing Symptoms of Multiple Sclerosis," appropriately admonishing that one must not forget this important art. Ludwig Kappos and Aaron Miller contribute the balanced articles "Interferons in Multiple Sclerosis" and "Glatiramer Acetate in the Treatment of Multiple Sclerosis," respectively. These first-generation immunomodulators are likely to remain active cornerstones of treatment for some time and set the standard by which newer therapies will be gauged. In this context, Paul O'Connor, in his article "Natalizumab and Other Monoclonal Antibodies," presages what may be the first of the second-generation therapies. Pivotal data on natalizumab is under active review by the US Food and Drug Administration, with approval for general use for the indication relapse reduction in relapsing forms of MS anticipated as early as 2005. Further on the horizon are representatives of at least six classes of mechanistically distinct, orally active molecules that have already entered phase I to phase III clinical trials. As developed by Lucchinetti and colleagues and elsewhere, neuroprotection and repair are increasingly emphasized as MS therapeutic goals. To be sure, control of pathogenetic aberrant immune responses can be considered a limited form of neuroprotection, but the concept is much broader. Hopefully, future issues devoted to MS will feature articles about neuroprotection and repair that are practical and not theoretical.

Unfortunately, the proportion of nonresponders to current-generation immunomodulators remains unacceptable. Therefore, escalating treatment to stabilize aggressive cases is frequently considered. In "Immunosuppressive Therapy for Multiple Sclerosis," Susan Gauthier, Guy Buckle, and Howard Weiner carefully review the rationale and available approaches. Harold Atkins and Mark Freedman consider the ultimate extensions of cytotoxic therapy in "Immunoablative Therapy as a Treatment for Aggressive Multiple Sclerosis." Although many clinicians view bone marrow transplantation as far too dangerous for the treatment of MS, it is carefully conceived trials that will determine its true limits.

Jerry S. Wolinsky, MD
Department of Neurology
The University of Texas Health Sciences Center at Houston
6431 Fannin Street
Houston, TX 77030, USA

E-mail address: jswolinsky@aol.com

ELSEVIER
SAUNDERS

Neurol Clin 23 (2005) 1–15

NEUROLOGIC
CLINICS

Clinical Features and Diagnosis of Multiple Sclerosis

Fred D. Lublin, MD

Mount Sinai Medical Center, Corinne Goldsmith Dickinson Center for Multiple Sclerosis, 5 East 98th Street, Box 1138, New York, NY 10029-6574, USA

The signs and symptoms of MS are the consequence of underlying neuropathologic changes that occur in the central nervous system (CNS). The primary mechanism of injury is inflammatory demyelination and, to a variable degree, axonal damage, which can occur early in disease course and concomitant with acute inflammation [1,2]. Either mechanism may produce clinical features. The role of axonal damage is clear-cut, disrupting conduction completely. Demyelination may result either in slowing of conduction or complete failure of transmission. The former produces symptoms when the slowing becomes critical. Because the pathologic damage may involve any area of the CNS, the location of the lesions also play a role in symptom production.

MS can produce any symptom or sign that might occur with damage to the CNS and, despite growing evidence for gray matter involvement [3], the clinical features best reflect damage mostly to white matter tracks. The most common findings include optic neuritis, weakness, sensory loss, ataxia, nystagmus, bladder dysfunction, and cognitive impairment; the full list is quite long.

Diagnosing multiple sclerosis

The diagnosis of MS is based on finding clinical evidence of lesions of the CNS that are disseminated in time and space. Dissemination in time suggests that there is more than one episode of CNS dysfunction. Dissemination in space suggests involvement of more than one area of the CNS. Diagnosis is accomplished through careful medical history and a detailed neurologic examination. Although all MS begins with a first attack, the essence of the

E-mail address: fred.lublin@mssm.edu

doi:10.1016/j.ncl.2004.09.003

clinical disease is the multiplicity of attacks. There have been several diagnostic criteria proposed in the past several decades, all affirming the need for dissemination, primarily white matter involvement, at a young age (20–50 years old) and including an important caveat: that there is no better diagnosis.

The diagnostic criteria for MS have been refined by Rose et al [4] and, penultimately, by the Poser criteria in 1982, which were developed by a committee established by the National Multiple Sclerosis Society (NMSS) [5]. The latter were established for use in clinical trials of MS. The categories proposed were clinically definite MS, laboratory-supported (dependent on positive cerebrospinal fluid [CSF] analysis) definite MS, probable MS (either clinically or laboratory supported), and possible MS. Because MRI scanning was relatively new at the time these criteria were developed, it was included as a paraclinical element (along with urodynamic testing and evoked potentials) but not defined further or quantified. The Poser criteria were used for almost 20 years but in the intervening years, there have been hundreds of studies better integrating MRI results into the diagnostic schema for MS and providing considerable knowledge of the importance of MRI in providing an in vivo view of the neuropathology of MS and the likelihood of developing MS [6].

In 2000, the NMSS convened a committee to update and revise the diagnostic criteria for MS, with the intention of increasing the role of MRI in the diagnostic schema. Other objectives for this revision were to simplify the categories and produce guidelines useful to practicing clinicians. The deliberations of that group then were reviewed by outside experts and published [7]. The need for this most current revision is underscored by the development of MS disease-modifying agents (DMAs) during the past decade. Since the advent of DMAs, the need for early, accurate diagnosis has become increasingly important, because the accumulated data suggest that the earlier treatment is started, the lower the risk for accumulating impairment or disability.

The general conclusions from the new criteria are that the diagnosis of MS requires objective evidence of lesions disseminated in time and space. MRI findings may contribute to determination of dissemination in time or space, and other supportive investigations include CSF analysis and visual evoked potential (VEP). The diagnostic categories are possible MS, MS, and not MS (the category of probable MS, used by Poser, had little practical value for clinicians, other than suggesting more certainty than possibility, and was of no value in clinical trials). The new guidelines reaffirmed the classical approach to diagnosing MS by clinical means only: the finding of evidence of lesions of the CNS; dissemination in time and space, based on a detailed history; and a complete neurologic examination. This schema allows for diagnosing MS in regions of the world where there is limited access to newer and more expensive technologies.

Most MS starts with an attack, relapse, or exacerbation (ie, an acute episode of CNS dysfunction lasting at least 24 hours [by convention], occurring in the absence of fever or metabolic derangement). All events occurring within 30 days of such an event are considered, also by convention, to be part of a single event, even though multiple areas of the CNS may be involved. The most common clinical course of MS follows a relapsing-remitting course of multiple attacks, as described later.

The role of MRI in the diagnosis of MS has been expanded considerably in this latest MS diagnostic guideline. After careful consideration of MRI studies of patients who had MS, the committee determined that the criteria of Barkhof et al [8], as modified by Tintore et al [9], provided the best combination of specificity and sensitivity, with emphasis on accuracy, as appropriate for a diagnostic guideline. For dissemination in space criteria, see criteria listed in Box 1 [8,9].

MRI also can be used to confirm dissemination in time (Box 2). If an MRI scan of the brain performed at 3 or more months after an initial clinical event demonstrates a new gadolinium-enhancing lesion, this indicates a new CNS inflammatory event, because the duration of gadolinium enhancement MS usually is less than 6 weeks. If there are no gadolinium-enhancing lesions but a new T_2 lesion (presuming there was an MRI at the time of the initial event), then a repeat MRI scan after another 3 months is needed with demonstration of a new T_2 lesion or gadolinium-enhancing lesion. The reason for the second scan to establish that a new T_2 lesion has occurred relates to the inclusion of all events within 30 days of an exacerbation as part of the initial exacerbation. A new T_2 lesion developing within 30 days after an exacerbation does not count as a new event, although it would show up as new on the first 3-month scan, thus necessitating a new T_2 lesion on the second 3-month scan. The 3-month interval was a consensus decision and is offered as a guideline.

Spinal fluid analysis also is useful for diagnosing MS but is not diagnostic by itself (because other conditions can produce similar abnormalities). The presence of immunoglobulin abnormalities in the CSF indicates the production of immunoglobulin by plasma cells or B cells within the CNS.

Box 1. New diagnostic criteria for MRI determination of dissemination in space

Three out of four of the following:

- At least one gadolinium-enhancing lesion or 9 T_2 hyperintense lesions
- At least one infratentorial lesion
- At least one juxtacortical lesion
- At least three periventricular lesions

A spinal cord lesion can substitute for any of the brain lesions. If there are immunoglobulin abnormalities in the CSF, then the MRI criteria are relaxed to only two T_2 lesions typical of MS.

Box 2. New diagnostic criteria for MRI determination of dissemination in time

- Gadolinium-enhancing lesion demonstrated on a scan performed at least 3 months after onset of a clinical attack at a site different from attack, or
- In the absence of gadolinium-enhancing lesions at the 3-month scan, follow-up scan after an additional 3 months showing a gadolinium-enhancing lesion or new T_2 lesion.

This is determined best by the finding of oligoclonal bands of immunoglobulin G (IgG) present in the CSF but not in serum. This is best assayed by using the isoelectric focusing technique. The finding of an elevated IgG index (a ratio of the IgG to protein in the serum and CSF) is equally helpful. The total protein in the CSF almost always is less than 100 mgdL in MS, and the finding of more than 50 white blood cells in the CSF is uncommon. A note of caution with the CSF interpretation: there is potential for false negative results as a result of laboratory variation and the potential for lack of quality control and standardization.

Evoked responses also can be used to provide evidence for dissemination in space. The most valuable is the VEP. The finding of a prolonged VEP in an individual who has no clinical evidence of an optic nerve lesion indicates subclinical involvement of the optic nerve. The other evoked responses were not found to be discriminative or sensitive enough to provide useful diagnostic information [10]. Concerns for quality control, similar to those mentioned for CSF analysis, exist for VEPs.

Putting these diagnostic guidelines into practice is straightforward but may require that the clinician review the MRI scans personally for the specific items delineated in the criteria. If a patient has had two or more attacks with objective evidence of involvement of two or more areas of the CNS and there is no better diagnosis, then the patient has met the criteria for dissemination in time and space. In this circumstance, additional studies are not necessary, an important issue in regions where access to MRI might be limited or nonexistent. If additional studies are undertaken, such as MRI or CSF analysis, they should yield consistent results, or the diagnosis should be questioned.

If there has been one attack and evidence of two lesions in the CNS, then evidence must be obtained for dissemination in time. This can be accomplished by the occurrence of a second attack or by evidence of dissemination in time with MRI scanning (see Box 2).

If there are two or more attacks but evidence on examination of involvement of only one area of the CNS, then it is necessary to establish dissemination in space. A second attack involving a new area of the CNS or changes on a subsequent MRI scan (see Box 1) fulfill this criterion.

If there has been one attack and evidence of only one area of CNS involvement (the clinically isolated syndrome or monosymptomatic presentation), then it is necessary to confirm dissemination in time and space. This can be accomplished clinically if there is a subsequent attack or by fulfilling the MRI criteria for dissemination for each (see Boxes 1 and 2).

In the case of insidious onset and progression of neurologic dysfunction suggestive of MS (usually primary progressive MS [PPMS]), it is necessary to find positive CSF and evidence of dissemination in time by MRI or continued progression for at least 1 year and dissemination in space by MRI (see Box 1) or two or more spinal MRI abnormalities or 4 to 8 cerebral MRI lesions and 1 spinal cord lesion or an abnormal VEP and 4 to 8 cerebral lesions on MRI or an abnormal VEP and less than four cerebral lesions plus one spinal cord lesion. These criteria were adapted from those published previously by Thompson et al [11]. Compared with other guidelines, investigators believed that CSF analysis was necessary to diagnose PPMS, because the risk for alternative diagnoses was greater than with other forms of MS. There is not an abundance of demographic data on pure PPMS, as defined currently. In the past, inclusion of patients who had relapses, often remote, has confounded this category. Analysis of recent clinical trials of PPMS should provide important data to support or modify the diagnostic guidelines.

Tables 1 and 2 outline the major features of the new criteria and are available on laminated cards from the NMSS. Initial studies show that the new criteria are highly sensitive and specific, leading to earlier diagnosis. Studies show more than twice the rate of conversion from a clinically isolated syndrome to MS using the new criteria versus the older criteria by Poser et al [12,13].

Clinical course of multiple sclerosis

The clinical course of MS is variable and nearly impossible to predict for an individual patient. There are several reasons. The disease is notoriously random in terms of frequency and severity of exacerbations and in extent and rate of progression and accrual of disability. MRI studies reveal that lesions occur much more frequently than recognized clinically. This may be because of the anatomic location of the lesion (perhaps occurring in an eloquent region) or because of the extent of damage produced by a given lesion (ie, if a lesion does not produce sufficient demyelination to slow or block conduction, then it may not be expressed clinically).

Further complicating this issue is whether or not MS is a single disease with several subtypes or a combination of different diseases with similar clinical features. The current data favor MS as a single disease, although this is by no means assured, especially in the case of PPMS. Although patients who have relapsing-remitting MS (RRMS) and secondary progressive MS (SPMS) usually have many lesions on cerebral MRI scans, patients who

Table 1
New multiple sclerosis diagnostic criteria

Clinical (attacks)	Objective lesions	Additional requirements to make diagnosis
2 or more	2 or more	• None; clinical evidence will suffice (additional evidence desirable but must be consistent with MS)
2 or more	1	• Dissemination in space by MRI *or* positive CSF and 2 or more MRI lesions consistent with MS *or* further clinical attack involving different site
1	2 or more	• Dissemination in time by MRI *or* second clinical attack
1 mono-symptomatic	1	• Dissemination in space by MRI or positive CSF and 2 or more MRI lesions consistent with MS AND • Dissemination in time by MRI or second clinical attack
0 (progression from onset)	1	• Positive CSF AND • Dissemination in space by MRI evidence of 9 or more T2 brain lesions *or* 2 or more cord lesions *or* 4–8 brain and 1 cord lesion *or* positive VEP with 4–8 MRI lesions *or* positive VEP with less than 4 brain lesions plus 1 cord lesion AND • Dissemination in time by MRI *or* continued progression for 1 year

Adapted from The National Multiple Sclerosis Society, 2001.

have PPMS tend to have fewer cerebral lesions. Similarly, CNS tissue from primary progressive patients tends to show less inflammation but qualitatively the pathologic process looks quite similar. There are no clear genetic differences between forms, and within families there may be cases of relapsing forms and the primary progressive form. This may be more a matter of gradations along a scale.

Currently the disease course is used to define the clinical subtypes of MS. At present, there are no biologic (eg, immunologic or genetic) markers or MRI characteristics that consistently indicate or predict the clinical course for an individual patient. The definitions that are used are derived from an international survey of individuals working in the field of MS [14]. The consensus results from that survey led to the following clinical course definitions.

RRMS (Fig. 1A) is characterized by clearly defined disease relapses with full recovery or with sequelae and residual deficit. Periods between disease relapses are characterized by a lack of disease progression. The defining elements of RRMS are episodes of acute worsening of neurologic function followed by a varying degree of recovery, with a stable course between attacks. This is the most common presenting form of MS. Most definitions of a relapse require that new symptoms or signs be present for at least 24 hours and that they not be associated with a fever, because elevated body

Table 2
Paraclinical evidence in MS diagnosis

What is a positive MRI? 3 out of 4 of the following: 1 Gd-enhancing lesion *or* 9 T2 hyperintense lesions if no Gd-enhancing lesion 1 or more infratentorial lesions 1 or more juxtacortical lesions 3 or more periventricular lesions Note: 1 cord lesion can substitute for 1 brain lesion	What provides MRI evidence of dissemination in time? A Gd-enhancing lesion demonstrated in a scan done at least 3 months following onset of clinical attack at a site different from attack, *or* In absence of Gd-enhancing lesions at 3 month scan, follow-up scan after an additional 3 months showing Gd-lesion or new T2 lesion.
	What is positive CSF? Oligoclonal IgG bands in CSF (and not serum) *or* elevated IgG index
What is positive VEP? Delayed but well-preserved wave form	

Adapted from The National Multiple Sclerosis Society, 2001.

temperature can unmask subclinical lesions. Patients who have RRMS may develop disability, even severe disability, in a stepwise fashion as a result of incomplete recovery from individual attacks. This should not be confused with the gradual, continual worsening that occurs in the progressive forms of MS (described later).

PPMS (see Fig. 1B) is defined as disease progression from onset with occasional plateaus and temporary minor improvements. The essential element in PPMS is a gradual, nearly continuously worsening baseline with minor fluctuations but no distinct relapses. Although near-continuous progression is required in this definition, it is recognized that progression at a constant rate throughout disease is unlikely and that accommodation must be made for variations in the rate of progression over time. PPMS is the form of MS that is most distinct from the others and the form most difficult to diagnose, as the gradually worsening course does not follow the classical time dissemination criteria. This form of MS tends to occur in an older age group compared with other forms and, unlike the other forms, afflicts males and females in approximately equal numbers. In addition, PPMS usually presents as a myelopathy and tends to have less cerebral MRI change than other forms.

SPMS (see Fig. 1C) is characterized by an initial relapsing-remitting disease course followed by progression with or without occasional relapses, minor remissions, and plateaus. SPMS may be considered a long-term outcome of RRMS, in that most patients who have SPMS begin with RRMS disease as defined here. Once the baseline between relapses begins to progressively worsen, however, the patient has switched from RRMS to SPMS. Even a single remote initial exacerbation followed many years later by a gradual progressive course falls within this definition. Approximately

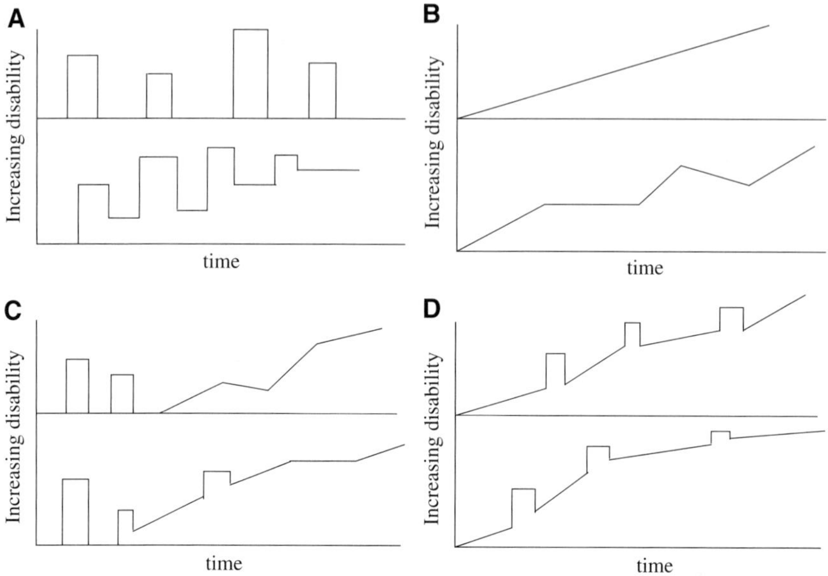

Fig. 1. (*A*) RRMS. There may be residual deficit from an attack, but the baseline between attacks remains stable until the next attack. (*B*) PPMS. There are no acute attacks, but a gradual, inexorable worsening over time. (*C*) SPMS. After an initial course of RRMS, the baseline deficit gradually worsens, with or without intervening acute attacks. (*D*) PRMS. Starts as primary progressive MS but has subsequent acute attacks at some point after onset.

50% or more of patients who have RRMS progress to SPMS. Patients who have SPMS tend to have greater disability than patients who have RRMS, and the disability develops from incomplete recovery from exacerbations and from gradual progression.

Progressive relapsing MS (PRMS) (see Fig. 1D) is defined as progressive disease from onset, with clear acute relapses, with or without recovery, with periods between relapses characterized by continuing progression. PRMS is an additional, albeit uncommon, clinical course that deserves a separate definition, as it was not included in the other definitions. This designation covers those patients who, after an initial progressive onset, go on to have superimposed acute attacks and gradual progression. From the author's initial studies, this form seems to resemble SPMS more than PPMS, even though these patients all start out with PPMS that changes to PRMS after the first true exacerbation.

Use of the term, relapsing progressive MS, is not recommended, as there is no consensus definition for it. Similarly, the term, chronic progressive MS, should be avoided, as there are three different forms of progressive MS, defined previously, with their own distinct clinical courses.

At the author's center, 68% of initial MS consultations resulted in a diagnosis of RRMS, 16% SPMS, 10% PPMS, and 6% PRMS. This is not a population-based sample, rather a highly selected referral group [15]. The New York State Multiple Sclerosis Consortium performed a survey of 3019 patients and found that 55% had RRMS, 31% SPMS, 9% PPMS, and 5% PRMS [16]. The disease course is a snapshot in time, however; because as many as 50% of patients who have RRMS eventually may develop SPMS and a percentage of patients who have PPMS could develop PRMS.

It should be emphasized that these terms are most useful in the context of research studies and should be used with care when communicating with affected individuals, family members, and third-party payers. These terms are useful for characterizing patients in clinical trials, where recruitment of homogenous groups of patients enhances the chance of discerning a treatment effect. The successful results of such trials usually are translated into approved therapies only for the subtype of MS tested. Such restrictions often do not make sense biologically.

In addition, the forms of MS can be characterized by severity. Two forms stand out, although both are uncommon.

Benign MS is a disease that allows patients to remain fully functional in all neurologic systems 15 years after disease onset. Although this form may comprise 10% to 15% of patients, diagnosis (thus, prognosis) is difficult, and by definition requires 15 years. Even then, relapses or progression can occur as late as 25 years later.

Malignant MS is a disease with a rapid, progressive course, leading to significant disability in multiple neurologic systems or death within a short time after disease onset. This is, fortunately, quite rare.

As discussed previously, because the disease course of most forms of MS is variable, prognosticating is difficult. There are some broad guidelines that can be followed with caution. Favorable indicators are listed in Box 3; unfavorable indicators are listed in Box 4.

Population studies reveal that patients who have frequent attacks and short interattack periods progress to serious disability more rapidly [17]. The individual attack rate is, however, variable and not predictable from one year to the next. In the RRMS interferon-β1b study, the rate for patients who were treated with placebo for 3 years was 1.21 attacks per year [18]. In the RRMS interferon-β1a weekly study [19], the group treated with placebo had an average of 0.82 attacks per year, and in the glatiramer acetate RRMS study [20], 0.84 attacks per year. These values probably are skewed toward higher attack rates, because patients were selected for these studies on the basis of high prestudy attack rates. In RRMS, the frequency of attacks tends to be greater earlier in the course of the disease. In the RRMS interferon-β1b study, the attack rate of the placebo group fell by approximately 40% from year 1 to year 5 [21]. The rate of progression in patients who had RRMS, as measured by a confirmed worsening of 1 point on the Kurtzke Expanded Disability Status Scale (EDSS), was 33% in the interferon-β1a at 2 years and 39% in the interferon-β1b study after 3 years. In the interferon-β1b SPMS study [22], nearly 50% of patients treated with

Box 3. Favorable prognostic indicators in multiple sclerosis

Early age of onset
Female sex
Optic neuritis as presenting episode
Sensory symptoms as presenting episode
Acute onset of symptoms
Little residual disability after each exacerbation (ie, excellent recovery)
Long interexacerbation period

placebo developed sustained worsening of at least 1 point on the Kurtzke EDSS scale by 33 months after entry into the study, demonstrating the greater degree of accrual of disability expected in SPMS compared with RRMS.

MRI scanning also has added to the ability to prognosticate. Several studies demonstrate that the presence of cerebral lesions on MRI scans performed at the time of a first attack of inflammatory demyelination (optic neuritis, acute myelopathy, or acute brainstem syndrome) greatly increases the chance of developing clinically definite MS over the successive 2 to 5 years [6]. The greater the lesion load at presentation, the greater the chance of increased disability [23].

Studies of a population of untreated patients who had MS revealed that approximately 50% of patients require assistance with ambulation within 15 years after diagnosis [24,25].

MS usually is not a lethal disease. Patients survive an average of 35 to 40 years from time of diagnosis, and the disease limits overall life span by approximately 7 years [26].

Mechanisms of production of clinical symptoms and signs in multiple sclerosis

Multiple sclerosis is a disorder of the immune system that has an impact on the CNS and thus can produce any constellation of symptoms and signs

Box 4. Unfavorable prognostic indicators in multiple sclerosis

Later age of onset
Progressive course from onset
Male sex
Frequent exacerbations
Poor recovery from exacerbations
Involvement of cerebellar or motor functions

that might occur from a lesion or lesions in areas of the brain, spinal cord, and optic nerves. Symptoms and signs in MS reflect primarily, but not exclusively, white matter involvement, although the body of data implicating neuronal injury is growing [27].

Variability of signs and symptoms—in type and in timing—is a hallmark of MS. A constellation of clinical problems, some more frequently seen than others, occurs in the disease; generally, they vary between individuals and are different over time in the same individual (Table 3).

Although generally it is not possible to attribute individual signs and symptoms to a specific type of CNS pathology, in many cases, the timing or persistence of such signs and symptoms may give clues to underlying pathology. For instance, some fleeting clinical problems—paroxysmal symptoms short in duration and unpredictable in onset and resolution—can be the result of short-term failure of conduction in nerve fibers because of elevated body temperature (from fever, exertion, or even weather). Longer term problems—true exacerbations that result in worsening of signs and symptoms for longer that 24 hours and with longer term resolution—may result from inflammation and demyelination, and resolution of such problems usually is the result of reduction of inflammation (natural or steroid-induced) and limited remyelination. Persistent disability, either after an acute exacerbation or as a consequence of slow progression of disease, is associated increasingly with damaged or severed nerve fibers, which cannot recover. Occasionally, modest recovery may be seen as a consequence of neuronal sprouting or neuronal circuit pathway changes, but the extent and significance of this process in MS is unclear.

Clinical features of multiple sclerosis

Although specific signs and symptoms may not be attributable to specific pathologies, nonetheless, the clinical features of MS are understood best in

Table 3
Multiple sclerosis: symptoms at presentation and during course

Deficit reported	Presenting	During course
Visual/oculomotor	49[a]	100
Paresis	42	88
Paresthesias	41	87
Incoordination	23	82
Genitourinary/bowel	10	63
Cerebral	4	39

[a] Expressed as a percentage. Because some patients had multiple symptoms, the total is greater than 100%.

From Whitaker JN, Mitchell GW. Clinical features of multiple sclerosis. In: Raine CS, McFarland HF, Tourtellotte WW, editors. Multiple sclerosis. Clinical and pathogenetic basis. London: Chapman and Hall Medical; 1997. p. 3–19.

the context of knowledge of the neurophysiologic and neuropathologic consequences of inflammatory, primarily demyelinating, disease.

Neurophysiology of multiple sclerosis clinical features

The clinical symptoms and signs in MS result from the failure of conduction in clinically relevant pathways in the CNS. Some lesions (detected primarily by paraclinical studies) may be clinically silent (ie, damage to CNS pathways is not reflected in frank symptoms or signs), but this may say more about the ability to measure clinical deficits than the clinical significance of various regions of the CNS. Demyelinating lesions in clinically eloquent areas produce signs only when there is an effect on the underlying conduction properties of the affected fibers [28]. Because the lesions of MS more often are inflammatory or demyelinating than necrotic, especially in earlier stages of lesion evolution, conduction often can be maintained through the underlying axon. Therefore, an inflamed or demyelinated nerve fiber may have no clinically discernable consequence because of maintained signal transmission through the safety factor of conduction, allowing the signal to jump the affected area, or no clinically discernable consequence because of slowed conduction in a fiber tract that is not sensitive to slowing of conduction. Conversely, clinical consequences may result from slowing in a speed critical fiber tract, fatigue of high-speed signaling, temporal dispersion, conduction block through a sufficiently long demyelinated segment, or conduction block resulting from a severed axon [29].

At a molecular level, the exposure of the potassium ion channel–rich regions of the internodal axon segment serves to impede conduction of signals through the demyelinated segment. Conversely, conduction, possibly slowed, may be maintained or restored in the demyelinated segment through upregulation of sodium ion channels, a mechanism for the rapid recovery of function seen after some exacerbations of MS [30].

Clinical patterns of multiple sclerosis

Although disease signs and symptoms are unpredictable in MS, there are certain clinical presentations that occur commonly in MS and are reflective of the primarily white matter location of most lesions. The production of signs occurs as a consequence of disruption of signal conduction through descending, ascending, or commissural pathways or the disconnection of neuronal pools.

At the initiation of disease, the majority of patients experience acute relapses and subsequent remissions of signs and symptoms, whereas a minority experience steady progression of disease from onset. The progressive impairment or disability that occurs over time with MS results from one of two mechanisms. There is either stepwise worsening as a result of accumulated deficits from residua of exacerbations or gradual, inexorable progressive disease, independent of the exacerbations. The relative roles of exacerbations and progressive disease in the accumulation of deficits are debated, but the data is clear that both have an impact on the long-term course of the illness. Recent data from a meta-analysis of several clinical trials studying MS demonstrate that residual deficit from exacerbations occurs after approximately 50% of attacks [31]. Later in the course of MS, progressive disease seems to contribute more strongly to the disability [32]. The relative importance of each may depend on the stage of the illness. Furthermore, it is unclear if the progressive form of the illness truly is a gradual worsening or the sum of many, small subclinical attacks. The pattern of lesion accrual seen on serial MRI scans suggests the latter.

The most common clinical manifestations of MS affect sensory pathways, motor function, cerebellar or brainstem structures, and autonomic function. There does not seem to be any predictable pattern either in the timing or location of lesions. Patients who have RRMS have an average of one to two exacerbations yearly, early in the course of the illness, with the number of attacks decreasing over time [17]. MRI studies, however, demonstrate a level of disease activity that is many times higher, although mostly subclinical [33]. MRI activity, as measured by new or gadolinium-enhancing lesions, follows a similar pattern, with more activity earlier in the disease course.

Some clinical presentations are distinctive of MS, for example, the combination of tremor, nystagmus, and scanning speech, know as Charcot's triad. The presence of bilateral internuclear ophthalmoplegia in a young adult is highly characteristic of MS. Initial attacks of MS frequently involve sensory pathways in the spinal cord; patients commonly present with complaints of numbness and paresthesias starting in the feet and rising over the course of a few days to waist level or higher. Another common initial event is optic nerve inflammation (optic or retrobulbar neuritis). Although this may occur as an isolated event, coincident abnormal brain MRI indicates a high risk for further attacks (ie, RRMS) [34,35].

Although individuals whose disease begins with characteristic relapses and remissions (RRMS) may present with any single or multiple signs or symptoms of CNS dysfunction, those whose disease begins with progression in the absence of clear relapses and remissions usually present with signs of myelopathy or cerebellar dysfunction.

References

[1] Trapp BD, Peterson J, Ransohoff RM, et al. Axonal transection in the lesions of multiple sclerosis. N Engl J Med 1998;338:278–85.

[2] Ferguson B, Matyszak MK, Esiri MM, et al. Axonal damage in acute multiple sclerosis lesions. Brain 1997;120(Pt 3):393–9.

[3] Inglese M, Ge Y, Filippi M, et al. Indirect evidence for early widespread gray matter involvement in relapsing-remitting multiple sclerosis. Neuroimage 2004;21:1825–9.

[4] Rose AS, Ellison GW, Myers LW, et al. Criteria for the clinical diagnosis of multiple sclerosis. Neurology 1976;26:20–2.
[5] Poser CM, Paty DW, Scheinberg L, et al. New diagnostic criteria for multiple sclerosis: guidelines for research protocols. Ann Neurol 1983;13:227–31.
[6] Frohman EM, Goodin DS, Calabresi PA, et al. The utility of MRI in suspected MS—report of the therapeutics and technology assessment subcommittee of the American Academy of Neurology. Neurology 2003;61:602–11.
[7] McDonald WI, Compston A, Edan G, et al. Recommended diagnostic criteria for multiple sclerosis: guidelines from the International Panel on the Diagnosis of Multiple Sclerosis. Ann Neurol 2001;50:121–7.
[8] Barkhof F, Filippi M, Miller DH, et al. Comparison of MRI criteria at first presentation to predict conversion to clinically definite multiple sclerosis. Brain 1997;120(Pt 11): 2059–69.
[9] Tintore M, Rovira A, Martinez MJ, et al. Isolated demyelinating syndromes: comparison of different MR imaging criteria to predict conversion to clinically definite multiple sclerosis. AJNR Am J Neuroradiol 2000;21:702–6.
[10] Gronseth GS, Ashman EJ. Practice parameter: the usefulness of evoked potentials in identifying clinically silent lesions in patients with suspected multiple sclerosis (an evidence-based review): report of the Quality Standards Subcommittee of the American Academy of Neurology. Neurology 2000;54:1720–5.
[11] Thompson AJ, Montalban X, Barkhof F, et al. Diagnostic criteria for primary progressive multiple sclerosis: a position paper. Ann Neurol 2000;47:831–5.
[12] Dalton CM, Brex PA, Miszkiel KA, et al. Application of the new McDonald criteria to patients with clinically isolated syndromes suggestive of multiple sclerosis. Ann Neurol 2002; 52:47–53.
[13] Tintore M, Rovira A, Rio J, et al. New diagnostic criteria for multiple sclerosis—application in first demyelinating episode. Neurology 2003;60:27–30.
[14] Lublin FD, Reingold SC. Defining the clinical course of multiple sclerosis: results of an international survey. National Multiple Sclerosis Society (USA) Advisory Committee on Clinical Trials of New Agents in Multiple Sclerosis. Neurology 1996;46:907–11.
[15] Oshinsky RJ, Elfont RM, Lublin FD. Incidence and clinical characteristics of the progressive relapsing form of MS. Neurology 1998;50:A209.
[16] Jacobs LD, Wende KE, Brownscheidle CM, et al. A profile of multiple sclerosis: the New York State Multiple Sclerosis Consortium. Multiple Sclerosis 1999;5:369–76.
[17] Weinshenker BG, Bass B, Rice GP, et al. The natural history of multiple sclerosis: a geographically based study. 2. Predictive value of the early clinical course. Brain 1989;112: 1419–28.
[18] The IFNB Multiple Sclerosis Study Group. Interferon beta-1b is effective in relapsing-remitting multiple sclerosis. I. Clinical results of a multicenter, randomized, double-blind, placebo-controlled trial. Neurology 1993;43:655–61.
[19] Jacobs LD, Cookfair DL, Rudick RA, et al. Intramuscular interferon beta-1a for disease progression in relapsing multiple sclerosis. The Multiple Sclerosis Collaborative Research Group (MSCRG). Ann Neurol 1996;39:285–94.
[20] Johnson KP, Brooks BR, Cohen JA, et al. Copolymer 1 reduces relapse rate and improves disability in relapsing-remitting multiple sclerosis: results of a phase III multicenter, double-blind placebo-controlled trial. The Copolymer 1 Multiple Sclerosis Study Group. Neurology 1995;45:1268–76.
[21] The IFNB Multiple Sclerosis Study Group and The University of British Columbia MS/MRI Analysis Group. Interferon beta-1b in the treatment of multiple sclerosis: final outcome of the randomized controlled trial. Neurology 1995;45:1277–85.
[22] Kappos L, Polman C, Pozzilli C, et al. Placebo-controlled multicentre randomised trial of interferon beta-1b in treatment of secondary progressive multiple sclerosis. Lancet 1998;352: 1491–7.

[23] Brex PA, Ciccarelli O, O'Riordan JI, et al. A longitudinal study of abnormalities on MRI and disability from multiple sclerosis. N Engl J Med 2002;346:158–64.

[24] Weinshenker BG, Bass B, Rice GP, et al. The natural history of multiple sclerosis: a geographically based study. I. Clinical course and disability. Brain 1989;112:133–46.

[25] Runmarker B, Andersen O. Prognostic factors in a multiple sclerosis incidence cohort with twenty-five years of follow-up. Brain 1993;116:117–34.

[26] Sadovnick AD, Ebers GC, Wilson RW, et al. Life expectancy in patients attending multiple-sclerosis clinics. Neurology 1992;42:991–4.

[27] Peterson JW, Bo L, Mork S, et al. Transected neurites, apoptotic neurons, and reduced inflammation in cortical multiple sclerosis lesions. Ann Neurol 2001;50:389–400.

[28] O'Riordan JI, Losseff NA, Phatouros C, et al. Asymptomatic spinal cord lesions in clinically isolated optic nerve, brain stem, and spinal cord syndromes suggestive of demyelination. J Neurol Neurosurg Psychiatry 1998;64:353–7.

[29] Smith KJ, McDonald WI. The pathophysiology of multiple sclerosis: the mechanisms underlying the production of symptoms and the natural history of the disease. Philos Trans R Soc Lond B Biol Sci 1999;354:1649–73.

[30] Waxman SG. Demyelinating diseases—new pathological insights, new therapeutic targets. N Engl J Med 1998;338:323–5.

[31] Lublin FD, Baier M, Cutter G. Effect of relapses on development of residual deficit in multiple sclerosis. Neurology 2003;61:1528–32.

[32] Confavreux C, Vukusic S, Moreau T, et al. Relapses and progression of disability in multiple sclerosis. N Engl J Med 2000;343:1430–8.

[33] O'Riordan JI, Thompson AJ, Kingsley DP, et al. The prognostic value of brain MRI in clinically isolated syndromes of the CNS. A 10-year follow-up. Brain 1998;121(Pt 3): 495–503.

[34] Beck RW, Cleary PA, Trobe JD, et al. The effect of corticosteroids for acute optic neuritis on the subsequent development of multiple sclerosis. The Optic Neuritis Study Group. N Engl J Med 1993;329:1764–9.

[35] Jacobs LD, Beck RW, Simon JH, et al. Intramuscular interferon beta-1a therapy initiated during a first demyelinating event in multiple sclerosis. CHAMPS Study Group. N Engl J Med 2000;343:898–904.

ELSEVIER
SAUNDERS

Neurol Clin 23 (2005) 17–38

NEUROLOGIC
CLINICS

Natural History of Multiple Sclerosis

Orhun H. Kantarci, MD, Brian G. Weinshenker, MD*

Department of Neurology, Mayo Clinic College of Medicine, Rochester, MN, USA

The natural history of multiple sclerosis (MS) has been reviewed extensively by various investigators, including one of the authors of this review in a prior volume of *Neurologic Clinics* [1,2]. Since the introduction of disease-modifying treatments, such as interferon-β [3], glatiramer acetate [4], and mitoxantrone [5], their use in the clinical setting has become more than an academic issue as it influences the decision as to whether or not and when to initiate these long-term treatments. Current understanding of MS pathogenesis suggests that axonal damage starts early in MS [6] and that early intervention promises the benefit of preventing long-term disability. Clinical trials of MS are limited in duration, however, given the time over which disability develops in MS. Long-term benefit from these treatments, considering robust measures of clinical disability, remains to be established. In general terms, long-term benefit with minimal toxicity is optimized by treating patients who are at highest risk for an adverse outcome and are most likely to respond to the best treatment at the optimal point in their disease course.

MS is part of a heterogeneous spectrum of idiopathic inflammatory demyelinating diseases (IIDDs) of the central nervous system (CNS). These syndromes vary in terms of the number and size of lesions and pathology (inflammation, demyelination, and axonal injury; degree of remyelination and repair). Some of the isolated IIDDs (optic neuritis [ON], transverse myelitis, and the fulminant Marburg form of MS) have the potential to convert to the prototypical relapsing-remitting form of MS (RRMS). RRMS often evolves into secondary progressive MS (SPMS). Neuromyelitis optica (NMO), alternatively, seems to remain distinct from MS and is associated with continued relapses throughout its clinical course. Hence, faced with a patient who has ON, a clinician cannot reliably know if the syndrome will remain clinically isolated indefinitely or is the precursor of

* Corresponding author. Department of Neurology, Mayo Clinic College of Medicine, 200 First Street, SW, Rochester, MN 55905.

E-mail address: weinb@mayo.edu (B.G. Weinshenker).

0733-8619/05/$ - see front matter
doi:10.1016/j.ncl.2004.10.002

MS, NMO, or recurrent ON with no evidence of dissemination beyond the optic nerves. If this could be predicted accurately, it would help with the decision as to whether or not to initiate and the specific agent with which to initiate long-term treatment. For example, there is growing evidence that certain subtypes of demyelinating disease, such as NMO, are managed best with immunosuppressive medication rather than standard immunomodulatory therapies that are used for MS, such as interferon-β and glatiramer acetate. This review addresses the natural history of MS and IIDDs, highlighting increasing appreciation of qualitative variation between different subgroups and quantitative variation within specific subgroups of the spectrum of the IIDDs of the CNS.

Natural history in idiopathic inflammatory demyelinating diseases

Disease course, impact of individual events throughout the course, and accumulating long-term disability collectively define disease severity and natural history in IIDDs. The spectrum of disease course may include an acute isolated attack without recurrence, recurrent exacerbations, or a progressive phase. Attacks and progression may occur in the same individual simultaneously or at different times during the evolution of the disease and may reflect different pathogenetic mechanisms. Although the impact of acute events is determined by the extent and severity of pathology, accumulating long-term disability is believed to be determined by the balance between demyelination, remyelination, and axonal loss; the mechanism of axon loss also is highly variable and includes cumulative episodes of acute axonal loss and gradual axonal degeneration in demyelinated tracts and, possibly, transsynaptic axonal degeneration.

The impact of all of these factors on the spectrum and natural history of IIDDs is illustrated in Fig. 1.

Isolated idiopathic inflammatory demyelinating diseases

IIDDs may present as clinically isolated syndromes with a wide variety of neurologic symptoms. Some patients do not experience recurrence (monophasic) (see Fig. 1), although some may have imaging or paraclinical (evoked potential studies) evidence of dissemination in space. Most patients, however, have clinical recurrence (polyphasic course). Recurrences may be restricted in distribution, as in the case of recurrent ON, recurrent acute transverse myelitis (ATM), and NMO. Recent data may suggest that these three syndromes are linked, in that a specific serologic marker for NMO frequently is positive in patients who have more limited syndromes of recurrent ON and recurrent ATM [7]. More often, patients experience relapsing multifocal inflammatory demyelinating attacks of the CNS (dissemination in time), such as in prototypic RRMS, or may develop an insidious, progressive course, most commonly of myelopathy (SPMS). This

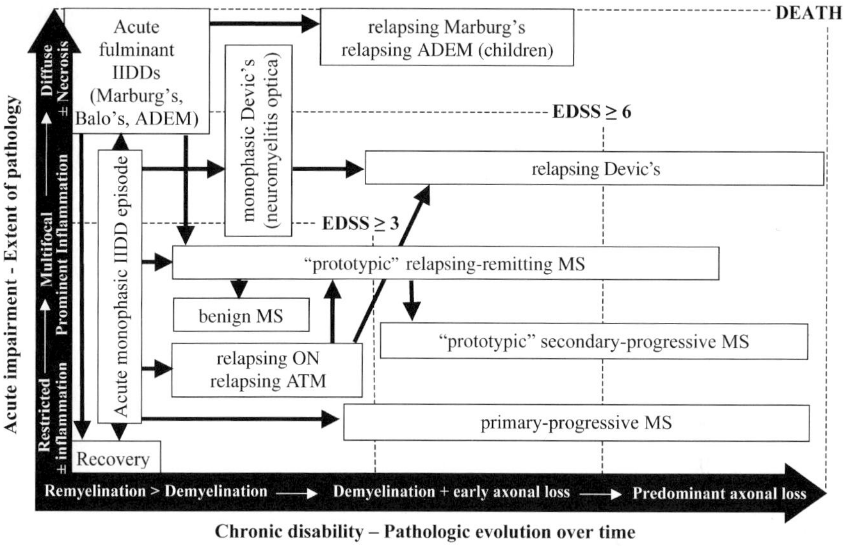

Fig. 1. The balance between inflammation and necrosis and the balance between demyelination, remyelination, and axonal loss on the natural history of IIDDs. (*Modified from* Kantarci OH, Weinshenker BG. Prognostic factors in multiple sclerosis. In: Stuart CD, editor. Handbook of multiple sclerosis. 3rd ed. New York: Marcel Dekker; 2001. p. 449–63; with permission).

phase, which follows one or more initial relapses, is indistinguishable from the course in patients who have MS and who have never had an isolated clinical episode (primary progressive MS [PPMS]). An international panel recently revised the Poser criteria [8] for diagnosis of RRMS, including imaging to expand the clinical definition of dissemination in space or time that is required to diagnose prototypic RRMS; the revised criteria commonly are referred to as the McDonald criteria [9]. This modification helps with earlier diagnosis of RRMS and yields a fourfold increase in the diagnosis of definite RRMS in the first 12 months after a clinically isolated event [10].

The immunopathologic mechanisms that determine evolution from a restricted monophasic syndrome to a multifocal polyphasic disease are incompletely understood. Predictors of conversion to MS in isolated IIDDs, however, have been investigated in several studies. Independent of the localization of the presenting syndrome, 88% of patients who had an initial brain MRI suggestive of MS at the presentation of an isolated IIDD (ON, ATM, or brainstem syndrome) developed clinically definite MS, as defined by the Poser criteria, within 14 years of onset, whereas only 19% who had normal MRI developed MS [11]. If follow-up MRIs were obtained at 18 months, 82% of patients showed new subclinical lesions and half of these patients developed clinically definite MS by Poser criteria [12]. At 18-months' follow-up, 84% of patients who had two or more enhancing lesions at presentation showed either clinical or radiologic evidence of temporal dissemination of disease activity and qualified as having RRMS, according to the McDonald criteria.

Among the isolated syndromes, ON is one that has been studied extensively. Long intracanalicular lesions of the optic nerve in MRI are associated with poor recovery from an ON attack [13]. In adults, 10-year risk of developing MS after any acute episode of ON is 38%. This risk increases to 56% if there is one or more typical lesions suggestive of MS in the MRI and is 22% if the MRI is normal [14]. In the latter group, male gender, absence of pain, presence of optic disk swelling, peripapillary hemorrhages, or retinal exudates are associated with lower risk of conversion to MS. The risk of conversion to MS is even lower in children: 13% in 10 years and 26% in 40 years after the initial attack [15]. A history of preceding infection within 2 weeks of ON onset decreases the risk, whereas recurrent or bilateral sequential ON increases the risk of conversion to MS. In the short term (average follow-up of 25 months, longest follow-up of 4.5 years) after an isolated attack of ON, the presence of oligoclonal bands in cerebrospinal fluid (CSF), in addition to three or more lesions suggestive of MS, predicts conversion to MS 63% of the time, whereas the absence of either invariably predicts no conversion to MS (negative predictive value of 100%) [16]. The presence of HLA-DR2 genotype has a positive predictive value of 44% and negative predictive value of 71% in determining conversion to definite MS [16]. Overall, these results suggest that natural history of ON is relatively benign compared with other isolated syndromes, because more than half of the patients do not develop MS 10 years into their disease [14], and if they do develop MS, they accumulate less long-term disability (see later discussion of natural history of prototypic MS). Hence, it is important to consider the relative risk of MS in these patients before starting any long-term treatment.

Complete ATM is a steroid-responsive, restricted monophasic syndrome of the spinal cord. In some patients it can evolve into NMO (discussed later). It is differentiated from spinal cord involvement of MS at presentation by the symmetric and combined sensory and motor involvement as opposed to the more restricted, asymmetric, and generally milder involvement seen in myelitis associated with MS (partial ATM) [17]. The sausage-shaped, swollen, and elongated enhancing spinal cord lesions have a characteristic appearance distinct from the multifocal lesions of MS [18]. In patients with partial ATM, the reported conversion to MS is between 58% to 80%. Sensory symptoms, posterolateral location of the lesion in the spinal cord, abnormal brain MRI, and oligoclonal bands in CSF predict conversion to MS [19,20].

Neuromyelitis optica (Devic's disease)

NMO is a distinct IIDD, which probably has a worse natural history than MS, although population-based studies are lacking and considerable variability may be seen in the outcome of NMO, as is the case in MS. NMO may be misdiagnosed as RRMS with existing clinical criteria at presentation, in that ON and myelitis may occur in either. It is a restricted syndrome of ON and myelitis, however, generally lacking the typical brain lesions seen in RRMS. The predilection of MS in Northern Europeans is less true for NMO [21,22], although the majority of cases reported in North American series are white Americans. The spinal cord lesions are longitudinally extensive and resemble those of complete ATM. CSF oligoclonal bands are uncommon, whereas a neutrophilic pleocytosis may occur occasionally during acute attacks. Attacks of NMO are more severe, less often steroid responsive, and often lead to significant morbidity and mortality from respiratory failure as a result of cervical myelopathy. For the one third who have a monophasic course, the mean survival is 90% in 5 years [23]. For the other two thirds, however, who have relapsing NMO, the survival rate after 5 years is 68%. Simultaneous ON and myelitis within 1 month predict a monophasic and relatively benign course, whereas a long interval between index events (relative risk increase of 2.2 per month), female sex (female versus male relative risk of 10.0), older age at onset (relative risk increase of 1.1 per year), and presence of other systemic autoimmune disease (relative risk of 4.2) predict a relapsing course and worse prognosis [24]. The pathology of NMO is relatively homogeneous and suggests a B-cell–mediated disorder with characteristics that are distinct from MS. NMO may be distinguished from MS by a specific autoantibody marker [7,25]. Distinguishing this disease from RRMS at presentation may have significant implications in terms of future management, although no medication is shown to change the natural history of this disease.

Fulminant idiopathic inflammatory demyelinating diseases

Acute fulminant monophasic syndromes with diffuse inflammatory demyelination of the CNS include acute disseminated encephalomyelitis (ADEM), Marburg variant of MS, Baló's concentric sclerosis, and other focal tumefactive demyelinating lesions that may simulate brain tumors (see Fig. 1). Distinction of these rare syndromes early in the course of disease has prognostic and treatment implications. Most patients who have isolated IIDDs recover from the attacks spontaneously or with corticosteroid treatment, whereas acute fulminant IIDDs or severe attacks of RRMS may be resistant to initial treatment with steroids but may respond dramatically to plasma exchange [26,27]. Early treatment with plasma exchange may lead to a moderate to marked functional improvement in 44% of patients who have an acute fulminant attack that has not been responsive to steroids, particularly in men and in those who have preserved reflexes at the onset of treatment [28]. No specific surrogate marker exists for the diagnosis of these disorders, but clinical, laboratory, and pathologic evidence in selected case may help distinguish these syndromes from other isolated IIDDs. (For a detailed review of pathologic features of these syndromes, see the article elsewhere in this issue by Lucchinetti et al.)

Innumerable, diffusely enhancing, subcortical, perivenous white matter lesions in MRI after a febrile illness in adolescents or children who have an absence of oligoclonal bands in CSF suggest ADEM. Pathology in such cases shows predominant perivascular inflammation with little evidence of confluent demyelination; demyelination is confined to sleeves of perivenous myelin. In many cases, distinction of ADEM from the first attack of RRMS may be difficult in children [29–33] and adults [34] without pathology support. Most patients who have ADEM recover, although relapses can occur in children and up to 20% mortality is described [35,36]. Given the lack of pathologic data from biopsy, clinical studies of the natural history of ADEM are of uncertain reliability, as the distinction between ADEM and fulminant forms of MS are difficult, if not impossible.

Confluent areas of enhancing hemispheric demyelination, typically asymmetric, on MRI in the absence of oligoclonal bands suggest the Marburg variant of MS [37]. Pathologically, the Marburg variant of MS is characterized by necrosis that is reflected in a more severe course. Patients who have the Marburg variant of MS may die, recover with significant morbidity, remain free of relapse, or develop clinical recurrences. The course of patients presenting with the Marburg variant of MS may evolve into prototypic RRMS after recovery from the initial attack [38].

Some patients may present with large tumor-like solitary demyelinating lesions. Baló's concentric sclerosis, the hallmark of which is a concentric whorled lesion, which may be identified on MRI scan in some cases, is reported to have a grave prognosis, although good response to corticosteroids is reported [39,40]. Other patients who have tumefactive lesions, however, respond to corticosteroids and have a more favorable course. The specificity and predictive value of the whorled appearance on MRI remains to be established. Many patients who have tumefactive lesions seem to have a monophasic course, but recurrent attacks typical of MS may develop in the future [41]. Brain biopsy often is necessary to differentiate acute tumefactive demyelinating lesions from tumors.

The long-term prognosis and natural history of fulminant IIDDs have not been well characterized, largely because of the limited number of patients and early morbidity and mortality resulting from these disorders. Should plasma exchange or other treatment modalities improve the outcome of the immediate attack, more patients may survive and recover, which will permit longer term follow-up of the long-term outcome, including evolution into prototypical MS.

Natural history of prototypical multiple sclerosis

The most common form of IIDD is RRMS. This prototypical disease evolves from an isolated demyelinating attack characterized by a multifocal inflammatory demyelination and varying degrees of accompanying axonal injury [42,43]. The disease has an asymptomatic period of unknown duration that precedes the initial presentation with an isolated syndrome [44]. After the presenting syndrome, patients have a variable course. Most continue to have relapses at a highly varying rate, some with complete remission and others with stepwise accumulation of deficit. SPMS evolves from RRMS after a highly variable period; the evolution is widely believed to be the result of the superimposition of progressive axonal injury that has exceeded the clinical threshold. Many natural history studies have examined the predictors of disease course in patients who have clinically definite MS as defined by Poser criteria. These studies may not apply directly to prediction of disease course in the asymptomatic period or initial presentation with an isolated demyelinating syndrome. Nevertheless, several predictors of long-term disability are identified consistently in populations regardless of ethnicity (discussed later as related to different endpoints).

Accumulating disability over time

Previous studies of natural history and prognostic factors in MS have used the Kurtzke Expanded Disability Status Scale (EDSS) to assess disability accumulating over time as an outcome measure [45]. EDSS is a sensitive scale of ambulatory disability, but it is an ordinal measure and is insensitive to cognitive dysfunction, which has an impact mainly on attention and fluency in 54% of patients even before a definite diagnosis of MS can be made [46]. Cognitive dysfunction seems to better correlate with the volume of MS lesions in the brain [47]. A task force sponsored by the National Multiple Sclerosis Society has proposed a new clinical assessment, the MS functional composite (MSFC), to address concerns about sensitivity, reproducibility, and detection of cognitive impairment [48]. Besides detecting cognitive impairment, MSFC correlates better than EDSS with hypointense T1- and hyperintense T2-weighted lesion volume, brain parenchymal fraction, and ventricular fraction volumes in MRI [49–51].

Despite some of the drawbacks of EDSS, several factors have been established consistently across ethnic barriers that predict a shorter time to reach more advanced levels of impairment (typically EDSS 6), including male gender; older age at onset (>40); motor, cerebellar, or sphincter symptoms at initial presentation; multifocal (polysymptomatic) disease at onset; frequent attacks within the first 5 years; short interval between the first two attacks; short time to reach an EDSS level 4; and a progressive course (Table 1) [52–61]. The EDSS score at 5 years correlates well with the long-term outcome, and the behavior of the disorder seems to be established by this time in most patients. Indeed, all the factors that seem to determine progression or accumulating disability over time seem to be operative until a disability level of EDSS 4 is reached. After this point the course is independent of baseline predictive factors [62]. Therefore, the course in the first 5 years usually predicts future outcome. This is not absolutely true, however, and seemingly benign cases may develop progressive disease [63].

Table 1
Predictors of natural history in prototypical relapsing-remitting multiple sclerosis with different endpoints

	Benign multiple sclerosis	Secondary progression	Long-term disability	Decreased survival
Demographic	Female gender Early age at onset	Male gender Older age at onset (>45)	Male gender Older age at onset (>45)	Male gender Higher socioeconomic status
Clinical	Optic neuritis or sensory symptoms at onset	Motor or sphincter symptoms at onset	Motor, cerebellar or sphincter symptoms or multifocal at onset	
	Long interattack interval—first 5 years (<3 attacks)	Recurrent motor or sphincter attacks	Short interattack interval—first 5 years (>3 attacks)	
	EDSS <3 in first 5 years	EDSS >4 in first 5 years	EDSS > 4 in first 5 years Progressive course	High early disability Progressive course
Radiologic			Brain atrophy correlates with long-term cognitive dysfunction	
Genetic	APOE*e2 allele		APOE*e4 allele	

Effect of pregnancy on natural history also has been studied. A dramatic decrease in relapse rate is observed throughout the pregnancy period, but patients seem to have an initial increase in the relapse rate post partum and follow their preconception disease course afterwards [64]. An earlier study suggests a significant decrease in the risk of a progressive course in women who became pregnant after onset of MS [65]. The decision to become pregnant, however, may be affected by disease course and a definite interpretation of the long-term effects of multiple pregnancies may be difficult to judge because of this bias.

MRI findings predicting conversion to definite MS have been used extensively as a surrogate marker of outcome in drug trials. The question can be raised as to how well MRI findings correlate with disease course and disability once a definite diagnosis of MS is established. Cross-sectional MRI analyses do not reliably predict the long-term outcome in MS. Conventional imaging studies fail to account for the extent of disease that is present in normal-appearing white matter and axonal damage at a given time [66]. Both these factors likely contribute to the long-term outcome in a given patient. Brain atrophy correlates with long-term cognitive dysfunction, which likely reflects predominant loss of axons and myelin [67]. The assessment of atrophy requires serial studies, however, which may help in follow-up of treatment effects but not in early prediction of disease course. Currently there is no initial MRI parameter that can be used by a clinician to predict the long-term natural history of MS once the diagnosis is established.

There has been recent interest in identifying genetic markers that predict long-term disease course and outcome in MS [68]. Genetic markers are particularly attractive and superior to most other biologic markers because they do not vary with disease stage or activity, as they are determined before the disease starts. Claims of association with disease course, however, are difficult to replicate. The most promising marker thus far is *APOE*; the presence of the e4 allele seems to be associated with worse prognosis and the presence of the e2 allele seems to be associated with a comparatively favorable disease course [68–70]. In contrast, the HLA DR1501 allele does not correlate with disease course, despite the fact that it increases susceptibility to MS [68]. A recent study challenges this notion, however, suggesting that there is a dose effect in the number of HLA DR1501 alleles and that homozygosity may be associated with more severe disease [71].

Recently, based on previous long-term studies, Scott et al [72] studied the short-term predictive value of six prognostic factors on disease progression as assessed by final EDSS and changes in EDSS between initial presentation and final follow-up. These factors were: age at onset (older versus younger than 40), symptoms at onset (motor or sensory plus motor versus isolated sensory or cranial nerve), interval between the first and second attacks (shorter than 2.5 years versus longer than 2.5 years), attack frequency in the first 2 years (greater than 2 versus less than or equal to 2), completeness of recovery from initial attacks as determined by EDSS at 1 year after the attack (greater than or equal to 2 versus less than 2), and MRI status (greater than three lesions accepted as suggestive of MS) at onset and at diagnosis of clinically definite MS. In this hospital-based cohort, the MRI findings did not predict short-term disease course or severity. When analyzed for time to an increase of a single digit in EDSS score, however, the patients who had four or more of these risk factors did significantly worse (mean of 34 months) than those who had four or fewer risk factors (mean of 87 months). This simplified and practical approach to incorporating conclusions from natural history studies into the decision-making about initiation of long-term treatment deserves further study and validation.

Development of secondary progression in multiple sclerosis

RRMS commonly evolves into a secondary progressive course, which is believed to represent the crossing of a threshold of axonal damage resulting from previous or ongoing inflammatory episodes that initially targeted myelin or oligodendrocytes. Although it may be difficult to determine when this happens clinically until it has already happened, and it may be difficult to use as an endpoint in drug trials, it is a relevant outcome measure that can be identified retrospectively. Three out of four patients in the population develop SPMS disease course by 25 years, whereas one remains with RRMS [57]. It has been established that male gender, older age at onset, polysymptomatic onset, and sphincter symptoms at onset predict conversion to SPMS [56,62,73,74]. Using a Bayesian model, considering all the information obtained during a longitudinal follow-up, early attainment of disability and higher attack rate of sphincter and motor symptoms predict conversion to SPMS, whereas frequent attacks of ON or other symptoms are less predictive as motor or sphincter attacks [74].

Benign versus nonbenign multiple sclerosis

Many studies attempt to classify disease course as benign versus nonbenign. The consensus for the definition of benign MS is that a patient remains fully functional in all neurologic systems 15 years after disease onset [75]. This definition, however, does not include any criteria for endpoint cut-off values, such as EDSS. Although no consensus exists for these cut-offs, several studies use definitions attempting to classify benign MS as an entity that is statically nonprogressive and does not result in accumulating disability. In the Turkish study, by 15 years' disease duration, one out of three individuals remained below an EDSS of 3 [58]. Almost half of the patients remained below an EDSS of 6 by 25 years [55,57,58]. In a population-based cohort [60] that was longitudinally followed and reassessed at 10 years, 68% (45 of 66) of the patients who had an EDSS less than 3 in the initial cohort (66 of 161 patients ascertained in 1991) remained fully functional at an EDSS less than 3 at 10-year follow-up, whereas only 17% developed an EDSS of 6 or higher [76]. In all the patients assessed initially in 1991, less than half (44%) remained below an EDSS of 6 by 2001. This study confirmed the presence of a benign disease course described in many of the earlier natural history studies. An untreated, completely ascertained MS cohort from Iceland was prospectively followed for 50 years. 75% of the patients had a relapsing-remitting or secondary progressive course and the remainder had a primary progressive disease course [77]. Of these patients, 76% remained at or below an EDSS of 3.5 after disease duration of greater than or equal to 15 years and 69% remained at or below an EDSS of 3.5 after 25 years.

Survival in multiple sclerosis

Survival is an easily replicable endpoint between studies, but 50% of MS patients die from causes other than MS [78] and mean survival is greater than 25 years after onset of disease [58,79–81]. Nevertheless, some of the factors that influence disability, such as gender, age at onset, initial symptoms, and socioeconomic status, also influence survival when large populations have been examined, presumably because death from MS largely is associated with advanced disability and progressive disease course

[82–84]. Therefore, factors that influence the rate of development of progressive disease course and the ability of disabled individuals to get high quality supportive care thereby influence survival rates.

Primary progressive multiple sclerosis

PPMS is the second most common form of IIDD after RRMS and represents approximately 7% of patients in a large hospital-based practice in California [85] and 20% of cases of MS in a population-based study from Ontario [86], using the published consensus definitions [75]. Disease course is one of insidious progression characterized by lack of clear-cut exacerbations and paucity of imaging (gadolinium-enhancing lesions), laboratory evidence, or, indeed, pathologic evidence of inflammation [87]. In this sense, it differs from other IIDDs and hence is discussed as a separate entity.

The insidious course typically leads to greater delay in patients seeking medical advice and diagnosis. By the time of diagnosis, patients often are mildly impaired (see Fig. 1). Patients later may recall an obscure attack that may have marked the beginning of the disease, thereby blurring the distinction between RRMS and PPMS. Older age of onset, lack of female preponderance, predilection to chronic progressive myelopathy, and paucity of intracranial lesions in MRI distinguish PPMS from the prototypical RRMS [88]. PPMS generally is included in the studies of natural history of MS and is the most robust predictor of a poor outcome, independent of any other demographic or clinical factor. Half of patients who have a progressive course from onset require at least unilateral gait assistance (EDSS $\geq$ 6) by 8 years [85,86]. Within the PPMS group, however, having three or more functional systems involvement (motor, cerebellar, sensory, or other) predicts a significantly worse outcome than having two or less systems involvement in the Ontario study [86]. Median time to EDSS 6, which marks moderate disability, is 5 years earlier, and median time to death is 13.5 years in the group where three or more functional systems are involved, versus the 33.2 years in the group where two or less functional systems are involved. The behavior of PPMS is found to be similar to that of SPMS when only the progressive phases are considered. These findings confirm the previous data from Sweden [57] and Turkey [58] suggesting that although PPMS has a worse prognosis, the median time to reach EDSS 6 is similar to that of SPMS, once the progressive phase of that group has begun; after 15 years, these forms of MS result in similar disability levels. One other finding that has emerged from previous studies is that PPMS and progressive relapsing MS follow the same course despite the superimposition of occasional attacks, such as ON, on top of the progressive course. Hence, there is no practical reason to differentiate these entities [85,86].

Because most of these studies use the Kurtzke EDSS, which is sensitive to ambulatory disability, it is no surprise that progressive disease defined by progressive motor dysfunction is associated with significant disability and high rates of unemployment with financial dependence [89].

Can we predict response to treatment in idiopathic inflammatory demyelinating diseases?

With the introduction of long-term disease-modifying therapies, an important outcome measure to consider is the modification of natural history of IIDDs. The overall effect of the new immunomodulatory agents on the evolution of MS-related disability in the MS population is unknown, but it is likely that there is substantial interindividual variation. Evaluation of predictors of individual response may facilitate cost-effective use of immunomodulation.

The impact of disease-modifying therapies on the natural history of multiple sclerosis

Current immunomodulatory therapies have an impact on many aspects of MS, principally inflammatory disease activity, as reflected by a reduction in attack frequency, attack severity, gadolinium-enhancing lesions, and T2 lesion burden. There is less convincing evidence that such treatments modify the neurodegenerative component of MS, as manifested by progression of disability in the absence of measurable inflammation, which applies to many patients who have SPMS and most patients who have PPMS, although interferon-β1a (Avonex, Biogen, Cambridge, Massachusetts, USA) may reduce the rate of brain atrophy [90].

The efficacy of long-term interventions has been shown in the context of short-term (2- to 5-year) randomized clinical trials. This has led to considerable speculation as to whether or not such treatments have longer-term clinical benefits. If this were the case, their use in all patients who have MS and at an early point in the illness, as advocated by some, would be easier to justify. The study of this issue is complicated enormously by factors that are partly generic to any long-term outcome study and also by factors specific to the analysis of the effects of therapies.

1. Patients are selected to receive treatment based on indications that are dependent on physician and patient opinions. Generally, physicians advise such treatments in those who have relapsing-remitting disease or some evidence of continuing, active inflammation in the context of SPMS. Some clinicians, however, initiate treatment in patients who have first presentation of demyelinating disease before dissemination in time and space is established (clinically isolated syndrome), whereas others do not initiate treatment except in those patients who have well-established evidence of continuing inflammatory disease activity. It is likely that individual patients chosen for therapy vary considerably in

prognosis and that the benefits of therapy will vary according to the reasons that treatment was initiated. Even in clinical trials that have homogeneous entry criteria, there probably is considerable variation in the application of the enrollment criteria based on individual opinions at the investigative sites of the need for long-term therapy in patients evaluated for participation.

2. The benefit experienced by individual patients may vary considerably, and the long-term benefit in terms of disability must be considered in light of intermediate or surrogate markers or endpoints that evaluate treatment benefit for individual patients. One of the major questions after demonstration of efficacy is prediction of individuals who are likely to benefit from long-term therapy. Currently available surrogate markers (gadolinium-enhancing lesions, MRI T2 lesion load, and MRI measurements of atrophy) and ultimate clinical measures for disease outcome (EDSS change and cognitive change) are weakly or not correlated, thereby compromising the use of such surrogates as strong indicators of ultimate outcome.
3. Long-term adherence to therapy is imperfect, in part because of lack of agreement on what constitutes treatment failure. Some interpret any evidence of continuing inflammatory disease activity (attacks or MRI lesions) as grounds for treatment failure and possibly modification of therapy. Others are more conservative and advise maintenance of a given therapy until robust indicators of treatment failure (major increase in disability or evolution to SPMS) are achieved. There is no standard treatment strategy that is applied widely to those who have treatment failure that would allow for an analysis of a specific combination of therapies administered in succession based on treatment failure from a first-line agent.
4. Patients who choose not to continue therapy or not to be followed usually do so because of perceived lack of efficacy. Hence, informative censoring, wherein there is a systematic bias in those discontinuing therapy or long-term follow-up, may influence the results of any long-term follow-up.
5. Benefit of treatments may change over time. To a large extent, this reflects the fact that the primary mechanism of disease evolution may change from inflammatory activity, generally reflected by attacks and new MRI lesions, to neurodegeneration, probably better reflected by cerebral atrophy and N-acetyl aspartate levels on magnetic resonance spectroscopy. Inflammatory and degenerative mechanisms seem to occur simultaneously in most patients, although the relative contribution of each may vary considerably. Another factor altering the benefit of treatment over time is development of neutralizing antibodies to interferon-β, which may mitigate some of the benefit of therapy in a sizable minority of patients, with variation according to the specific preparation of interferon-β used.

The strategies that theoretically may be applied to study the impact of disease-modifying therapies on the natural history of MS include the following:

1. Extend clinical trials of therapeutic agents for long periods of time (ie, 10 years or more) and concentrate on less expensive but more robust measures, such as major change in disability, or milestones, such as attainment of EDSS 6 (requires a cane) or EDSS 8 (wheelchair confined).
2. Conduct long-term follow-up of individual patients who receive treatment or participate in a clinical trial, concentrating on robust outcomes as noted previously. Patients in clinical trials have good quality baseline data. As is typical of recent studies, patients are compared with those who originally had been randomized to placebo. Because of the short duration of such studies, patients commonly take placebo for only 2 to 3 years, after which many switch to open-label therapy. Hence, the benefits of therapy may be underestimated, should the active-treatment-from-onset group be compared with the placebo-from-onset group; the placebo group may receive treatment for a substantial part of the follow-up period. The outcomes in patients in such trials could be compared with data from natural history studies on a data set matched for important prognostic variables, such as disease duration, baseline disability, and possibly others. Such an approach would be highly dependent on adherence to therapy, the following of all patients, and the adequacy of matching to natural history controls. The problems of informative censoring are discussed previously. If adequately powered, however, informative sensoring would be able to detect differences in select subgroups of patients who might benefit, even if many patients do not. Such follow-up studies may measure surrogate markers and robust clinical markers and would have the advantage of correlating change over time in such surrogates with robust ultimate indicators. Bayesian principles are ideal for such an approach [74,91].
3. Survey communities with complete ascertainment and well-characterized disability profiles, concentrating on overall changes in robust indicators, such as the proportion wheelchair confined or institutionally-confined. Although this is the ultimate measure of success for such therapies, and concerns about bias would be mitigated by the complete ascertainment approach, the success of such a strategy depends on having an adequate proportion of patients exposed to and adhering to therapy. Such a strategy still may miss a beneficial effect on an important minority of patients by studying the change over time in the entire cohort.

There are no available examples of lengthy long-term clinical trials (approach 1 above). Few pharmaceutical companies are able to underwrite such an effort. Also, it is difficult to have patients accept a randomized trial, particularly a placebo-controlled study of this duration.

There have been community-wide assessments of disability (approach 3 above) in a limited number of population-based studies that have evaluated the change in spectrum of disability in a single community over time [76]. The proportion of patients in such communities who have been treated with long-term therapies, however, has been small. In a study in Olmsted County, Minnesota, in 2000 involving a cross-sectional analysis of disability, 25% of patients had received one of the standard disease-modifying therapies for MS (interferon-β1b or -β1a or glatiramer acetate) [76]. Of patients receiving treatment, the mean duration of treatment was 13 to 15 months for the specific agent that they were taking, and 44% of those who had been started on treatment had stopped their initial treatment. Of those discontinuing therapy, fewer than 50% started taking an alternative agent. Thus, these considerations provide low power for using the community survey approach to assess the overall impact of such agents on the profile of disability in the community. Although this may not reflect the proportion of patients taking these agents in other communities, the Olmsted County community is among the most intensively studied for the spectrum of disability since the early 1990s.

Attempts have been made to obtain long-term follow-up studies of patients in the glatiramer acetate and interferon-β1a (Avonex and Rebif, Serono, Serono International S.A., Geneva, Switzerland) clinical trials of patients who have RRMS. In fact, there have been long-term cross-sectional evaluations at 8 years in patients who participated in the major pivotal trials that led to FDA approval of these three agents. None have been published as full manuscripts, and only abstract data are available. Sufficient data in abstract form are available for two preparations of interferon-β1a, which are summarized in Table 2. The adequacy of these studies is highly dependent on completeness of follow-up and absence of informative censoring. Ninety three percent completion of follow-up was achieved for the interferon-β1a (Avonex) clinical trial study (Rudick et al., personal communication, 2004) versus 68% for the interferon-β1a (Rebif) clinical trial [92]. Comparisons of placebo groups and active groups seem to show a benefit in favor of those initially randomized to active therapy. An attempt has been made to compare the results in the interferon-β1a long-term follow-up study to those expected from natural history studies. This approach is one that must be undertaken and, when fully exploited, might allow comparison of prognostic factors and factors potentially predictive of disease response that can be determined at enrollment to stratify the analysis appropriately. An independent body performing such data analyses would be ideal considering the proprietary interests of industry and the need for a consistent matching approach based on available data. Cooperation between industry and independent investigative agencies with wide support and credibility is essential to this process.

Table 2
Long-term follow-up studies of clinical trials in relapsing-remitting multiple sclerosis

	Rebif (interferon-β1a) PRISMS [92]			Avonex (interferon-β1a) Avonex Pivotal Study[a]	
Treatment arm	Placebo	44 μg tiw	22 μg tiw	Placebo	30 μg qweekly
N eligible	184	189	187	87[a]	85[b]
Duration of blinded study (y)		2			2
Follow-up interval (y)		8			8
N followed (% randomized)	123 (67)	136 (74)	123 (65)	81 (93)	79 (93)
% Followed on original treatment at follow-up		74	70		
Mean time on study active agent (y)	5.2+	7.3+	7.2+	3.4	2.9
EDSS at enrollment (mean ± SD)	2.4 ± 1.2	2.5 ± 1.3	2.5 ± 1.2	2.3 ± 0.1	2.4 ± 0.1
EDSS change at follow-up					
Median time to 1-point worsening	3.9	7.2	5.2		
% Worsened to original endpoint	55[c]	42[c]	55[b]		
First quartile to 2-point worsening	3.8	6.5	6		
% at EDSS 6 or worse		20		42	29

[a] (Rudick et al., personal communication, 2004.)
[b] Completed 2-year follow-up at study termination.
[c] At 7 years; 1 EDSS point for EDSS < 6, 0.5 for EDSS > 6; estimated from graph.

Predictors of early response to treatment in multiple sclerosis

As discussed previously, long-term outcome assessment of disease-modifying effects of treatments in prototypical RRMS is limited. Even with short-term responses, however, one problem that plagues the analysis of response to therapy is the inconsistent definition of responder versus nonresponder in different drug trials. Typically, treatment failure is defined in absolute terms (eg, "Is there continuing evidence of attacks?" "Has SPMS supervened?"). A more reasonable approach may involve a consideration of the difference between a period of baseline clinical and possible MRI activity and the activity while on treatment. A preference for an absolute over relative definition is dependent on the clinician's estimate of the value of current immunomodulatory therapies and the standard to which these treatments should be held. If near-complete suppression is believed to be the standard, then an absolute definition may be appropriate but may be unrealistic given current therapy and may lead to excessive switching of treatment or discontinuation of effective therapy.

Although the short-term follow-up in the CHAMPS study suggests that conversion to definite MS is delayed with early treatment in clinically isolated IIDDs, the long-term benefit on natural history or predictors of prevention of conversion to definite MS are unknown [93]. In recent post hoc analyses of this study, the benefit from interferon-β1a is more evident in an isolated spinal cord syndrome than a brainstem-cerebellar syndrome; in the case of isolated ON, the effect is marginal [94]. If the patients were stratified into a high-risk group using a more stringent definition of having at least nine T2-weighted hyperintense lesions and at least one enhancing lesion in the initial MRI, a two-thirds reduction was predicted in conversion to definite MS in 2 years [95]. Even in this group, however, almost half the patients (44%) did not convert to definite MS in 2 years without any treatment. Results from this study suggest that, at least in the short term, interferon-β may slow down the natural history of isolated IIDDs in terms of conversion to MS but the benefit is more predictable in patients who have a spinal cord syndrome at onset or more disease activity as evidenced by the higher MRI lesion load.

Some short-term predictors of response to interferon-β therapy in clinically definite RRMS or SPMS are older age at onset, long disease duration, and higher relapse rate the year before initiation of treatment [96–99]. Recently, early and sustained induction of soluble serum TNF-related apoptosis inducing ligand (TRAIL) levels has been associated with good response and no induction is associated with poor response to treatment with interferon-β [100]. Development of neutralizing antibodies through the course of the disease dampened the TRAIL response and persistence of clinical response. In one study, the HLA DRB1*1501 genotype was associated with response to copolymer but not interferon-β treatment [101]. If confirmed, the results from the latter two studies may provide biologic markers to predict early and short-term response to disease-modifying treatments. Recent unconfirmed attempts to use genetic expression profiling of responders versus nonresponders to interferon treatment has provided limited information. However, this type of discovery approach may be a feasible method in large well characterized patient series that have sufficient power and long-term follow-up to provide a biologic marker that will predict response to treatment. It may ultimately enhance the future understanding of the MS disease process [102].

Summary

The natural history of prototypical MS at the population level is well established. Conversion to definite MS in patients who have clinically isolated demyelinating events is the subject of great interest in the context of several large clinical trials, and reasonable stratification of individual risk is possible in this context. The natural history of some of the more rare forms of IIDDs only recently are being elucidated. Most of the predictors of outcome are individually weak but a combination of initial demographic and clinical findings with measures of early disease activity and course evaluated clinically and with imaging can be used to predict outcome. Inasmuch as practicing clinicians need to be aware of the existence of benign cases and isolated IIDDs that never convert to definite MS, they also need to realize that for patients who have early deterioration, the long-term course likely is unfavorable and an aggressive approach to application of proven therapies is appropriate.This review emphasizes the importance of evaluating patient-specific factors to predict outcome and tailor therapy for the individual. But considering the imperfection of any of the current predictors of disease outcome, it is necessary to monitor patients with standard clinical measurements and, in research contexts, with increasingly sophisticated imaging and other tools. Hopefully, some of these newer modalities may prove more sensitive and predictive of clinically important consequences. There have been some promising developments in terms of predicting treatment response; they are limited, however, to short-term responses; predictors of long-term response have not yet been established. The MS community still is in need of better surrogate markers and predictors of treatment response and long-term outcome that can be instituted cost effectively into clinical management pathways. Research in the areas of genetics, immunology, and pathology of IIDDs promises to provide us with such markers in the future.

References

[1] Weinshenker BG. The natural history of multiple sclerosis. Neurol Clin N Am 1995;13: 119–46.

[2] Confavreux C, Vukusic S. Natural history of multiple sclerosis: implications for counselling and therapy. Curr Opin Neurol 2002;15:257–66.

[3] The IFNβ Multiple Sclerosis Study Group. Interferon beta-1b is effective in relapsing-remitting multiple sclerosis. I. Clinical results of a multicenter, randomized, double-blind, placebo-controlled trial. Neurology 1993;43:6655–61.

[4] Johnson KP, Brooks BR, Cohen JA, et al. Copolymer I reduces relapse rate and improves disability in relapsing-remitting multiple sclerosis: results of a phase III multicenter, double-blind, placebo-controlled trial. Neurology 1995;45:1268–76.

[5] Hartung HP, Gonsette R, König N, et al. Mitoxantrone in progressive multiple sclerosis: a placebo-controlled, double-blind, randomized, multi-center trial. Lancet 2002;360: 2018–25.

[6] Trapp BD, Peterson J, Ransohoff RM, et al. Axonal transection in the lesions of multiple sclerosis. N Engl J Med 1998;338:278–85.

[7] Weinshenker BG, Fujihara K, Pittock SJ, et al. The Asian optico-spinal form of multiple sclerosis is the same entity as Neuromyelitis Optica in Caucasians: insights from a novel serum marker. Neurology 2004;62:A480–1.

[8] Poser CM, Paty DW, Scheinberg LC, et al. New diagnostic criteria for multiple sclerosis: guidelines for research protocols. Ann Neurol 1983;13:227–31.

[9] McDonald IW, Compston A, Edan G, et al. Recommended diagnostic criteria for multiple sclerosis: Guidelines from the international panel on the diagnosis of multiple sclerosis. Ann Neurol 2001;50:121–7.

[10] Tintore M, Rovira A, Rio J, et al. New diagnostic criteria for multiple sclerosis: application in first demyelinating episode. Neurology 2003;60:27–30.

[11] Brex PA, Ciccarelli O, O'Riordan JI, et al. A longitudinal study of abnormalities on MRI and disability from multiple sclerosis. N Engl J Med 2002;346:158–64.
[12] CHAMPS Study Group. MRI predictors of early conversion to clinically definite MS in the CHAMPS placebo group. Neurology 2002;59:998–1005.
[13] Miller DH, Newton MR, Van der Poel JC, et al. Magnetic resonance imaging of the optic nerve in optic neuritis. Neurology 1998;38:175–9.
[14] Optic Neuritis Study Group. High- and low-risk profiles for the development of multiple sclerosis within 10 years after optic neuritis. Experience of the optic neuritis treatment trial. Arch Opthalmol 2003;121:944–9.
[15] Lucchinetti CF, Kiers L, O'Duffy A, et al. Risk factors for developing multiple sclerosis after childhood optic neuritis. Neurology 1997;49:1413–8.
[16] Söderström M, Ya-Ping J, Hillert J, et al. Optic neuritis: prognosis for multiple sclerosis from MRI, CSF and HLA findings. Neurology 1998;50:708–14.
[17] Scott TF, Bhagavatula K, Snyder PJ, et al. Transverse myelitis. Comparison with spinal cord presentations of multiple sclerosis. Neurology 1998;50:429–33.
[18] Campi A, Filippi M, Comi G, et al. Acute transverse myelopathy: spinal and cranial MR study with clinical follow-up. Am J Neuroradiol 1995;16:115–23.
[19] Cordonnier C, de Seze J, Breteau G, et al. Prospective study of patients presenting with acute partial transverse myelopathy. J Neurol 2003;250:1447–52.
[20] Ford B, Tampieri D, Francis G. Long-term follow-up of acute partial transverse myelopathy. Neurology 1992;42:250–2.
[21] Shibasaki H, Kuroda Y, Kuriowa Y. Clinical studies of multiple sclerosis in Japan: classical multiple sclerosis and Devic's disease. J Neurol Sci 1974;23:215–22.
[22] O'Riordan JI, Gallagher GL, Thompson AJ, et al. Clinical, CSF and MRI findings in Devic's neuromyelitis optica. J Neurol Neurosurg Psychiatry 1996;60:382–7.
[23] Wingerchuk DM, Hogencamp WF, O'Brien PS, et al. The clinical course of neuromyelitis optica (Devic's disease). Neurology 1999;53:1107–14.
[24] Wingerchuk DM, Weinshenker BG. Neuromyelitis optica: clinical predictors of a relapsing course and survival. Neurology 2003;60:848–53.
[25] Weinshenker BG. Neuromyelitis optica: what it is and what it might be. Lancet 2003;361: 889–90.
[26] Weinshenker BG, O'Brian PC, Petterson TN, et al. A randomized trial of plasma exchange in acute central nervous system inflammatory demyelinating disease. Ann Neurol 1999;46: 878–86.
[27] Weinshenker BG. Therapeutic plasma exchange for acute inflammatory demyelinating syndromes of the central nervous system. J Clin Apheresis 1999;14:144–8.
[28] Keegan M, Pineda AA, McClelland RL, et al. Plasma exchange for severe attacks of CNS demyelination: predictors of response. Neurology 2002;58:143–6.
[29] Duquette P, Murray TJ, Pleines GC, et al. Multiple sclerosis in childhood: clinical profile in 125 patients. J Pediatr 1987;111:359–63.
[30] Ghezzi A, Deplano V, Faroni J, et al. Multiple sclerosis in childhood: clinical features of 149 cases. Mult Scler 1997;3:43–6.
[31] Kesselring J, Miller DH, Robb SA, et al. Acute disseminated encephalomyelitis: MRI findings and distinction from multiple sclerosis. Brain 1990;113:291–302.
[32] Tenembaum S, Chamoles N, Fejerman N. Acute disseminated encephalomyelitis: a long-term follow-up study of 84 pediatric patients. Neurology 2002;59:1224–31.
[33] Hartung HP, Grossman RI. ADEM: distinct disease or part of the MS spectrum? Neurology 2001;56:1257–60.
[34] Schwarz S, Mohr A, Knauth M, et al. Acute disseminated encephalomyelitis: a follow-up study of 40 adult patients. Neurology 2001;56:1313–8.
[35] Dale RC, de Sousa C, Chong WK, et al. Acute disseminated encephalomyelitis, multiphasic disseminated encephalomyelitis and multiple sclerosis in children. Brain 2000;123: 2407–22.

[36] Hynson JL, Kornberg AJ, Coleman LT, et al. Clinical and neuroradiological features of acute disseminated encephalomyelitis in children. Neurology 2001;56:1308–12.
[37] Johnson MD, Lavin P, Whetsell WO Jr. Fulminant monophasic multiple sclerosis, Marburg's type. J Neurol Neurosurg Psychiatry 1990;53:918–21.
[38] Giubilei F, Sarrantonio A, Tisei P, et al. Four-year follow-up of a case of acute multiple sclerosis of the Marburg type. Ital J Neurol Sci 1997;18:163–6.
[39] Revel MP, Valiente E, Gray F, et al. Concentric MR pattern in multiple sclerosis: report of two cases. J Neuroradiol 1993;20:252–7.
[40] Bolay H, Karabudak R, Tacal T, et al. Balo's concentric sclerosis: report of two patients. J Neuroimaging 1996;6:98–103.
[41] Kepes JJ. Large focal tumor-like demyelinating lesions of the brain: Intermediate entity between multiple sclerosis and acute disseminated encephalomyelitis—a study of 31 patients. Ann Neurol 1993;33:18–27.
[42] Lucchinetti C, Bruck W, Parisi J, et al. Heterogeneity of multiple sclerosis lesions: implications for the pathogenesis of demyelination. Ann Neurol 2000;47:707–17.
[43] Lucchinetti C, Bruck W, Noseworthy J. Multiple sclerosis: recent developments in neuropathology, pathogenesis, magnetic resonance imaging studies and treatment. Curr Opin Neurol 2001;14:259–69.
[44] Allen IV. Asymptomatic multiple sclerosis: what does it mean? In: Siva A, Kesselring J, Thompson A, editors. Frontiers in multiple sclerosis, vol. II. London: Martin Dunitz; 1999. p. 11–5.
[45] Kurtzke JF. Rating neurological impairment in MS: an Expanded Disability Status Scale (EDSS). Neurology 1983;33:1444–52.
[46] Achiron A, Barak Y. Cognitive impairment in probable multiple sclerosis. J Neurol Neurosurg Psychiatry 2003;74:443–6.
[47] Hohol MJ, Guttmann CR, Orav J, et al. Serial neuropsychological assessment and magnetic resonance imaging analysis in multiple sclerosis. Arch Neurol 1997;54:1018–25.
[48] Rudick R, Antel J, Confavreux C, et al. Clinical outcomes assessment in multiple sclerosis. Ann Neurol 1996;40:469–79.
[49] Kalkers NF, Bergers L, de Groot V, et al. Concurrent validity of the MS functional composite using MRI as a biological disease marker. Neurology 2001;56:215–9.
[50] Rudick RA, Cutter G, Baier M, et al. Use of the Multiple Sclerosis Functional Composite to predict disability in relapsing MS. Neurology 2001;56:1324–30.
[51] Kalkers NF, Bergers E, Castelijns JA, et al. Optimizing the association between disability and biological markers in MS. Neurology 2001;57:1253–8.
[52] Kurtzke JF, Beebe GW, Nagler B, et al. Studies on the natural history of multiple sclerosis. Early prognostic features of the later course of the illness. J Chronic Dis 1977;30:819–30.
[53] Confavreux C, Aimared G, Devic M. Course and prognosis of multiple sclerosis assessed by computerized data processing of 349 patients. Brain 1980;103:281–300.
[54] Phadke JG. Clinical aspects of multiple sclerosis in north-east Scotland with particular reference to its course and prognosis. Brain 1990;113:1597–628.
[55] Weinshenker BG, Rice GP, Noseworthy JH, et al. The natural history of multiple sclerosis: a geographically based study. III. Multivariate analysis of predictive factors and models of outcome. Brain 1991;114:1045–56.
[56] Riise T, Gronning M, Fernandez O, et al. Early prognostic factors for disability in multiple sclerosis, a European multicenter study. Acta Neurol Scand 1992;85:212–8.
[57] Runmarker B, Andersson O. Prognostic factors in a multiple sclerosis incidence cohort with 25 years follow-up. Brain 1993;116:117–34.
[58] Kantarci O, Siva A, Eraksoy M, et al. Survival and predictors of disability in Turkish MS patients. Neurology 1998;51:765–72.
[59] Myhr KM, Riise T, Vedeler C, et al. Disability and prognosis in multiple sclerosis: demographic and clinical variable important for the ability to walk and awarding of disability pension. Mult Scler 2001;7:59–65.

[60] Rodriguez M, Siva A, Ward J, et al. Impairment, disability and handicap in multiple sclerosis: a population based study in Olmsted County, Minnesota. Neurology 1994;44: 28–33.
[61] Levic ZM, Dujmovic I, Pekmezovic T, et al. Prognostic factors for survival in multiple sclerosis. Mult Scler 1999;5:171–8.
[62] Confavreux C, Vukusic S, Moreau T, et al. Relapses and progression of disability in multiple sclerosis. N Engl J Med 2000;343:1430–8.
[63] Thompson AJ. Benign multiple sclerosis. J Neurol Neurosurg Psychiatry 1999;67:138.
[64] Confavreux C, Hutchinson M, Hours MM, et al. Rate of pregnancy-related relapse in multiple sclerosis. N Engl J Med 1998;339:285–91.
[65] Runmarker B, Andersen O. Pregnancy is associated with a lower risk of onset and a better prognosis in multiple sclerosis. Brain 1995;118(Pt 1):253–61.
[66] Miller DH, Thompson AJ, Filippi M. Magnetic resonance studies of abnormalities in the normal appearing white matter and grey matter in multiple sclerosis. J Neurol 2003;250: 1407–19.
[67] Zivadinov R, Sepcic J, Nasuelli D, et al. A longitudinal study of brain atrophy and cognitive disturbances in the early phase of relapsing-remitting multiple sclerosis. Neurol Neurosurg Psychiatry 2001;70:773–80.
[68] Kantarci OH, de Andrade M, Weinshenker BG. Identifying disease modifying genes in multiple sclerosis. J Neuroimmunol 2002;123:144–59.
[69] Schmidt S, Barcellos LF, DeSombre K, et al. Multiple Sclerosis Genetics Group. Association of polymorphisms in the apolipoprotein E region with susceptibility to and progression of multiple sclerosis. Am J Hum Genet 2002;70:708–17.
[70] Kantarci OH, Hebrink DD, Achenbach SJ, et al. Association of *apoE* polymorphisms with disease severity in MS is limited to women. Neurology 2004;65:811–4.
[71] Barcellos LF, Oksenberg JR, Begovich AB, et al. HLA-DR2 dose effect on susceptibility to multiple sclerosis and influence on disease course. Am J Hum Genet 2003;72:710–6.
[72] Scott TF, Schramke CJ, Novero J, Chieffe C. Short-term prognosis in early relapsing-remitting multiple sclerosis. Neurology 2000;55:689–93.
[73] Trojano M, Avolio C, Manzari C, et al. Multivariate analysis of predictive factors of multiple sclerosis course with a validated method to assess clinical events. J Neurol Neurosurg Psychiatry 1995;58:300–6.
[74] Bergamaschi R, Berzuini C, Romani A, et al. Predicting secondary progression in relapsing-remitting multiple sclerosis; a Bayesian analysis. J Neurol Sci 2001;189:13–21.
[75] Lublin FD, Reingold SC. Defining the clinical course of multiple sclerosis: results of an international survey. Neurology 1996;50:423–8.
[76] Pittock SJ, Mayr WT, McClelland RL, et al. Change in MS-related disability in a population-based cohort: a 10-year follow-up study. Neurology 2004;62:51–9.
[77] Benedikz J, Stefansson M, Guomundsson J, et al. The natural history of untreated multiple sclerosis in Iceland. A total population-based 50 year prospective study. Clin Neurol Neurosurg 2002;104:208–10.
[78] Sadovnick AD, Eisen K, Ebers GC, et al. Cause of death in patients attending multiple sclerosis clinics. Neurology 1991;41:1193–6.
[79] Phadke JG. Survival pattern and cause of death in patients with multiple sclerosis. Results from an epidemiological survey in North East Scotland. J Neurol Neurosurg Psychiatry 1987;50:523–31.
[80] Riise T, Gronning M, Aarli JA, et al. Prognostic factors for life expectancy in multiple sclerosis analyzed by Cox models. J Clin Epidemiol 1988;41:1031–6.
[81] Poser S, Kurtzke JF, Poser W, Schlaf G. Survival in multiple sclerosis. J Clin Epidemiol 1989;42:159–68.
[82] Bronnum-Hansen H, Koch Henriksen N, Hyllested K. Survival of patients with multiple sclerosis in Denmark: a nationwide, long-term epidemiologic survey. Neurology 1994;44: 1901–7.

[83] Pekmezovic T, Jarebinski M, Drulovic J, et al. Survival of multiple sclerosis patients in the Belgrade population. Neuroepidemiology 2002;21:235–40.
[84] Wallin MT, Page WF, Kurtzke JF. Epidemiology of multiple sclerosis in US veterans. VIII. Long-term survival after onset of multiple sclerosis. Brain 2000;123(Pt 8):1677–87.
[85] Andersson PB, Waubant E, Gee L, Goodkin DE. Multiple sclerosis that is progressive from the time of onset: clinical characteristics and progression of disability. Arch Neurol 1999;56: 1138–42.
[86] Cottrell DA, Kremenchutzky M, Rice GP, et al. The natural history of multiple sclerosis: a geographically based study: 5. The clinical features and natural history of primary progressive multiple sclerosis. Brain 1999;122:625–39.
[87] Revesz T, Kidd D, Thompson AJ, et al. A comparison of the pathology of primary and secondary progressive multiple sclerosis. Brain 1994;117:759–65.
[88] McDonnell GV, Hawkins SA. Primary progressive multiple sclerosis: increasing clarity but many unanswered questions. J Neurol Sci 2002;199(1–2):1–15.
[89] McDonnell GV, Hawkins SA. Clinical study of primary progressive multiple sclerosis in Northern Ireland. J Neurol Neurosurg Psychiatry 1998;64:451–4.
[90] Fischer JS, Priore RL, Jacobs LD, et al. Neuropsychological effects of interferon beta-1a in relapsing multiple sclerosis. Multiple Sclerosis Collaborative Research Group. Ann Neurol 2000;48:885–92.
[91] Weinshenker BG. Bayesian analysis: What does it add to studies of the natural history of MS? J Neurol Sci 2001;189:1–2.
[92] Paty D, Kappos L, Moraga MS, et al. Long-term observational efficacy and safety follow-up of the PRISMS cohort. Mult Scler 2003;(Suppl 1):P555.
[93] Jacobs LD, Beck RW, Simon JH, et al. Intramuscular interferon beta-1a therapy initiated during a first demyelinating event in multiple sclerosis. CHAMPS Study Group. N Engl J Med 2000;343:898–904.
[94] Beck RW, Chandler DL, Cole SR, et al. Interferon beta-1a for early multiple sclerosis: CHAMPS trial subgroup analyses. Ann Neurol 2002;51:481–90.
[95] O'Connor P, CHAMPS. The effects of intramascular interferon beta-Ia in patients at high risk for development of multiple sclerosis: a post hoc analysis of data from CHAMPS. Clin Ther 2003;25:2865–74.
[96] Kracke A, von Wussow P, Al-Masri A, et al. Mx proteins in blood leukocytes for monitoring interferon beta-1b therapy in patients with MS. Neurology 2000;54:193–9.
[97] Kappos L, Polman C, Pozzilli C, et al. Final analysis of the European multicenter trial on IFNB-1b in secondary progressive MS. Neurology 2001;57:1969–75.
[98] Roullet E, Pez D, Le Canuet P, et al. Application of different criteria for clinical response to beta-interferon in relapsing-remitting MS. Neurology 2003;(Suppl 1):A168.
[99] Waubant E, Vukusic S, Gignoux L, et al. Clinical characteristics of responders to interferon therapy for relapsing MS. Neurology 2003;61:184–9.
[100] Wandinger KP, Lunemann JD, Wengert O, et al. TNF-related apoptosis inducing ligand (TRAIL) as a potential response marker for interferon-beta treatment in multiple sclerosis. Lancet 2003;361:2036–43.
[101] Fusco C, Andreone V, Coppola G, et al. HLA-DRB1*1501 and response to copolymer-1 therapy in relapsing-remitting multiple sclerosis. Neurology 2001;57:1976–9.
[102] Sturzebecher S, Wandinger KP, Rosenwald A, et al. Expression profiling identifies responder and non-responder phenotypes to interferon-beta in multiple sclerosis. Brain 2003;126(Pt 6):1419–29.

ELSEVIER
SAUNDERS

Neurol Clin 23 (2005) 39–60

NEUROLOGIC
CLINICS

Gender Issues

Patricia K. Coyle, MD*

Multiple Sclerosis Comprehensive Care Center, School of Medicine, SUNY at Stony Brook, Stony Brook, NY, USA

Gender is involved in both characteristic presentations of multiple sclerosis (MS): the young woman of childbearing age who has episodic neurologic dysfunction and the older man who has progressive myelopathy. MS is a prototype for neurologic disease which benefits from a gender-based approach, because sex influences virtually every aspect of the disorder (Table 1). This article reviews the multifaceted impact of gender and sex on MS.

Basic biology

Perhaps the strongest justification for a gender-based approach to human diseases is the fact that body organs (and in particular the nervous, endocrine, and immune systems) differ anatomically and physiologically by sex [1]. Certainly the nervous system is recognized as sexually dimorphic [2,3]. Men and women show intrinsic differences in density of neurons; size of regional brain areas and cell clusters; cell receptor expression; neurotransmitter systems; cerebral blood flow patterns; response to stress, hunger, and satiety; and cortical activation patterns.

Neuroimaging studies in healthy control patients, using 4-Tesla (strength level) MRI, confirm sex-based differences [4]. Global brain white matter water content is higher in women. Women have smaller white matter volumes, but larger gray matter volumes, than men. Men's brains do not age as well as women's, with greater increases in white matter water content and reported greater losses of gray matter volume, than women. A recent study of the spinal cord reports that men have larger upper cervical cord volumes than women [5].

* Department of Neurology, School of Medicine, SUNY at Stony Brook, HSC, T12, Room 020, Stony Brook, NY 11794-8121.

E-mail address: pcoyle@notes.cc.sunysb.edu

doi:10.1016/j.ncl.2004.10.003 *neurologic.theclinics.com*

Table 1
Gender and sex aspects of multiple sclerosis

Demographic factors
Disease is most common in young, postpubertal women
Men are preferentially affected by progressive subtype, with perimenopausal onset
Men have a worse prognosis
Etiologic factors
Linked genes may differ based on gender
Disease onset generally at puberty or perimenopause
Disease activity
Disease activity suppressed during pregnancy, temporarily increased post partum; pregnancy may have a long-term disease benefit
Symptoms, signs, and MRI lesion activity show a relationship to the menstrual cycle
Breastfeeding may affect disease activity
Therapy
Use of disease-modifying therapies is limited by pregnancy and breastfeeding
Sex hormone therapy and prophylactic postpartum therapies under evaluation
Certain drugs have sex-specific side effects and considerations
Disease features
Sexual dysfunction is common symptom of MS
Diagnosis more likely to be delayed in women
General issues
Female/male health maintenance issues often are neglected in a chronic disease, such as MS
Specific psychosocial issues (domestic violence or parenting/spousal/vocational/self-image issues) are distinct based on patient gender

The endocrine system includes the gonadal organs that distinguish the sexes. The major link between the endocrine and central nervous system (CNS) is the hypothalamic-pituitary-adrenal gland (HPA) axis. This axis involves regulatory (positive and negative) feedback loops. The hypothalamus secretes a small peptide, gonadotropin-releasing hormone, in a pulsatile fashion, which is influenced by the menstrual cycle. Gonadotropin-releasing hormone regulates release of the gonadotropins, follicle-stimulating hormone (FSH), and luteinizing hormone (LH) by the anterior pituitary gland. The pituitary also releases lactotropins, in particular prolactin. FSH and LH promote development of ova and stimulate sex hormone secretion by the ovaries. The ovary also secretes inhibin, a peptide hormone that suppresses FSH release. Cortisone and corticosterone, important hormones in the HPA axis, are higher in women than in men. There is growing appreciation of complex interactions between the HPA axis and the immune system [6]. In fact, HPA axis dysfunction is implicated as a fundamental factor in development of autoimmune and immune-mediated diseases.

The immune system also is sexually dimorphic. Females of all species, vertebrates and invertebrates, show stronger immune responses [7]. Women have higher baseline immunoglobulin levels, higher CD4+ T-cell numbers, greater production of Th1 cytokines, and more sustained responses to antigenic challenge [8]. In a recent study, women, in particular those who did not have MS, showed a higher rate of T-cell reactivity to immunodominant proteolipid protein peptides [9]. The heightened immune response of women is not explained by sex hormones, because invertebrates lack such hormones.

Sex has a strong impact on diseases that are considered autoimmune. There are more than 80 such disorders. Among the estimated 8.5 million Americans who have autoimmune disease, almost 80% are women. Most autoimmune diseases show female predominance, and some are affected by hormonal states. Rheumatoid arthritis and psoriasis are believed to improve during pregnancy [10], although systemic lupus erythematosus may worsen [11]. Symptom fluctuation connected to the menstrual cycle is reported in systemic lupus erythematosus and rheumatoid arthritis, whereas post-menopausal rheumatoid arthritis patients are believed to improve with estrogen replacement therapy [11].

The preferential involvement of women in autoimmune disorders is not understood fully. Although their intrinsic stronger immune responses likely play a role, microchimerism also has been implicated. Microchimerism refers to the small population of cells and DNA in a person from a genetically distinct individual [12]. This can occur naturally (in exchanges of fetal/maternal, twin/twin, or sib/sib cells), or iatrogenically (by transplantation or transfusion). Such foreign cells and DNA can persist for decades. Fetal and maternal microchimerism is a common feature in pregnancy, and healthy individuals often show low levels of maternal microchimerism. Fetal microchimerism is implicated in disorders such as systemic sclerosis, thyroid disease, and primary biliary cirrhosis. Maternal microchimerism is implicated in systemic sclerosis, dermatomyositis, and neonatal lupus. Tissue-specific microchimerism may contribute to targeted autoimmunity, and the specific HLA genes and HLA relationships between cell populations likely will be important in determining negative, positive, or null effects of microchimerism.

Sex hormones

The three major classes of sex hormones share the same precursor, cholesterol (Table 2) [11]. All three classes are present and play important roles in both sexes and are secreted by many tissues in addition to the gonads. End-stage hormones and their intermediate metabolites are active, with final hormone products determined by local tissue enzymes. Sex hormones have many surprising and complex actions, including important effects on the nervous and immune systems (Table 3). Estrogens, for example, help masculinize the brain [10]. Sex hormones modulate immune responses and the HPA axis. They have genomic and nongenomic effects and often have more than one receptor, the best studied of which is the estrogen receptor, which, in contrast to progestin and androgen receptors, is distributed fairly widely in the CNS. There are at least two estrogen

Table 2
Sex hormones

Estrogens
Estrone (E1)
Estradiol (E2): predominant menstrual cycle estrogen
Estriol (E3): placental (pregnancy) estrogen
Progestins
Progesterone
Androgens
Testosterone
DHEA: intermediate metabolite

receptors, α and β, which are present on microglia [13]. A third receptor, x, recently has been discovered [14].

Hormones may act synergistically. For example, the effect of estrogen plus progesterone is greater than either one alone. Hormones may show concentration effects, with opposite actions at low and high levels. Although estrogens facilitate immune responses at low concentration, they suppress responses at high concentrations. Sex hormones are involved in feedback loops that inhibit their own production. Links between the endocrine and immune systems are reinforced by the multiple and diverse effects of sex hormones on the immune system. In turn, glucocorticoids suppress sex hormone production and actions [8].

Prolactin is a hormone and cytokine, with isotype and multiple receptor subunits [15–17]. It is secreted by the pituitary gland and certain lymphocytes. Levels are affected by immune factors and cognitive stimuli. Prolactin receptors are found on T and B lymphocytes. Prolactin is immunostimulatory and promotes Th1 phenotype, natural killer cell activity, and production of cytokines, such as interleukin 1 (IL-1) and interferon-γ (IFN-γ).

Sex steroid hormones form a complex network. Other hormones, such as growth hormone and insulin-like growth factor, also show sexual dimorphism [8]. The full sex-related effects of all these hormones are not yet understood.

Animal models

Sex plays a key role in animal models of MS. Theiler's murine encephalomyelitis virus is a picornavirus model of CNS demyelination. Inoculation of virus into susceptible mice produces biphasic CNS disease. The first stage is acute encephalitis, whereas the second stage is a chronic immune-mediated demyelinating myelitis, driven by persistent infection of glial cells and CNS macrophages [18]. Female animals are more susceptible to disease and show more severe encephalitis [19]. During early infection they display a more pronounced response of Th1 cytokines, resulting in high levels of proinflammatory cytokines. In contrast, males show a Th2 response, with appropriate high levels of regulatory cytokines. Anticytokine

Table 3
Sex hormone actions

Reproduction related
Menses
Pregnancy
Sexual activity
Nervous system
Increased axon growth, myelination
Neurotransmission
Neural remodeling, increase in synapses, spine density, astrocyte volume
Motor coordination
Enhanced cognitive performance
Increased transcription of neurotrophic factor (neuroprotective) genes
Regulation of brain apoptosis (via activation of glycogen kinase 3 enzyme)
Inhibition of nitric oxide production by microglia [97]
Amplifies excitotoxic damage to oligodendrocytes (testosterone)
Immune system
Estrogens
Receptors on CD8+ T cell
Cytokine effects (T2 phenotype, modulation of stimulated production) [Gilmore et al, 1997]
Increased foxP3 expression, CD4+ CD25+ regulatory T cells
Suppression of antigen-specific T-cell proliferation, delayed type hypersensitivity, natural killer cell activity, macrophage differentiation, B-cell proliferation, granulocyte inflammation
Potentiation of mitogen-induced B-cell stimulation
Increased transcription of endothelial nitric oxide synthase gene [98]
Progestins
Synergistic with estrogens
Favors Th2 phenotype (increased IL-4)
Mast cell degranulation
Androgens
Decreased B-cell precursors
Blunted response to glucocorticoids
Th1 to Th2 ratio regulated by DHEA to cortisol ratio increased natural killer cell activity, lipopolysaccharide-stimulated monocyte toxicity (DHEA)

therapy with IL-4 and IL-10 is successful in females but not in males. In the chronic infection stage, male animals actually develop worse disease [18]. Female mice, with milder disease, show higher antiviral antibody levels and less infectious virus.

Experimental allergic encephalomyelitis (EAE) is produced in mice, rats, and primates by immunization with myelin or its components (myelin basic protein, myelin oligodendrocyte glycoprotein, and proteolipid protein) or by adoptive transfer of pathogenic CD4+ T cells. Disease manifestations vary based on animal strain and species. The EAE model has several profound sex-specific effects, including the protective effect of sex hormones (estrogens and androgens) (Table 4) [10,20–24]. Although testosterone is converted to 17β-estradiol in vivo, its protective effect in EAE is not dependent on estrogens [21]. In the EAE model, sex-based differences involve changes in immune

Table 4
Sex-specific effects in experimental allergic encephalomyelitis

Females
More susceptible to EAE
More severe disease
Pregnancy is protective
Exogenous estrogens ameliorate disease
Oophorectomy worsens disease
Exogenous estrogens can change treatment nonresponder to responder
Males
Less susceptible to EAE
Milder disease
Exogenous estrogens or testosterone ameliorates disease
Castration increases disease susceptibility, worsens disease
Castration changes disease pattern from male to female
Testosterone levels decrease during relapses

Data from Gilmore W, Weiner LP, Correale J. Effect of estradiol on cytokine secretion by proteolipid protein-specific T cell clones isolated from multiple sclerosis patients and normal control subjects. J Immunol 1997;158:446–51.

factors, such as the animal's cytokine profile (with quantitative decreases in proinflammatory cytokines and chemokines), in the degree of cerebrospinal fluid inflammation and in the extent of nitric oxide production [25].

Recent studies implicate leptin, a pleiotropic cytokine-like hormone, in sex-related EAE vulnerability [26,27]. Leptin levels are higher in females than in males. This hormone has several actions and affects food intake and body weight, basal metabolism, hematopoiesis, inflammation, and the immune response to pathogens. Leptin is produced by neurons, activated T cells, and local inflammatory cells. Immune effects of leptin include increasing CD4+ Th1 cells, costimulating proliferation of naive T cells, and increasing certain cytokines (IFN-γ and -α) while decreasing others (IL-4). Leptin-deficient mice are resistant to development of EAE but become susceptible when they are treated with recombinant leptin. One of the most popular EAE models involves SJL/J mice. Typically, EAE can be induced only in female mice, which have much higher leptin levels than male mice. Recombinant leptin treatment makes SJL/J males susceptible to EAE and increases female vulnerability. In two distinct EAE models (for relapsing and progressive disease), serum leptin surges precede clinical disease onset. Hormone levels correlate with inflammation-related anorexia, weight loss, and EAE susceptibility. Acute starvation lowers leptin levels. Animals starved before EAE onset show decreased disease severity, with suppression of the pathologic Th1 response.

Multiple sclerosis demographics

Women make up 70% to 75% of all patients who have MS. This strong sex preference, which is most pronounced in populations with the highest prevalence rates [28], likely involves immune, hormonal, and genetic factors. Several studies report immune differences in patients who have MS based on sex. Men showed higher levels of in vitro tumor necrosis factor α (TNF-α) production by T cells [29]. Peripheral blood T cells, which produce IFN-γ, correlate with the EDSS of women (but not men) who had MS. In response to proteolipid protein, women who had MS secreted higher levels of IFN-γ but lower levels of IL-5 than men [30].

Age of onset suggests a link to hormonal factors. Risk for MS begins at puberty. Less than 1% of cases show disease onset before age 10. In this unusual subset, the sex ratio is equal. Pediatric MS (onset before age 16) makes up only 5% of all cases. Peak onset is post puberty, in the early 20s, with the average age of onset of relapsing MS at around 28 to 30 years. Risk for relapsing MS seems to decline with perimenopause. This clearly is a young person's disease; 90% of patients are between 15 and 50 years of age. Although no consistent sex hormone abnormalities are reported, in one study, 25% of premenopausal patients show low estradiol levels [31].

In contrast to the other clinical subtypes, primary progressive MS shows an equal sex ratio. Patients who are progressive from onset have disease starting at around ages 38 to 41, a decade later than typical patients who have relapsing MS. In essence, this subtype preferentially affects men. It is almost as though risk for MS for men increases at their perimenopause, coincident with decreasing testosterone [21]. Endogenous testosterone levels begin to fall at age 30. In a recent study, 24% of men who had MS had low testosterone levels compared with matched control patients [31]. In another study, four men who had MS and sexual dysfunction were found to have abnormally low testosterone levels, believed to be on a hypothalamic basis [32]. The dysfunction improved with testosterone therapy. In patients who have primary progressive MS, men show an older age of onset and reach disability faster [33]. This is consistent with the worse prognosis for men, even accounting for their greater risk for a progressive course and older age at disease onset, both poor prognosis factors. It is not known why men have a worse prognosis. Testosterone makes oligodendrocytes more vulnerable to excitotoxic death [34]. This does not, however, explain the postulated protective effect of testosterone in MS.

Sex influences certain genes linked to MS. The major histocompatibility class II HLA-DR2 DQ6 haplotype, a susceptibility gene, is more common in female than male patients [35,36]. Several studies report a relationship between MS and polymorphisms in the estrogen receptor gene [37–39], although not in all populations [40]. In Sardinians, a polymorphic intronic CA repeat in the IFN-γ gene (on chromosome 12g14) protects against MS, but only in men [41]. In the Olmsted County (Rochester, Minnesota) population, two CD95 polymorphisms account for 28% of the risk for MS in women but 0% in men [42]. Because CD95 and its ligand mediate activation-induced apoptosis, this may be an important factor for MS occurrence in women. In another recent study, a specific APOE polymorphism (the E4* ε2 allele) is associated with a milder disease course, but only in women [43].

There may be sex-related MRI differences. One study finds that women have a significantly greater number of enhancing lesions [44]. This needs to be confirmed in independent and larger studies.

With regard to epidemiology, MS seems to be on the rise [45]. This is not unique to MS and is true also for several major allergic and immune-mediated disorders. Such diseases become more common as early infectious exposures decline. This occurs in developed countries, which have decreases in early infections as a result of vaccination programs and improved public hygiene measures. In at least one study, increase in MS cases is limited to women [46].

Pregnancy

Pregnancy is the single most important gender issue in MS and the focus of many studies and reports [47–53]. There are two broad areas of concern: the effects of MS on pregnancy and the effects of pregnancy on MS. It is now well established that MS has no effect on fertility, the ability to conceive, or the pregnancy state. There is no increase in spontaneous abortions or fetal defects. Although MS does not affect pregnancy, the reverse is not true.

Pregnancy does not increase risk for MS, but onset of the disease is less likely to occur during pregnancy. The major effect of pregnancy on MS is a decrease in disease activity. This is not surprising, because pregnancy is an immunosuppressive state produced by several factors, such as changes in hormones, pregnancy-related factors, and a shift favoring Th2 responses (Table 5) [54,55]. A pregnancy-related condition, such as pre-eclampsia, however, with its associated blood-brain barrier disruption, may make patients who have MS more vulnerable to lesion formation [56].

Table 5
Immunosuppressive factors in pregnancy

Increase in hormones (estrogen, progesterone, glucocorticoids)
Increase in human chorionic gonadotropin
Increase in norepinephrine
Increase in vitamin D3
Shift from Th1 to Th2 (decrease in cell-mediated immunity and increase in humoral immunity, immune complexes, and blocking antibodies)
Increase in pregnancy-related immunoregulator proteins (γ-fetoprotein, pregnancy-specific glycoproteins, early pregnancy factor)
Cytokine changes: increases in IFN-τ (ruminants), IL-10, and IL-4; decreases in IL-2, IL-12, TNF-α, and IFN-γ (including inhibitory plasma factor)
Maternal/fetal MHC class II disparity (no class II expression by trophoblast layer, suppression of antipaternal MHC-specific T cells)
Increase in CD4+ CD25+ regulatory T cells [22]

Perhaps the most informative study to date has been the Pregnancy in MS (PRIMS) trial [57], a 2-year prospective analysis of a European database involving 254 women who had MS and 269 pregnancies. All but 8 of the women had relapsing MS. Annual relapse rate fell during pregnancy, particularly in the third trimester when the rate was 70% below the prepregnancy baseline. Relapse rate then rebounded in the postpartum period to 70% above the prepregnancy level before returning to baseline after 3 months. There were no further significant fluctuations over the succeeding 2 years. Increased prepregnancy and intrapregnancy relapse rates and higher disability score at onset of pregnancy correlated with occurrence of postpartum relapse [58]. The PRIMS study left some unanswered questions, such as those regarding the nature of the postpartum relapses. Although several studies show a decrease in relapses during pregnancy, only one small study confirms suppression of MRI lesion activity in the later stages of pregnancy [59]. The immediate postpartum period is one of the clearest risk factors for disease activity, because 20% to 40% of women who are post partum experience relapse [60].

Another important aspect of pregnancy in MS involves genetic counseling. Risk for MS in white populations approximates 0.2%. With an affected parent, risk to the child increases to 3% to 5%. Risk may be greater with an affected father, consistent with greater genetic loading [61]. When both parents have MS, risk to the child increases to 30.5%. In a recent Canadian study of twins, concordance rate for MS was 25.3% in monozygotic and 5.4% in dizygotic twins [28]. Monozygotic concordance was almost completely accounted for by female twins, who made up 22 of 24 concordant pairs.

There has been controversy as to whether or not pregnancy affects long-term prognosis. Until the early 1950s, women who had MS were advised not to get pregnant because it would worsen their disease [62]. Some physicians recommended abortion. Accumulating data led to a complete reversal of this position. There is no evidence that pregnancy is detrimental to relapsing MS. In fact, studies suggest pregnancy is associated with a more favorable long-term prognosis [50,51]. Anecdotal observations suggest that patients who have progressive MS do not do well during pregnancy. Because most pregnant patients have relapsing disease, this must be addressed in future studies using large databases.

Another issue is whether or not the type of anesthesia used at delivery has an impact on subsequent MS course. The PRIMS study analyzed the effect of epidural anesthesia and found no impact on relapse rate or disability at 2 years. There are case studies associating spinal anesthesia (used for general procedures rather than for childbirth) with subsequent relapses. This has led to the common recommendation that spinal anesthesia be avoided in patients who have MS.

The fact that the postpartum period is recognized as carrying a high risk for relapse raises prophylactic treatment issues. One issue is when to resume conventional immunomodulator therapy. Provided patients do not breastfeed, treatment can be resumed immediately. The second issue is specific prophylactic treatment regimens. These have involved largely postpartum use of intravenous immunoglobulin (IVIG). One study evaluated nine pregnant patients who had MS and who had experienced a total of 13 prior postpartum relapses within 2 to 9 weeks of delivery [63]. They received IVIG 0.4 g/kg daily for 5 days, followed by 0.4 g/kg at 6 and 12 weeks. There were no relapses in the 6 months post partum, with three relapses at 8 to 10 months. Another study evaluated 15 patients who had MS during pregnancy and 6 months post partum. IVIG was given within 1 to 3 days of delivery (0.4 g/kg daily for 5 days), followed by booster doses of 0.4 g/kg daily at 6 and 12 weeks. None of the 14 patients who received postpartum IVIG relapsed after delivery, whereas one untreated patient had an attack at 5 weeks [60]. In another study, eight women treated with IVIG post partum were compared with 18 untreated women. Ten patients in the untreated group relapsed post partum compared with only one patient in the treated group [64]. In a fourth study, 50 patients received a 60-g IVIG load after giving birth, followed by 10 g monthly for 6 months. Their postpartum relapse rate was 33% lower than that predicted by the PRIMS study. A follow-up prospective study of pulsed IVIG therapy (the GAMPPT trial) recently has been completed in Europe, in which 173 patients were randomized to either a 10-g or 60-g IVIG load given over a maximum of 3 days after delivery, followed by 10 g monthly for 6 months [65]. Both protocols resulted in relapse suppression, with a trend toward a better effect with the higher IVIG load. Patients are being followed an additional year in this study. A recent retrospective analysis of 108 pregnant patients who had relapsing MS analyzed 3 groups. Group I (N = 39) was untreated control patients; Group II (N = 41) received IVIG post partum for 5 days (0.4g/kg/d) in the first week, with booster doses at 6 and 12 weeks post partum; and Group III (N = 28) was treated during gestation (after weeks 6 to 8) and post partum [66,67]. The investigators conclude that IVIG therapy decreased relapse rates during pregnancy and in the postpartum period. Group I showed no decrease in relapses during pregnancy until the third trimester.

In addition to IVIG, prophylactic pulse intravenous methylprednisolone (IVMP) has been evaluated. Twenty-two postpartum control patients who had MS were compared with 20 patients treated with IVMP monthly for 6 months. The relapse rate in the first 3 months post partum was 2 ± 0.7 control patients and 0.8 ± 0.4 (P = 0.015) for patients treated with MS. From months 4 to 11, the two groups showed no significant difference in relapse rate (1.3 ± 06 and 1 ± 0.5) [68].

In summary, several studies suggest that postpartum prophylactic treatment with IVIG and possibly IVMP can decrease postpartum relapses. Resumption of immunomodulator therapy, although not formally studied, is expected to do the same.

Breastfeeding

Data on the impact of breastfeeding is so limited that no recommendation can be made. Studies have found either no effect from breastfeeding on reducing relapse rate or a decrease in relapses [57,69,70]. The decision of whether or not to breastfeed is important because it has implications for therapy (see later discussion of Therapy Considerations).

Menstrual cycle

The menstrual cycle is a hormonal state that reflects integrated actions between the hypothalamus, pituitary gland, ovarian follicle, and endometrium [71]. The normal cycle lasts 28 days. By convention, bleeding starts on day 1. It typically lasts 3 to 7 days, with a total blood loss of up to 80 mL. Day 14 marks ovulation, coincident with a brief surge in FSH and LH. Estrogen levels peak mid cycle, followed by progesterone. Falling estrogen and progesterone levels induce bleeding. Immunologic changes are reported in association with the menstrual cycle [72].

Up to 80% of patients who have MS report disease fluctuations around their cycle [73–75]. This may be more pronounced for patients who have relapsing MS versus those who have progressive MS. Most common is increase in symptoms or signs in the week before or during the week of menstruation. Worsening symptoms include fatigue, myalgias, depression, and endurance. Worsening signs include spasticity; weakness; incoordination; and abnormalities in gait, sensation, vision, and sphincter function. Rare patients report relapses associated with specific phases of the menstrual cycle [76]

Several studies use MRI to explore the relationship between MS and the menstrual cycle. They suggest a relationship between sex hormone levels and MRI changes. In one study, 10 women (five who had MS and five control patients) underwent MRI scans weekly. Increases in brain water content, consistent with increased blood-brain barrier permeability, correlate with plasma estradiol levels [77]. Another study performed a single MRI per patient in 30 women who had MS, either in the early follicular (days 1 to 3), late follicular (days 14 to 16), or luteal (days 21 to 23) phase of their cycle [78]. Brain lesion activity was greatest when estradiol levels were high and progesterone levels were low. In a small study of eight women who had relapsing MS, MRI was performed during the follicular (days 3 to 9) and luteal phase (days 21 to 28). Although there was no difference in MRI activity in the two cycles, during the luteal phase, higher progesterone to estradiol ratios correlated with increased number and volume of contrast brain lesions [79]. In a follow-up study of 17 patients who had relapsing MS, contrast brain MRI was performed in the follicular and luteal phases. Again, there was no difference in contrast lesion activity between the phases, but the progesterone to estradiol ratio during the luteal phase was associated with contrast lesion formation. In addition, women who had MS showed lower testosterone levels than matched control patients. Testosterone levels were higher in the patients who did not have MRI activity, and plasma dehydroepiandrostenedione (DHEA) levels correlated with lack of T2 lesion development [80]. This study supports the protective effect of testosterone in MS.

Contraceptive use

There is limited data on oral contraceptives in MS. Contraceptives seem not to increase risk for development of MS or worsen overall disease course. In fact, use is associated with fewer symptoms, less disability, and lower risk for developing MS [81–83]. Patients who take contraceptive therapy are less likely to experience menstrual worsening of signs or symptoms [75]. One study found that patients who had MS and were on the pill and who had a pregnancy before onset of MS showed greater disability [81]. In summary, the available data does not suggest any problem in use of oral contraceptives in patients who have MS.

Hormone replacement therapy

Hormone replacement therapy is used infrequently in MS. There are no convincing studies to document benefit, but MS is not a contraindication to therapy. Up to 75% of women who note menstrual cycle worsening report symptomatic improvement with hormone replacement therapy.

Miscellaneous

One study suggests a relationship between MS and endometriosis, but patients were preselected [84]. In a 1998 survey of 3680 women who had a history of surgical treatment for endometriosis, there was increased risk for MS ($P < 0.0001$) and connective tissue disorders, allergies, chronic fatigue syndrome, hypothyroidism, and asthma.

There is virtually no information on menopause and MS. In one small study, 50% of patients report worsening disability at menopause [82]. Perimenopause is the time when primary progressive MS often begins and when patients transition from relapsing to progressive MS. From a practical viewpoint, perimenopause is a time of greater bone loss and, therefore, carries increased risk for osteoporosis.

Therapy considerations

Therapeutic considerations with implications based on gender can be divided into three major areas (Table 6). The first area deals with disease-

Table 6
Gender and sex consideration in therapy for multiple sclerosis

Disease-modifying therapies
Pregnancy, attempts to become pregnant, and breastfeeding considered contraindications to therapy
Use of contraception recommended for women of childbearing age on therapy
Injection site reactions (including redness, induration, fibrosis, and lipoatrophy) may be cosmetic considerations; lipoatrophy risk for women
Flu-like reactions more likely in patients who are young and have small body mass
Potential impact on menstrual cycle, fertility
Possible differential efficacy based on sex
Glucocorticoids
Implications of use in pregnancy and breastfeeding
Adverse effects, including cosmetic (striae, acne, fat redistribution, bone disturbances, and cataracts)
Symptomatic therapies
Implications of use in pregnancy and breastfeeding
Interactions between drugs (eg, oral contraceptives)
Adverse effects, including cosmetic, sexual dysfunction, and gender preferential
Sex hormone therapy
Use of estriol, estradiol/progestin in women who have relapsing MS
Use of androgens (testosterone patch or DHEA) in men who have MS

modifying therapies (DMTs). These drugs revolutionized management of MS by making it a treatable disease. They are categorized somewhat differently regarding pregnancy risk and gender concerns (Table 7). The Food and Drug Administration and the National Multiple Sclerosis Society consensus guidelines indicate that DMTs should not be used in patients who have MS and who are pregnant, trying to become pregnant, or breastfeeding.

Table 7
Gender and sex issues with the disease-modifying therapies

Disease-modifying therapy	Pregnancy risk	Sex considerations
Interferon-β	C	Abortofacients in some animal models (no negative fetal effects documented) Can cause menstrual disturbances Flu-like reactions more common in young individuals who have small body mass Subcutaneous injection associated with site reactions
Glatiramer acetate	B	Site reactions; occasional lipoatrophy (in females)
Mitoxantrone	D	Cytotoxic agent with potentially deleterious fetal effects Menstrual disturbances (up to 60%) amenorrhea (up to 43%), rare azoospermia, rare permanent sterility Hair thinning

Justification for these strict guidelines is based on two issues. DMTs are not proven safe in pregnancy, and it is not known if they are present in breast milk. A large pregnancy database (245 pregnancies) has been reported for glatiramer acetate [85]. There were 66% healthy live births, 20% spontaneous abortions, 11% elective abortions, 2.9% congenital anomalies, 0.4% ectopic pregnancies, and 0.4% stillbirths. These results compare favorably to pregnancy data from the United States and do not suggest any adverse fetal effects. A smaller IFN-β database of 30 pregnancies reports similar results (45% healthy live births, 27.6% spontaneous abortions including one fetal death, 21% elective abortions, 6.9% prenatal births, and one pregnancy lost to follow-up) [86]. A recent Spanish database evaluated 36 pregnancies in 31 patients exposed to IFN-ß [87]. There were 27 satisfactory deliveries and 9 spontaneous abortions. There have been many births in women exposed to MS immunomodulators, with no definable fetal damage syndromes recognized to date.

Mitoxantrone therapy raises fertility and pregnancy concerns. This anthracenedione is a chemotherapy agent, which intercalates into DNA and inhibits DNA repair. Use of mitoxantrone in young patients raises issues regarding banking of ova and sperm for use in future pregnancies. Permanent amenorrhea can occur when treating perimenopausal women (typically age 40 or older).

There is no clear-cut policy on how long patients should be off DMT before trying to become pregnant. Most often 1 month is recommended [88]. Regarding resumption of therapy after pregnancy, the only limiting factor is breastfeeding. If patients choose not to breastfeed, DMT can be restarted immediately.

There is no documented differential response to DMT based on gender. Two studies suggest, however, that this may need to be looked at more carefully. In a secondary progressive study of subcutaneous IFN-β1a, women responded better than men [89]. In the post hoc analysis of primary progressive MS PROMiSe trial, men (but not women) showed significantly less progression with glatiramer acetate therapy [90].

A second treatment issue involves glucocorticoids. Glucocorticoids most often are used short term to treat relapses and hasten recovery. They are not used in the first trimester of pregnancy, when a negative effect on organogenesis has devastating consequences. They can be used to treat second- and third-trimester relapses, although overuse may slow postnatal growth, and they are associated with birth defects in some animal models. Glucocorticoids are excreted in breast milk, so breastfeeding is contraindicated during their use. Among the potentially negative effects of glucocorticoids are aseptic necrosis of the femoral head/osteonecrosis and osteoporosis (decrease in bone density). Therapeutic measures involve early morning dosing of the glucocorticoid, supplementation with calcium and vitamin D, regular physical activity, bone density monitoring, and specific osteoporosis therapy when indicated.

The final therapeutic area involves symptom management. MS is associated with several symptoms that need treatment. Pharmacotherapy for symptoms can have implications based on gender. As a general rule, use of any drugs in pregnant or breastfeeding patients is kept to a minimum. Potential interactions between drugs that patients who have MS may use, such as the effect of carbamazepine or phenytoin on decreasing oral contraceptives, must be appreciated. Certain therapies may be more likely to produce side effects based on gender; women are at greater risk for amantadine-related livedo reticularis. Some drugs may produce sexual dysfunction as a side effect, such as those that increase serotonin levels.

The impact of sex hormones on the immune and nervous systems, on animal models of MS, and on the MS disease process itself has stimulated interest in using them to treat MS. In one study of 12 women who had MS (six had relapsing and six secondary progressive), oral estriol was used at 8 mg daily [91]. This dose duplicates levels achieved in the second trimester of pregnancy. The trial involved a crossover study design, with frequent MRI scans. No benefit was found for secondary progressive MS. Patients who had relapsing MS showed a decrease in the number and size of contrast-enhancing brain lesions during therapy, an increase when off therapy, and a positive response to retreatment with use of estriol plus progesterone. T2 brain lesion volume stabilized during therapy, increased during therapy, and improved during retreatment. Treatment decreased delayed hypersensitivity responses to tetanus and peripheral blood mononuclear cell IFN-γ messenger RNA production, consistent with a shift away from Th1 responses. This immune shift was confirmed in stimulation studies using mitogens and recall antigens [92]. Although patient numbers are small, there was improvement in the Paced Auditory Serial Addition Test (PASAT), a cognitive processing speed test. More definitive estriol studies are being pursued in a multicenter trial. DHEA has been used in a limited fashion to treat MS, and testosterone gel therapy is being evaluated in a small group of men who have MS. Progesterone therapy also has been discussed, based on its neurotrophic properties. POPARTMUS is a double-blind, placebo-controlled European multicenter trial evaluating postpartum oral progestin plus a weekly estradiol patch for postpartum MS [93]. Treatment is during 12 weeks, followed by 12 weeks' blinded observation.

The use of sex hormones to treat MS raises issues regarding combination therapy versus monotherapy, the use of an estrogen with progesterone to avoid uterine problems, and development of synthetic designer hormones, which may have the desired effects for MS without ancillary feminization or masculinization concerns. Selective estrogen receptor modulators also are under development.

Multiple sclerosis symptoms

The two major MS symptoms that benefit from an approach based on patient gender are bladder dysfunction and sexual dysfunction (Table 8).

Table 8
Gender and sex-related aspects of multiple sclerosis sexual and bladder dysfunction

- Sexual dysfunction
  - Unusual early (<5%), common late (70%–90%)
  - Shared disorders
    - Sexual desire disorders (hypoactive sex drive, sexual aversions)
    - Sexual arousal disorder
    - Orgasmic disorder
    - Decreased sensation
    - Fatigue
  - Male disorders
    - Erectile dysfunction
    - Ejaculatory disorders
  - Female disorders
    - Vaginal dryness
    - Sexual pain disorder (dyspareunia, vaginismus)
  - Evaluation
    - General approach: identify sexual symptoms, role of MS, couple's relationship, orgasmic capacity, interests/attitudes; address associated problems (bladder/bowel, pain, depression, fatigue, and so forth)
    - Men: assess nocturnal/diurnal erections, ejaculations (normal, premature, delayed, or absent)
    - Women: vaginal lubrication
  - Treatment
    - Open communication
    - Sex devices/vibrators
    - Alternative techniques, stimulation, positions
    - Lubricating gels
    - Oral agents (sildenafil citrate)
    - Injection/intraurethral therapy (prostaglandin E1)
    - Vacuum devices, prostheses
- Bladder dysfunction
  - Unusual early, common late (75%), often fluctuates over time
  - Three types of neurogenic bladder
    - Detrusor hyperreflexia (50%–90%)
    - Detrusor sphincter dyssynergia (25%–45%)
    - Detrusor hyporeflexia (20%)
  - Complications include negative impact on quality of life and social activities; infection, sepsis; vesicoureteral reflux; hydronephrosis; kidney, bladder stones; renal failure; bladder carcinoma
  - Urinary tract infections in men require renal system imaging
  - Evaluation
    - Urinalysis, ± culture/sensitivity
    - Postvoid residual
    - Urodynamics (cystometrogram)
    - Imaging (ultrasound, intravenous pyelogram)
  - Treatment
    - Voiding schedule
    - Controlled fluid intake (sufficient to minimize risk for infection; restricted at night)
    - Bedside commonde/urinal
    - Regular emptying techniques (crede maneuver, tapping, straining)
    - Pelvic floor exercises
    - Pads/special undergarments

Table 8 (*continued*)

Catheterization (intermittent, chronic)
Avoidance of caffeine, alcohol, aspartame
Oral agents (anticholinergics, tricyclic antidepressants, vasopressin analogues, alpha-adrenergic antagonist, cholinergic agonists, antispasticity agents)
Intravesical agents (anticholinergics, vanilloids, botulinum toxin)
Patch (oxybutinin)
Electromyography biofeedback, neuromuscular electrical stimulation
Surgical procedures (implants, sphincterotomy, diversion procedures)

These symptoms are correlated [94]. Both are unusual early but more common over time in MS. Up to 90% of men and 72% of women are believed to experience sexual problems, and up to 75% experience bladder difficulties. Sexual dysfunction requires engaging not only patients, but also their partners, to optimize symptom management.

Wellness and psychosocial issues

Gender has an impact on many health maintenance and psychosocial issues. Because neurologists often assume the role of principal care provider for patients who have MS, they must be aware of health maintenance. This often is neglected in chronic diseases, such as MS (Table 9) [95,96].

As a disease that affects young people, and which has an unpredictable course, MS has a profound impact on psychosocial issues (Table 10). These issues differ somewhat for women and men, so gender must be taken into account [97–99].

Summary

Gender issues in MS encompass basic pathogenesis and clinical, therapeutic, and psychosocial aspects of the disease. Future research in

Table 9
Health maintenance/preventive healthcare issues in multiple sclerosis

Shared
Regular medical checkups
Cancer prevention screening: colon evaluation, stool guaiac
Good nutritional practices
Regular exercise program
Appropriate sleep hygiene
Appropriate weight
Minimize abuse potentials: no use of tobacco, moderate alcohol use
Women
Annual gynecologic examination and Papanicolaou smear
Regular manual breast examination, periodic mammography
Bone density studies
Hormone replacement therapy consideration
Men
Annual prostate evaluation
Regular testicular examination

Table 10
Psychosocial aspects of multiple sclerosis with gender implications

Economic and vocational issues
Ability to maintain job or career; job discrimination
Ability to financially support oneself and the family unit/household
Insurance coverage
Access to care
Social and family issues
Domestic violence (physical, mental)
Role as spouse, parent, or child
Social isolation, impact on daily activities
Dependency
Marriage stressors
Mobility limitations
Limiting symptoms (cognitive/bladder/sexual dysfunction, spasticity, pain)
Psychologic issues
Denial of illness
Unstable disease course, uncertain future
Self-image and self worth

this area should lead not only to better insights into the nature of MS but also to improved treatment and management strategies.

References

[1] Legato MJ. Women's health: not for women only. Int J Fertil 1998;43;2:65–72.
[2] De Vries GJ, Boyle PA. Double duty for sex differences in the brain. Behav Brain Res 1998; 92:205–13.
[3] Patchev VK, Almeida OFX. Gender specificity in the neural regulation of the response to stress. Mol Neurobiol 1998;16:63–77.
[4] Rooney WD, Li X, Telang FW, et al. Age and sex: effects on brain properties assessed by $^{1}H_2OT_1$ histograms. Proc Int Soc Mag Reson Med 2003;11:1087.
[5] Rashid W, Davies GR, Chard DT, et al. Gender and intracranial volume effects appear to influence upper cervical cord size more than disease effects in early relapsing-remitting [abstract]. Mult Scler 2004;10:S225–6, Poster 523.
[6] Da Silva JAP. Sex hormones and glucocorticoids: interactions with the immune system. Ann N Y Acad Sci 1999;876:102–18.
[7] Kurtz J, Wiesner A, Gotz P, et al. Gender differences and individual variation in the immune system of the scorpionfly Panorpa vulgaris (Insecta: Mecoptera). Dev Comp Immunol 2000; 24:1–12.
[8] Whitacre CC. Sex differences in autoimmune disease. Nat Immunol 2001;2:777–80.
[9] Greer JM, Csurhes PA, Pender MP, et al. Effect of gender on T-cell proliferative responses to myelin proteolipid protein antigens in patients with multiple sclerosis and controls. J Autoimmun 2004;22:345–52.
[10] Palaszynski KM, Liu H, Loo KK, et al. Estriol treatment ameliorates disease in males with experimental autoimmune encephalomyelitis: implications for multiple sclerosis. J Neuroimmunol 2004;149:84–9.
[11] Gilmore W, Weiner LP, Correale J. Effect of estradiol on cytokine secretion by proteolipid protein-specific T cell clones isolated from multiple sclerosis patients and normal control subjects. J Immunol 1997;158:446–51.

[12] Adams KM, Nelson JL. Microchimerism. An investigative frontier in autoimmunity and transplantation. JAMA 2004;291:1127–31.
[13] Drew PD, Chavis JA, Bhatt R. Sex steroid regulation of microglial cell activation. Relevance to multiple sclerosis. Ann N Y Acad Sci 2003;1007:329–34.
[14] Adams JU. Scratching the surface for estrogen's effects. Scientist 2004;28–30.
[15] Chikanza IC. Prolactin and neuroimmunomodulation: iIn vitro and in vivo observations. Ann N Y Acad Sci 1999;876:119–30.
[16] McMurray RW. Bromocriptine in rheumatic and autoimmune diseases. Semin Arthritis Rheum 2001;31:21–32.
[17] Mellai M, Giordano M, D'Alfonso S, et al. Prolactin and prolactin receptor gene polymorphisms in multiple sclerosis and systemic lupus erythematosus. Hum Immunol 2003; 64:274–84.
[18] Alley J, Khasabov S, Simone D, et al. More severe neurologic deficits in SJL/J male than female mice following Theiler's virus-induced CNS demyelination. Exp Neurol 2003;180: 14–24.
[19] Hill KE, Pigmans M, Fujinami RS. Gender variations in early Theiler's virus induced demyelinating disease: differential susceptibility and effects of IL-4, IL-10 and combined IL-4 with IL-10. J Neuroimmunol 1998;85:44–51.
[20] Fillmore PD, Blankenhorn EP, Zachary JF, et al. Adult gonadal hormones selectively regulate sexually dimorphic quantitative traits observed in experimental allergic encephalomyelitis. Am J Pathol 2004;164:167–75.
[21] Kim S, Liva SM, Dalal MA, et al. Estriol ameliorates autoimmune demyelinating disease. Neurology 1999;52:1230–8.
[22] Palaszynski KM, Loo KK, Asjpiro KF, et al. Androgens are protective in experimental autoimmune encephalomyelitis: implications for multiple sclerosis. J Neuroimmunol 2004; 146:144–52.
[23] Polanczyk MJ, Carson BD, Subramanian S, et al. Cutting edge: estrogen drives expansion of the CD4+ CD25+ regulatory T cell compartment. J Immunol 2004;173: 2227–30.
[24] Voskuhl RR, Palaszynski K. Sex hormones in experimental autoimmune encephalomyelitis: implications for multiple sclerosis. Neuroscientist 2001;7:258–70.
[25] Voskuhl RR, Pitchekian-Halabi H, MacKenzie-Graham A, et al. Gender differences in autoimmune demyelination in the mouse: implications for multiple sclerosis. Ann Neurol 1996;39:724–33.
[26] Ding M, Wong JL, Rogers NE, et al. Gender differences of inducible oxide production in JSJ/J mice with experimental autoimmune encephalomyelitis. J Neuroimmunol 1997;77: 99–106.
[27] Matarese G, Sanna V, Di Giacomo A, et al. Leptin potentiates experimental autoimmune encephalomyelitis in SJL female mice and confers susceptibility to males. Eur J Immunol 2001;31:1324–32.
[28] Sanna V, Di Giacomo A, La Cava A, et al. Leptin surge precedes onset of autoimmune encephalomyelitis and correlates with development of pathogenic T cell responses. J Clin Invest 2003;111:241–50.
[29] Willer CJ, Dyment DA, Risch NJ, et al. Twin concordance and sibling recurrence rates in multiple sclerosis. Proc Natl Acad Sci USA 2003;100:12877–82.
[30] Nguyen LT, Ramanathan M, Weinstock-Guttman B, et al. Sex differences in in vitro proinflammatory cytokine production from peripheral blood of multiple sclerosis patients. J Neurol Sci 2003;209:93–9.
[31] Pelfrey C, Cotleur A, Lee J, et al. Sex differences in cytokine responses to myelin peptides in multiple sclerosis. J Neuroimmunol 2002;130:211.
[32] Wei T, Lightman SL. The neuroendocrine axis in patients with multiple sclerosis. Brain 1997;120:1067–76.

[33] Foster SC, Daniels C, Bourdette DN, et al. Dysregulation of the hypothalamic-pituitary-gonadal axis in experimental autoimmune encephalomyelitis and multiple sclerosis. J Neuroimmunol 2003;140:78–87.
[34] Confavreux C, Vukisic S, Adeleine P. Early clinical predictors and progression of irreversible disability in multiple sclerosis: an amnesic process. Brain 2003;126:770–82.
[35] Caruso A, Gerevini VDG, Castiglione M, et al. Testosterone amplifies excitotoxic damage of cultured oligodendrocytes. J Neurochem 2004;88:1179–85.
[36] Celius EG, Harbo HF, Egeland T, et al. Sex and age at diagnosis are correlated with the HLA-DR2, DQ6 haplotype in multiple sclerosis. J Neurol Sci 2000;178:132–5.
[37] Duquette P, Pleines J, Girard M, et al. The increased susceptibility of women to multiple sclerosis. Can J Neurol Sci 1992;19:466–71.
[38] Kikuchi S, Fukazawa T, Niino M, et al. Estrogen receptor gene polymorphism and multiple sclerosis in Japanese patients: interaction with HLA-DRB1*1501 and disease modulation. J Neuroimmunol 2002;128:77–81.
[39] Mattila KM, Luomala M, Lehtimaki T, et al. Interaction between ESR1 and HLA-DR2 may contribute to the development of MS in women. Neurology 2001;56:1246–7.
[40] Nino M, Kikuchi S, Fukazawa T, et al. Estrogen receptor gene polymorphism in Japanese patients with multiple sclerosis. J Neurol Sci 2000;179:70–5.
[41] Savettieri G, Cittadella R, Valentino P, et al. Lack of association between estrogen receptor 1 gene polymorphisms and multiple sclerosis in southern Italy in humans. Neurosci Lett 2002; 327:115–8.
[42] Goris A, Heggarty S, Marrosu MG, et al. Linkage disequilibrium analysis of chromosome 12q14–15 in multiple sclerosis: delineation of a 118-kb interval around interferon-gamma (IFNG) that is involved in male versus female differential susceptibility. Genes Immun 2002; 3:470–6.
[43] Kantarci OH, Hebrink DD, Achenbach SJ, et al. CD95 polymorphisms are associated with susceptibility to MS women: a population-based study of CD95 and CD95L in MS. J Neuroimmunol 2004;146:162–70.
[44] Kantarci OH, Hebrink DD, Achenbach SJ, et al. Association of APOE polymorphisms with disease severity in MS is limited to women. Neurology 2004;62:811–4.
[45] Weatherby SJM, Mann CLA, Davies MB. Pilot study of the relationship between gadolinium-enhancing lesions, gender effect and polymorphisms of antioxidant enzymes in multiple sclerosis. J Neurol 2000;247:467–70.
[46] Bach JF. Mechanisms of disease: the effect of infections on susceptibility to autoimmune and allergic diseases. N Engl J Med 2002;347:1080–6.
[47] Wynn DR, Kurland LT, Rodriguez M. A reappraisal of the epidemiology of multiple sclerosis in Olmsted County, Minnesota. Neurology 1990;40:780–6.
[48] Abramsky O. Pregnancy and multiple sclerosis. Ann Neurol 1994;36:S38–41.
[49] Bernardi S, Grasso MG, Bertollini R, et al. The influence of pregnancy on relapses in multiple sclerosis: a cohort study. Acta Neurol Scand 1991;84:403–6.
[50] Birk K, Rudick R. Pregnancy and multiple sclerosis. Arch Neurol 1986;43:719–26.
[51] Damek DM, Shuster E. Pregnancy and multiple sclerosis. Mayo Clin Proc 1997;72: 977–89.
[52] Runmarker B, Andersen O. Pregnancy is associated with a lower risk of onset and a better prognosis in multiple sclerosis. Brain 1995;118:253–61, 285–91.
[53] Sadovnick AD, Eisen K, Hashimoto SA, et al. Pregnancy and multiple sclerosis. A prospective study. Arch Neurol 1994;51:1120–4.
[54] Thompson DS, Nelson LM, Burns A, et al. The effects of pregnancy in multiple sclerosis: a restrospective study. Neurology 1987;36:1097–9.
[55] Elenkov IJ, Wilder RL, Bakalov VK, et al. IL-12, TNF-alpha, and hormonal changes during late pregnancy and early postpartum: implications for autoimmune disease activity during these times. J Clin Endocrinol Metab 2001;86:4933–8.

[56] Marzi M, Vigano A, Trabattoni D, et al. Characterization of type 1 and type 2 cytokine production profile in physiologic and pathologic human pregnancy. Clin Exp Immunol 1996;106:127–33.

[57] Boster A, Gebarski S, Mikol D. Does disruption of the blood brain barrier in pre-eclamptic MS patients predispose to increased disease activity? [abstract]. Mult Scler 2004;10:S188, Poster 381.

[58] Confavreux C, Hutchinson M, Hours MM, et al. Rate of pregnancy-related relapses in multiple sclerosis. N Engl J Med 1998;339:285–91.

[59] Vukusic S, Hutchinson M, Hours M, et al. Pregnancy and multiple sclerosis (the PRIMS study): clinical predictors of post-partum relapse. Brain 2004;127:1353–60.

[60] Van Walderveen MA, Tas MW, Barkhof F, et al. Magnetic resonance evaluation of disease activity during pregnancy in multiple sclerosis. Neurology 1994;44:327–9.

[61] Orvieto R, Achiron R, Rotstein Z, et al. Pregnancy and multiple sclerosis: a 2-year experience. Eur J Obstet Gynecol Reprod Biol 1999;82:191–4.

[62] Kantarci OH, Barcellos LF, Oxenberg JR, et al. Men with MS transmit the disease more often to their children than women: the carter effect [abstract]. Mult Scler 2004;10:S203, Poster 440.

[63] Coyle PK. Multiple sclerosis. In: Kaplan PW, editor. Neurologic disease in women. New York: Demos Vermande. p. 251–64.

[64] Achiron A, Rotstein Z, Noy S, et al. Intravenous immunoglobulin treatment in the prevention of childbirth-associated acute exacerbations in multiple sclerosis: a pilot study. J Neurol 1996;243:25–8.

[65] Tagaris GA, Tenzoudi M, Panagopoulos G, et al. Intravenous immunoglobulin in childbirth-related exacerbations of multiple sclerosis. J Neurol 1999;52:A133–44.

[66] Haas J. Presentation of results of the GAMPPT trial: gammaglobulins post pregnancy in multiple sciences for prevention of exacerbations after delivery. Charcot Foundation Satellite Symposium. Vienna (Austria): European Committee for Treatment and Research in Multiple Sclerosis (Ectrims); 2004.

[67] Achiron A, Kishner I, Dolev M, et al. Effect of intravenous immunoglobulin treatment on pregnancy and postpartum related relapses in multiple sclerosis. J Neurol 2004;251:1133–7.

[68] Confavreux C. Intravenous immunoglobulins, pregnancy and multiple sclerosis. J Neurol 2004;251:1138–9.

[69] De Seze J, Chapelotte M, Delalande S, et al. Intravenous corticosteroids in the postpartum period for reduct acute exacerbations in multiple sclerosis. Mult Scler 2004;10:596–7.

[70] Nelson LM, Franklin GM, Jones MC, et al. Risk of multiple sclerosis exacerbation during pregnancy and breast-feeding. JAMA 1988;259:3441–3.

[71] Worthington J, Jones R, Crawford M, et al. Pregnancy and multiple sclerosis-a 3-year prospective study. J Neurol 1994;241:228–33.

[72] Case AM, Reid RL. Effects of the menstrual cycle on medical disorders. Arch Intern Med 1998;158:1405–12.

[73] Angstwurm MWA, Gartner R, Ziegler-Heitbrock HWL. Cyclic plasma IL-6 levels during normal menstrual cycle. Cytokine 1997;9:370–4.

[74] Smith R, Studd JWW. A pilot study of the effect upon multiple sclerosis of the menopause, hormone replacement therapy and the menstrual cycle. J R Soc Med 1992;85:612–3.

[75] Wilson S, Donnan P, Swingrem R, et al. A serial observational study on hormonal influences in MS symptoms [abstract]. Mult Scler 2004;10:S188–9, Poster 382.

[76] Zordrager A, DeKeyser J. Menstrually related worsening of symptoms in multiple sclerosis. J Neurol Sci 1997;149:95–7.

[77] Zorgdrager A, DeKeyser J. Premenstrual exacerbations of multiple sclerosis. J Neurol Neurosurg Psychiatry 1998;65:279–80.

[78] Rooney WD, Coyle PK, Li X, et al. Sex differences of brain $^{1}H_2OT_1$ values in controls and MS subjects: the role of estradiol. Proc Intel Soc Mag Reson Med 2003;11:123.

[79] Bansil S, Lee HS, Jindal S, et al. Correlation between sex hormones and magnetic resonance images lesions in multiple sclerosis. Acta Neurol Scand 1999;99:91–4.
[80] Pozzilli C, Falaschi P, Mainero C, et al. MRI in multiple sclerosis during the menstrual cycle: relationship with sex hormone patterns. Neurology 1999;53:622–4.
[81] Tomassini V, Giugni E, Mainere C, et al. Relationship between sex hormones and MRI activity in relapsing-remitting multiple sclerosis. Neurology 2001;56:A254.
[82] Poser S, Raun NE, Wikstrom J, et al. Pregnancy, oral contraceptives and multiple sclerosis. Acta Neurol Scand 1979;59:108–18.
[83] Smith R, Studd JW. A pilot study on the effect upon multiple sclerosis of the menopause, hormone replacement therapy and the menstrual cycle. J R Soc Med 1992;85:612–3.
[84] Villard-Mackintosh L, Vessey MP. Oral contraceptives and reproductive factors in multiple sclerosis incidence. Contraception 1993;47:161–8.
[85] Sinaii N, Cleary SD, Ballweg ML, et al. High rates of autoimmune and endocrine disorders, fibromyalgia, chronic fatigue syndrome and atopic diseases among women with endometriosis: a survey analysis. Hum Reprod 2002;17:2715–24.
[86] Coyle PK, Johnson K, Pardo L, et al. Pregnancy outcomes in patients with multiple sclerosis treated with glatiramer acetate (Copaxone). Neurology 2003;60(Suppl 1):A60.
[87] Sandberg-Wollheim M. Outcome of pregnancy during treatment with interferon-beta-1a (rebif) in patients with multiple sclerosis. Neurology 2002;58:A455.
[88] Heras V, Tintore M, Tellez N, et al. Study on pregnancy and multiple sclerosis therapies [abstract]. Mult Scler 2004;10:S188, Poster 380.
[89] Coyle PK, Christie S, Fodor P, et al. MS gender issues: clinical practices of women neurologists. Mult Scler 2004;10:582–8.
[90] Li DKB, Zhao GJ, Paty DW. Randomized controlled trial of interferon-beta-1a in secondary progressive MS. Neurology 2001;56:1505–13.
[91] Wolinsky JS, Houston TX, Pardo L, et al. Effect of glatiramer acetate on primary progressive multiple sclerosis: initial analysis of the completed PROMISE Trial. Neurology 2004;62:A97.
[92] Sicotte NL, Liva SM, Klutch R, et al. Treatment of multiple sclerosis with the pregnancy hormone estriol. Ann Neurol 2002;52:421–8.
[93] Soldan SS, Retuerto AI, Sicotte NL, et al. Immune modulation in multiple sclerosis patients with the pregnancy hormone estriol. J Immunol 2003;171:6267–74.
[94] Vukusic S, El-Etr M, Cornie C, et al. POPARTMUS: a European multicenter trial of post-partum progestin and estriol in multiple sclerosis [abstract]. Mult Scler 2004;10:S271, Poster 688.
[95] DasGupta R, Fowler CJ. Sexual and urological dysfunction in multiple sclerosis: better understanding and improved therapies. Curr Opin Neurol 2002;15:271–8.
[96] Shabas D, Weinreb H. Preventive healthcare in women with multiple sclerosis. J Women's Health Gender-Based Medicine 2000;9:389–95.
[97] Stuifbergen AK, Roberts GJ. Health promotion practices of women with multiple sclerosis. Arch Phys Med Rehabil 1997;78(Suppl 5):S3–9.
[98] Drew PD, Chavis JA. Female sex steroids: effects upon microglial cell activation. J Neuroimmunol 2000;111:77–85.
[99] Kleinert H, Wallerath T, Euchenhofer C, et al. Estrogens increase transcription of the human endothelial NO synthase gene analysis of the transcription factors involve. Hypertension 1998;31:582–8.

ELSEVIER
SAUNDERS

Neurol Clin 23 (2005) 61–75

NEUROLOGIC
CLINICS

Genetics of Multiple Sclerosis

Jorge R. Oksenberg, PhD*, Stephen L. Hauser, MD

Department of Neurology, University of California at San Francisco, School of Medicine, San Francisco, CA, USA

Multiple sclerosis is a complex genetic disease

The cause of multiple sclerosis (MS) is unknown, but it is widely believed to be an autoimmune disease occurring in genetically susceptible individuals after exposure to as-yet undefined environmental factors. The genetic etiology is indicated foremost by the recurrence risk in family members of the affected individual [1,2]. One measure of familial aggregation is the λ_s statistic, defined as the ratio of the lifetime risk to siblings of affected individuals (Ks) to the population prevalence (K) of the disease (λ_s = Ks/K). A $\lambda_s = 1$ indicates nonfamilial clustering of cases; for MS, the total λ_s is between 20 (0.02/0.001) and 40 (0.04/0.001) [3]. Recurrence is higher in the children of conjugal pairs who have MS than in offspring of single affected individuals; concordant siblings tend to share age of symptom onset rather than year of onset, and second- and third-degree relatives of patients who have MS also are at increased risk for MS. Observations seem to confirm that genetics, rather than a common environmental exposure, is primarily responsible for familial aggregation. Studies of half-siblings [4] and adoptees [5] also are in agreement with the conclusion that genetic sharing rather than the family microenvironment is the key factor for familial aggregation of the disease. Twin studies from different populations consistently indicate that a monozygotic twin of a patient who has MS is at higher risk (25%–30% concordance) for MS than is a dizygotic twin (2%–5%) [6,7], providing additional evidence for a significant genetic etiology. Twin concordance seems to exhibit gender dimorphism and mirror disease prevalence [7].

The authors are supported by the National Multiple Sclerosis Society, the National Institutes of Health, and the Nancy Davis and Montel Williams Foundations.

* Corresponding author. Department of Neurology, School of Medicine, University of California, San Francisco, 513 Parnassus Avenue, S-256, San Francisco, CA 94143-0435, USA.

E-mail address: oksen@itsa.ucsf.edu (J.R. Oksenberg).

0733-8619/05/$ - see front matter
doi:10.1016/j.ncl.2004.09.006 *neurologic.theclinics.com*

Neither the recurrence rate nor twin concordance data support the presence of a mendelian trait, however. Modeling of the available data predicts that the MS-prone genotype requires the allelic interaction, either programmed or stochastic, of multiple genes, each exerting a small or, at most, a moderate effect on the overall risk and several postgermline events. These include genes that rearrange from their position in the genome to encode a vast variety of T-cell receptors and immunoglobulins, somatic mutations, post-transcriptional regulatory mechanisms, and incorporation of retroviral sequences. In addition, it is likely that interactions with infectious, nutritional, climatic, and other environmental influences affect genetic susceptibility considerably (Box 1).

Narrowing the search and identifying the multiple sclerosis genes

On February 15, 2001, the International Human Genome Sequencing Consortium and the company Celera simultaneously reported the completion of the first draft of the human genome sequence. This historic scientific milestone provided a direct way to connect a chromosomal region with its DNA sequence and gene content and dramatically changed the ability to examine genetic variation as it relates to human disease. An early gain of the Human Genome Project was the development of detailed maps of highly polymorphic markers (ie, microsatellites) for all chromosomes, facilitating comprehensive genome-wide screenings. Some investigators proposed that a reasonable approach to gene discovery in complex disorders involves first determining the chromosomal region of the genomic effect by means of linkage analysis. The establishment of genetic linkage requires the collection of family pedigrees with more than one affected member to track, with the help of the DNA markers, the inheritance of discrete chromosomal segments that deviate from independent segregation and cosegregate with the disease (Fig. 1). Once these regions in linkage with the trait are identified and confirmed, a narrow and well-defined list of candidate genes can be

Box 1. Model of genetic contributions in multiple sclerosis

1. Multiple genes of moderate and cumulative affect that dictate susceptibility and influence disease course.
2. No major gene/locus with the exception of the MHC.
3. Postgenomic (transcriptional/translational) mechanisms.
4. Unidentified nonheritable (environmental) factors.
5. Unknown genetic parameters and mode of inheritance.
6. Complex gene-gene and gene-environment interactions.
7. Gender effect in susceptibility and transmission.
8. Genetic heterogeneity may result in clinical isoforms.

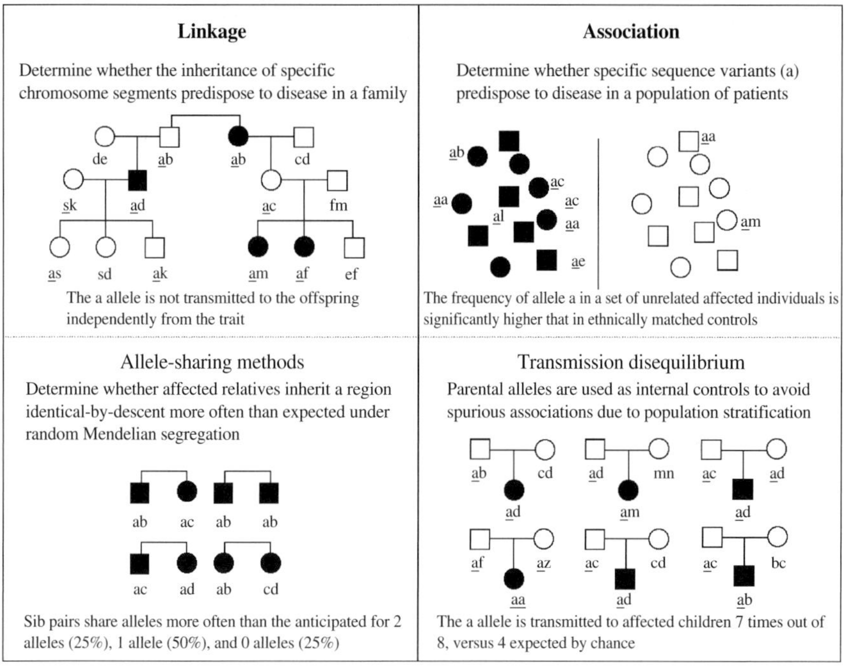

Fig. 1. Methods of genetic analysis.

compiled for analysis, even in the absence of a unifying model of pathogenesis. The potential of linkage mapping for gene identification in complex diseases was highlighted in a study of type 2 diabetes. The investigators followed original linkage data that implicated the distal long arm of chromosome 2 and identified a disease-associated intronic polymorphism in calpain-10, a ubiquitously expressed member of the calpain-like family of cysteine proteases [8]. In a second example, the identification of a locus linked to Crohn's disease on chromosome 16 resulted in the discovery of a frameshift mutation in *NOD2*, a member of the Apaf-1/Ced-4 superfamily of apoptosis regulators, a frameship mutation associated with disease susceptibility [9,10].

Linkage studies in multiple sclerosis

The three pivotal whole genome screens performed in multiple affected families that have MS were completed and published by American, Canadian, and United Kingdom researchers almost a decade ago [11–13]. Since then, follow-up screenings in confirmatory and additional data sets also have been completed. The studies confirmed the known association with the *HLA* class II *DR2* haplotype (*HLA-DRB1*1501-DQA1*0102-DQB1*0602*) but failed to find other major loci in MS. Altogether, the screens identified approximately 60 candidate genomic regions that have a potential involvement in disease susceptibility, consistent with the long-held view that MS is a polygenic disorder but total, or even predominant, replication between the different screens was not present. This is in part because of the strategy of reporting all peaks suggestive of linkage with the recognition that false positives are generated along with the true positives. It also is possible that the study design in each case overestimated the power and underestimated the confounding influence of disease heterogeneity and the limitations of parametric methods of statistic analysis. Because each study used a somewhat overlapping but different set of genetic markers and different clinical inclusion criteria, however, direct comparison of results is not straightforward. Nevertheless, the analysis of the composite published data identified partially overlapping regions, including 1p36-p33, 2p23-p21, 3p14-p13, 3q22-q24, 4q31-qter, 5p14-p12, 5q12-q13, 6p21-22, 6q22-27, 6q22-27, 7q21-q22, 17q22, 18p11, and 19q12-13 [14]. In addition, meta-analysis of the raw and published data from the original genomic scans singled out discrete common MS-susceptibility loci at chromosomes 5, 6, 16, 17, 19, and 22 [15,16]. A more recent meta-analysis combined the raw genotyping data from nine populations with a total of 719 families [17]. Strong evidence of linkage was observed only in the major histocompatibility complex (MHC) region on chromosome 6p21, confirming that this region represents the strongest MS susceptibility locus in the genome. Additional suggestive linkage was seen in 17q21 and 22q13.

In summary, evidence for linkage exceeding the threshold for genome-wide statistic significance is seen in the MHC region on chromosome 6p21.3. Additional regions were identified, but the overall data provide support primarily for chromosomes 19q13 and 17q21. Consensus is emerging to consider them bona fide MS loci and designate the *HLA* region at 6p21.3, 19q13, and 17q21 as MS loci 1, 2, and 3, respectively. Although these efforts represent real progress toward the development of a unifying model of pathogenesis, current understanding of the genetic basis of MS remains rudimentary and further work is necessary to define fully the complete set of disease loci and genes.

MS1, chromosome 6p21.3, the major histocompatibility complex

The human MHC (the human leukocyte antigen [*HLA*] system) consists of linked gene clusters located at 6p21.3, spanning almost 4 million base pairs (Fig. 2). HLA molecules are cell-surface glycoproteins whose primary role in an immune response is to display and present short antigenic peptide fragments to peptide/MHC-specific T cells. Many of the *HLA class I* and *II* genes are highly polymorphic, resulting in the generation of enormously diverse numbers of different genotypic combinations or haplotypes. The polymorphic residues that define an *HLA* allele are constrained to exons 2

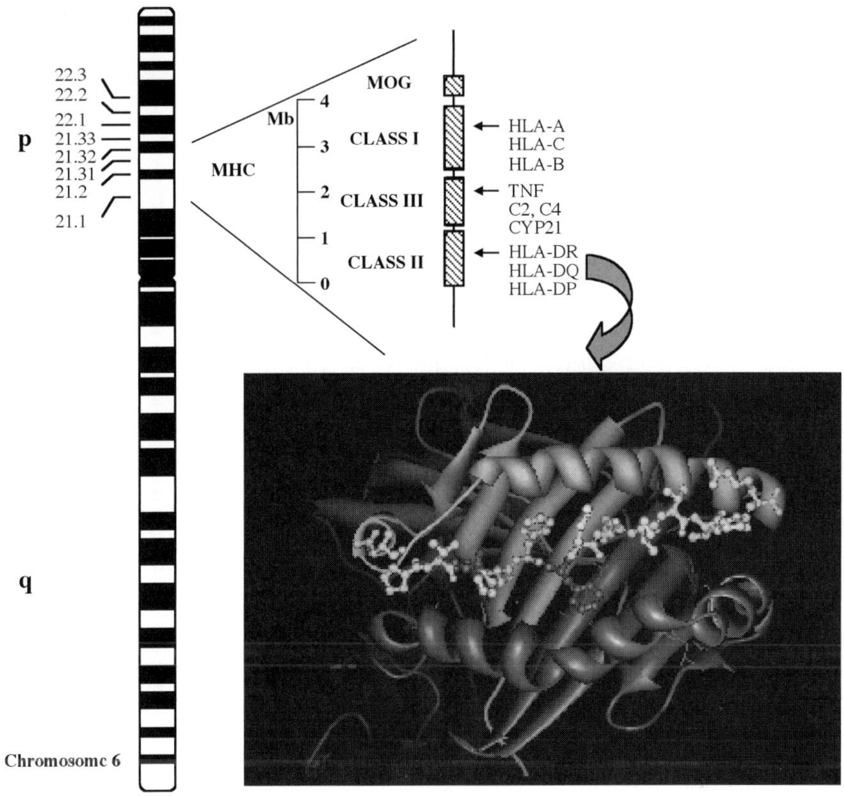

Fig. 2. The 6p21-23 region. The full sequence of the MHC region was completed and reported in 1999. From 224 identified loci, 128 are predicted to be expressed and approximately 40% to have immune-response functions. The diagram shows the relative positions of class I and II loci involved in antigen presentation. Other genes mapped in the MHC region include complement proteins, genes for the 21-hydroxylase, tumor necrosis factor, and heat-shock proteins, collectively known as class III. The graphic representation of the crystal structure is a top view of *HLA-DRA*0101, DRB*1501* in complex with a putative MS autoantigen, the MBP peptide 85-99.

and 3 for *class I* and exon 2 for *class II* and are clustered in the antigen-peptide–binding groove of the molecule, suggesting that polymorphism developed in response to evolutionary pressures. At the population level, this heterogeneity ensures, for example, that even if a portion of individuals succumbed to a new pathogen because of their inability to mount an efficacious immune response, others bearing distinct MHC molecules are resistant. Hence, the ability to respond to an antigen, either foreign or self, and the nature of that response are to a large extent determined by the unique amino acid sequences of *HLA* alleles, an observation that powered the rationale for focusing on genetic associations between *HLA* genotypes and susceptibility to autoimmune diseases, including MS [18].

The genetic association of MS with *HLA* genes, specifically the *HLA-DR2* (*DRB1*1501, DQB1*0602*) haplotype, has been known for more than 30 years [19,20] (Box 2). This association has been a consistent finding across most MS populations, the only exceptions being the association with different haplotypes, *DR3* and *DR4*, in patients who have MS and are from Sardinia [21], for which a founder effect was claimed [22], and perhaps no *DRB1* association in some Asian populations who have a restricted disease, termed neuromyelitis optica, in which optic nerve or spinal cord involvement predominates [23]. The strength of the association between primary progressive MS (PPMS) and *HLA-DR2* is uncertain. Several small studies fail to show any association between PPMS and *DR2*, although a larger study from Northern Ireland seems to show the association [24]. The association with *DR2* also is characteristic of juvenile (onset at or later than 16 years) MS [25]. Using family data, the proportion of the total genetic susceptibility explained by the *HLA* locus can be estimated; at the lower end, under an additive model, it could explain as little as 15% and at the upper end, under a multiplicative genetic model, the *HLA* association can explain as much as 60% of the genetic etiology of MS [26].

Box 2. Genetic contributions of the *HLA* locus to multiple sclerosis

1. Linkage scores > 3.0 and highly significant allelic association with the *HLA-DRB1*1501-DQB1*0602* haplotype have established that the strongest genetic determinant maps to the *MHC* region, explaining 15% to 60% of MS genetic susceptibility.
2. The *HLA-DRB1* gene constitutes the centromeric boundary of the class-II association with MS.
3. Linkage restricted to families segregating the *HLA-DRB1*1501* allele. Locus heterogeneity may not be present in all populations.
4. There is a dose effect of the *DRB1*1501* haplotype on susceptibility.
5. No significant effect on:
   Early clinical manifestations
   Age of onset
   Response to IFNB
6. *HLA- DRB1*1501* positive patients may progress faster to EDSS ≥6
7. There is a paucity of benign or mild MS and an increase of severe MS in individuals homozygous for the *DRB1*1501* haplotype.

Attempts to identify the primary susceptibility gene in the *HLA-DRB1*1501-DQB1*0602* haplotype have not provided consensus. The identification of the true predisposing gene or genes within the haplotype is made more complex by the extensive linkage disequilibrium (LD) across the region and by the presence of many other potential candidate genes that have roles in immune function within this superlocus. LD refers to the presence of alleles at neighboring loci segregating together more frequently than expected. When the effect of *DRB1*1501* is removed from the *DR2* haplotype, inconclusive evidence against [27] or in favor [28,29] of a primary role for *DQB1*0602* in MS susceptibility is reported. There also is debate as to the role of non-HLA genes mapping to this region [30]. Results suggesting that genes of interest exist within the *class III* [31,32] or telomeric to the *class I* regions also are reported [21,33–36]. Associations with genetic markers telomeric to the *MHC* also were detected in type 1 diabetes, celiac disease [37], inflammatory bowel disease [38], and rheumatoid arthritis [39,40].

Because patterns of genomic disequilibrium differ between populations, the most direct and practical approach to resolve this complex genetic obstacle is to scrutinize and compare a large number of MS haplotypes in well-characterized data sets from distinct populations. Compared with the white population, African Americans are at low risk for MS [41], but some combinations in cis of *DRB1* and *DQB1* alleles are unique in African Americans. Specifically, the *DRB1*1501, DQB1*0602* haplotype does not display the rigidity and high degree of LD in African Americans that is characteristic of whites. For example, in African Americans, *DQB1*0602* is found in association with *DRB1*11012* (the fifth digit makes this allele African only) and other DRB1 genes. Studies of *HLA* and MS in low-risk ethnic groups generally have used small cohorts and the results are inconclusive or conflicting, but case-control and family-based association studies recently were performed for *DRB1* and *DQB1* loci in a large and well-characterized African American MS cohort [42]. A selective association with *HLA-DRB1*15* was revealed, indicating a primary role for the *DRB1* locus in MS independent of *DQB1*0602*, although a modulating influence for *DQB1* on clinical outcome cannot be excluded and warrants further investigation. It then is likely that *HLA-DRB1* constitutes the centromeric boundary of the class II *DR-DQ* association in MS. Surprisingly, a substantial proportion of the susceptibility chromosomes from African American patients who have MS displayed haplotypes consistent with an African origin. The haplotypic features of these *DRB1*15*-positive chromosomes indicate an older African origin for the HLA-associated MS susceptibility gene(s), predating the divergence of human ethnic groups, rather than a genetic admixture in people of European descent. Positive selection for *DRB1*1501* seems to have occurred in Europeans but not in Africans, and although the factors that drove this selection, presumably infectious pathogens, are unknown, one possible consequence was a heightened susceptibility to MS, a disorder almost nonexistent in Africa. The low prevalence of MS in Africa likely is the result of additional protective genetic or environmental factors.

A primary role for *HLA-DRB1* in susceptibility to MS is consistent with a pathogenesis model, which involves a T-cell–mediated autoimmune response against the 85-99 peptide of myelin basic protein (MBP) [43–46]. The crystal structure of DRβ1501 differs from other non–DR2-related DRβ molecules in that aromatic residues in the ligand are preferred in the large hydrophobic P4 pocket of the peptide binding domain [47]. For MBP, this pocket is occupied primarily by the aromatic side chain Phe92, which acts as an important primary anchor and accounts for its high-affinity binding to the HLA-DRα0101/DRβ1501 heterodimer. The polymorphic residue at DRβ 71 also is critically important in creating the necessary space for Phe92 of MBP, and Ala at this position has been observed only for *DR15* alleles (*DRB1*1501-DRB1*1506*) and *DRB1*130,* but not for *DRB1*0301. HLA-DRB1*1501*, *DRB1*150,3* and *DRB1*0301* alleles, alternatively, all share a critical Val residue at position 86, where the HLA-DRβ chain also is polymorphic, and can encode either Val or Gly. DRβVal86 at the base of the P1 pocket results in a smaller pocket than that observed for DR1 and DR4 (Gly), for example, influencing not only binding and presentation of a number of self antigens including MBP but also DRαβ dimer stability [47–49]. The Val86/Val86 genotype has been implicated in association studies of Swedish and Australian populations that have MS [27,50].

An effect of *HLA-DR2* copy number on disease risk has been suggested [51,52]. These observations were unexpected because if HLA-DR2 molecules confer susceptibility by presenting an encephalitogenic peptide, then a dominant effect is expected. In EAE, a single copy of a disease-associated *MHC* haplotype, when present in the context of an appropriate genetic background, generally is sufficient for the induction of susceptibility. Alternatively, the penetrance of the trait could be modified by competition for the peptide with other MHC molecules, which present it benignly, or by the effect of a neighboring non-HLA modifier gene.

HLA-DR2 is reported to be associated with an earlier age of disease onset, female gender, and severe, relapsing-remitting, and mild MS courses [53–57], or to have no influence on disease course [58–62]. The effect of *HLA-DR2* genotype on clinical phenotypes, including age of onset, disease course, and severity, recently was tested in a well-characterized familial data set [52]. In the mild or benign patient group that had MS, *DR2* homozygotes were significantly less frequent compared with patients classified as having nonmild MS. Here, mild MS was defined as maintaining an Extended Disability Status Scale (EDSS) score of less than 3 for at least 10 years. When a more stringent definition of mild MS was applied, in which disease duration of at least 15 years was imposed, no *DR2* homozygotes were present in this subgroup. Both observations provide strong support for *HLA-DR2* as a disease modifier. Several studies suggesting the influence of non-*HLA* genes (*IL-1R*, *TNF*, *TGFB*, *APOE*, *CTLA4*, and *CCR5*, among others) on disease course and severity in MS have been reported and await confirmation.

MS2, chromosome 19q13

Genomic screens have shown support for linkage to this region and a meta-analysis [16] of all four pivotal genomic screens identified 19q13 as a significant disease locus. Additional evidence for this region came from allelic association and from follow-up studies [63–66]. Overall, the effect of the 19q13 locus likely is moderate, with an estimated locus-specific $\lambda_s = 1.5$, thus accounting for 4% to 6% of the overall genetic component in MS. On chromosome 19q13, the minimal critical region spans approximately 70 to 80 cM. This region contains 380 genes, including many attractive disease candidates. The well-documented involvement of apolipoprotein E (apoE) in neurologic disease, for example, makes this gene an interesting candidate for MS studies. The apoE protein long has been associated with regeneration of axons and myelin after lesions of central and peripheral nervous tissue, and its isoforms have been shown to have differential effects on neuronal growth. Several studies excluded *APOE* as a susceptibility factor in MS but reported an association between the apolipoprotein (*APOE*)-4 allele and more severe disease [67–70]. Another study reported some evidence for a protective effect of the *APOE-2* allele, observing that the time to reach secondary progression for patients whose initial disease type was relapsing-remitting was significantly longer for *APOE-2/3* genotypes compared with *APOE-3/3* and *-3/4* genotypes [71]. In a multicase data set, the proportion of *APOE-4* carriers was significantly higher in the severe disease group than the nonsevere group [66]. Alternately, the proportion of *APOE-2* carriers was significantly higher in the mild disease group than the nonmild group. Some biologic support for the *APOE-4* association with disease progression was suggested by an MRI investigation, which revealed more extensive tissue destruction or less efficient repair in MS *APOE-4* carriers [72]. Additional suggestive candidate genes in the 19q13 extended region include *TGFB1*, immunoglobulin-like transcripts *(ILT)*, killer-cell inhibitory receptors *(KIR)*, the leukocyte-associated inhibitory receptors *(LAIR)*, the *Fc receptor IL-11*, the heavy chain of the *MHC class I–like Fc receptor*, and *APOC4*.

MS3, chromosome 17q21-23

The chromosomal segment 17q21 was highlighted first in the genome scan performed in MS pedigrees collected in the United Kingdom [13] and confirmed in Finish families [73]. On chromosome 17q21, the minimal critical region spans between 36 and 46 cM and includes 331 genes. Further support for chromosome 17q21 was detected in follow-up studies in both populations [74–76] in association screening in several European and migrant European populations (http://www.mrc-bsu.cam.ac.uk/Msgenetics/GAMES) and in as-yet unpublished data in Canadian sibling pairs. No evidence of linkage to this region was detected in French or American families that had MS [65,77]. In a recently published analysis of 22 multicase Finish families, the putative MS locus in chromosome 17q was mapped to a less than 4-cM region covering approximately 2.5 Mb at 17q22-23 [75]. Biologically relevant genes, such as *MPO, ICAM2*, and *PECAM1*, map in the immediate vicinity.

Future directions

Although genetic components in MS clearly are present, the lack of an obvious and homogeneous mode of transmission has prevented the efficient application of classical genetic epidemiologic techniques. When a disease results from highly penetrant genomic variants, genetic linkage is a powerful method for significantly reducing the chromosomal regions that need to be examined for gene discovery. The power of linkage analysis to detect multiple signals of modest strength is limited, however. It has been argued that because of the low relative risk of any MS gene-variant, incomplete penetrance, and relative high frequency in the population at large, the linkage approach will not provide evidence for the location of the disease gene except in the case of unrealistically large samples available for analysis [78]. Alternatively, association studies of well-selected candidate genes may be more powerful for the detection of susceptibility alleles in complex disorders. Allelic association refers to a significantly increased or decreased frequency of a marker allele in individuals carrying a disease trait and represents deviation from the random occurrence of the allele with respect to disease phenotype. Candidate genes are defined as genes that are logical possibilities to play a role in a disease; for immune-mediated diseases, candidate genes might encode cytokines, immune receptors, and proteins involved in pathogen clearance. Multiple polymorphisms within each candidate locus, however, must be tested in adequately powered data sets to ensure that any true effect is identified. Unfortunately, the direct testing by association of possibly relevant candidate genes, identified by speculation based on concepts of pathogenesis, generally has been unproductive for gene identification in MS and other complex disorders. Progress in understanding the fundamental architecture of the human genome suggests that the tools finally may be at hand to achieve this elusive but important goal.

A powerful recent discovery is the finding that long-range disequilibrium exists in the human genome and, consequently, single nucleotide polymorphisms (SNPs) tend to exist as discrete segments of strong LD, the so-called "haplotype blocks" [79]. The maintenance of these blocks with their limited number of haplotypes most likely is the result of the nonuniform distribution of recombination, which tends to occur at hot spots demarcating one block from the next. In simple terms, these blocks can be considered the basic unit of inheritance. Therefore, rather than considering each individual chromosome as carrying a unique combination of SNP alleles, human chromosomes may be regarded as mosaics comprising blocks of SNP alleles with common patterns. These blocks are consistently large in size across the genome, show no evidence of historical recombination, and have low haplotype diversity. On average, significant SNP associations are seen at distances in the range of 20 to 100 kilobases (kb), with only 2 to 4 common patterns of variation (ie, haplotypes) observed for any given block [80,81]. Furthermore, between the genomic blocks are short intervals where recombination apparently is most active in creating assortments of these patterns. The immediate implication of these observations is that the blocks allow the efficient testing of all genetic variation within this region, regardless of whether or not all variants have been discovered. It may be possible, therefore, to use only a representative fraction of the total genetic variation as an adequate test for the extended chromosomal region under investigation. Recognizing that the study of these blocks would enable efficient identification of genes determining susceptibility to MS, the authors established a multidisciplinary research team that aggregates clinical and basic science efforts across six institutions, the International MS Genetic Consortium, to use and, in some cases, generate, detailed haplotype maps in relevant regions of the genome for the purpose of disease gene identification (https://chgr.mc.vanderbilt.edu/ms/).

Summary

Compelling epidemiologic and molecular data indicate that genes play a primary role in determining who is at risk for developing MS, how the disease progress, and how someone responds to therapy. The genetic component of MS etiology is believed to result from the action of allelic variants in several genes. Some loci may be involved in the initial pathogenic events, whereas others could influence the development and progression of the disease. Their incomplete penetrance and moderate individual effect probably reflect interactions with other genes, post-transcriptional regulatory mechanisms, and significant environmental influences. Equally significant, it also is likely that genetic heterogeneity exists, meaning that specific genes influence susceptibility and pathogenesis in some who are affected but not in others.

The past few years have seen progress in the development of laboratory and analytic approaches to study nonmendelian complex genetic disorders and in defining the pathologic basis of demyelination, setting the stage for the final characterization of the genes involved in MS susceptibility and pathogenesis. Large-scale molecular genetics explorations have become routine. The careful and methodic mining of data could lead to the identification of coregulated genes and characterization of genetic networks that underlie specific cellular process. This complex organization ultimately is what defines the function and, therefore, the phenotype. With the aid of high-capacity technologies, the combined analysis of genomic, transcriptional, proteomic, and phenotypic information will define a useful conceptual model of pathogenesis and a framework for understanding the mechanisms of action of existing therapies for this disorder and the rationale for novel curative strategies.

References

[1] Robertson NP, Fraser M, Deans J, et al. Age-adjusted recurrence risks for relatives of patients with multiple sclerosis. Brain 1996;119:449–55.
[2] Sadovnick AD, Yee IM, Ebers GC. Factors influencing sib risks for multiple sclerosis. Clin Genet 2000;58:431–5.
[3] Risch N. Corrections to linkage strategies for genetically complex traits. III. The effect of marker polymorphism on anlaysis of affected relative pairs. Am J Hum Genet 1992;51: 673–5.
[4] Sadovnick AD, Ebers GC, Dyment DA, et al. Evidence for genetic basis of multiple sclerosis. Lancet 1996;347:1728–30.
[5] Ebers GC, Sadovnick AD, Risch NJ. A genetic basis for familial aggregation in multiple sclerosis. Nature 1995;377:150–1.
[6] Mumford CJ, Wood NW, Kellar-Wood H, et al. The British Isles survey of multiple sclerosis in twins. Neurology 1994;44:11–5.
[7] Willer CJ, Dyment DA, Risch NJ, et al. Twin concordance and sibling recurrence rates in multiple sclerosis. Proc Natl Acad Sci USA 2003;100:12877–82.
[8] Horikawa Y, Oda N, Cox NJ, et al. Genetic variation in the gene encoding calpain-10 is associated with type 2 diabetes mellitus. Nat Genet 2000;26:163–75.
[9] Hugot JP, Chamaillard M, Zouali H, et al. Association of NOD2 leucine-rich repeat variants with susceptibility to Crohn's disease. Nature 2001;411:599–603.
[10] Ogura Y, Bonen DK, Inohara N, et al. A frameshift mutation in NOD2 associated with susceptibility to Crohn's disease. Nature 2001;411:603–6.
[11] Ebers GC, Kukay K, Bulman DE, et al. A full genome search in multiple sclerosis. Nat Genet 1996;13:472–6.
[12] Haines JL. A complete genomic screen for multiple sclerosis underscores a role for the major histocompatibility complex. Nat Genet 1996;13:469–71.
[13] Sawcer S, Jones HB, Feakes R, et al. A genome screen in multiple sclerosis reveals susceptibility loci on chromosome 6p21 and 17q22. Nat Genet 1996;13:464–8.
[14] Oksenberg JR, Baranzini SE, Barcellos LF, et al. Multiple sclerosis: genomic rewards. J Neuroimmunol 2001;113:171–84.
[15] The Transatlantic Multiple Sclerosis Genetics Cooperative. A meta-analysis of genomic screens in multiple sclerosis. Mult Scler 2001;7:3–11.
[16] Wise LH, Lanchbury JS, Lewis CM. Meta-analysis of genome searches. Ann Hum Genet 1999;63:263–72.
[17] GAMES and the Transatlantic Multiple Sclerosis Cooperative. A meta-analysis of whole genome linkage screens in multiple sclerosis. J Neuroimmunol 2003;143:39–46.
[18] Begovich AB, Oksenberg JR. Variation in genes regulating the immune system and relationship to disease. In: Miller MS, Cronin M, editors. Genetic polymorphisms and susceptibility to disease. London: Francis and Taylor; 2000. p. 139–74.
[19] Bertrams J, Kuwert E, Liedtke U. HLA antigens and multiple sclerosis. Tissue Antigens 1972;2:405–8.

[20] Jersild C, Fog T, Hansen GS, et al. Histocompatibility determinants in multiple sclerosis. Lancet 1973;ii:1221–5.
[21] Marrosu MG, Murru R, Murru MR, et al. Dissection of the HLA association with multiple sclerosis in the founder isolated population of Sardinia. Hum Mol Genet 2001;10:2907–16.
[22] Marrosu MG, Lai M, Cocco E, et al. Genetic factors and the founder effect explain familial MS in Sardinia. Neurology 2002;58:283–8.
[23] Kira J, Kanai T, Nishimura Y, et al. Western versus Asian types of multiple sclerosis: immunogenetically and clinically distinct disorders. Ann Neurol 1996;40:569–74.
[24] McDonnell GV, Hawkins SA. Clinical study of primary progressive multiple sclerosis in Northern Ireland, UK. J Neurol Neurosurg Psychiatry 1998;64:451–4.
[25] Boiko AN, Gusev EI, Sudomoina MA, et al. Association and linkage of juvenile MS with HLA-DR2(15) in Russians. Neurology 2002;58:658–60.
[26] Multiple Sclerosis Genetic Group. Clinical demographics of multiplex families with multiple sclerosis. Ann Neurol 1998;43:530–4.
[27] Allen M, Sandberg-Wollheim M, Sjogren K, et al. Association of susceptibility to multiple sclerosis in Sweden with HLA class II DRB1 and DQB1 alleles. Hum Immunol 1994;39: 41–8.
[28] Spurkland A, Ronningen K, Vandvik B, et al. HLA-DQA1 and HLA-DQB1 genes may jointly determine susceptibility to develop multiple sclerosis. Hum Immunol 1991;30: 69–75.
[29] Boon M, Nolte IM, Bruinenberg M, et al. Mapping of a susceptibility gene for multiple sclerosis to the 51 kb interval between G511525 and D6S1666 using a new method of haplotype sharing analysis. Neurogenet 2001;3:221–30.
[30] Ligers A, Dyment DA, Willer CJ, et al. Evidence of linkage with HLA-DR in DRB1*15-negative families with multiple sclerosis. Am J Hum Genet 2001;69:900–3.
[31] de Jong BA, Huizinga TW, Zanelli E, et al. Evidence for additional genetic risk indicators of relapse-onset MS within the HLA region. Neurology 2002;59:549–55.
[32] Palacio LG, Rivera D, Builes JJ, et al. Multiple sclerosis in the tropics: genetic association to STR's loci spanning the HLA and TNF. Mult Scler 2002;8:249–55.
[33] Shinar Y, Pras E, Siev-Ner I, et al. Analysis of allelic association between D6S461 marker and multiple sclerosis in Ashkenazi and Iraqi Jewish patients. J Mol Neurosci 1998;11: 265–9.
[34] Fogdell-Hahn A, Ligers A, Gronning M, et al. Multiple sclerosis: a modifying influence of HLA class I genes in an HLA class II associated autoimmune disease. Tissue Antigens 2000; 55:140–8.
[35] Rubio JP, Bahlo M, Butzkueven H, et al. Genetic dissection of the human leukocyte antigen region by use of haplotypes of Tasmanians with multiple sclerosis. Am J Hum Genet 2002; 70:1125–37.
[36] Lie BA, Akselsen HE, Bowlus CL, et al. Polymorphisms in the gene encoding thymus-specific serine protease in the extended HLA complex: a potential candidate gene for autoimmune and HLA-associated diseases. Genes Immun 2002;3:306–12.
[37] Lie BA, Sollid LM, Ascher H, et al. A gene telomeric of the HLA class I region is involved in predisposition to both type 1 diabetes and coeliac disease. Tissue Antigens 1999;54:162–8.
[38] Hampe A, Coriton O, Andrieux N, et al. A 356-Kb sequence of the subtelomeric part of the MHC Class I region. DNA Seq 1999;10:263–99.
[39] Zanelli E, Jones G, Pascual M, et al. The telomeric part of the HLA region predisposes to rheumatoid arthritis independently of the class II loci. Hum Immunol 2001;62:75–84.
[40] Jawaheer D, Li W, Graham RR, et al. Dissecting the genetic complexity of the association between human leukocyte antigens and rheumatoid arthritis. Am J Hum Genet 2002;71: 585–94.
[41] Kurtzke JF, Beebe GW, Norman JE. Epidemiology of multiple sclerosis in US veterans: 1. Race, sex, and geographic distribution. Neurology 1979;29:1228–35.

[42] Oksenberg JR, Barcellos LF, Cree BA, et al. Mapping multiple sclerosis susceptibility to the HLA-DR locus in African Americans. Am J Hum Genet 2004;74:160–7.
[43] Allegretta M, Nicklas JA, Sriram S, et al. T cells responsive to myelin basic protein in patients with multiple sclerosis. Science 1990;247:718–21.
[44] Pette M, Fujita K, Kitze B, et al. Myelin basic protein specific T cell lines from MS patients and healthy individuals. Neurology 1990;40:1770–6.
[45] Oksenberg JR, Panzara MA, Begovich AB, et al. Selection for T-cell receptor Vβ-Dβ-Jβ gene rearrangements with specificity for a myelin basic protein peptide in brain lesions of multiple sclerosis. Nature 1993;362:68–70.
[46] Krogsgaard M, Wucherpfennig KW, Canella B, et al. Visualization of myelin basic protein T cell epitopes in multiple sclerosis lesions using a monoclonal antibody specific for the human histocompatibility leukocyte antigen (HLA)-DR2-MBP 85–99 complex. J Exp Med 2000; 191:1395–412.
[47] Smith KJ, Pyrdol J, Gauthier L, et al. Crystal structure of HLA-DR2 (DRA*0101, DRB1*1501) complexed with a peptide from human myelin basic protein. J Exp Med 1998; 188:1511–20.
[48] Verreck FA, Termijtelen A, Koning F. HLA-DR beta chain residue 86 controls DR alpha beta dimer stability. Eur J Immunol 1993;23:1346–50.
[49] Wucherpfennig KW, Sette A, Southwood S, et al. Structural requirements for binding of an immunodominant myelin basic protein peptide to DR 2 isotypes and for its recognition by human T cell clones. J Exp Med 1994;179:279–90.
[50] Teutsch SM, Bennetts BH, Buhler MM, et al. The DRB1 Val86/Val86 genotype associates with multiple sclerosis in Australian patients. Hum Immunol 1999;60:715–22.
[51] Rasmussen TE, Hallett JW Jr, Tazelaar HD, et al. Human leukocyte antigen class II immune response genes, female gender, and cigarette smoking as risk and modulating factors in abdominal aortic aneurysms. J Vasc Surg 2002;35:988–93.
[52] Barcellos LF, Oksenberg JR, Begovich AB, et al. HLA-DR2 dose effect on susceptibility to multiple sclerosis and influence on disease course. Am J Hum Genet 2003;72:710–6.
[53] Engell T, Raun NE, Thomsen M, et al. HLA and heterogeneity of multiple sclerosis. Neurology 1982;32:1043–6.
[54] Duquette P, Decary F, Pleines J, et al. Clinical sub-groups of multiple sclerosis in relation to HLA: DR alleles as possible markers of disease progression. Can J Neurol Sci 1985;12: 106–10.
[55] Madigand M, Oger JJ, Fauchet R, et al. HLA profiles in multiple sclerosis suggest two forms of disease and the existence of protective haplotypes. J Neurol Sci 1982;53:519–29.
[56] Masterman T, Ligers A, Olsson T, et al. HLA-DR15 is associated with lower age at onset in multiple sclerosis. Ann Neurol 2000;48:211–9.
[57] Hensiek AE, Sawcer SJ, Feakes R, et al. HLA-DR 15 is associated with female sex and younger age at diagnosis in multiple sclerosis. J Neurol Neurosurg Psychiatry 2002;72:184–7.
[58] Celius EG, Harbo HF, Egeland T, et al. Sex and age at diagnosis are correlated with the HLA-DR2, DQ6 haplotype in multiple sclerosis. J Neurol Sci 2000;178:132–5.
[59] McDonnell GV, Mawhinney H, Graham CA, et al. A study of the HLA-DR region in clinical subgroups of multiple sclerosis and its influence on prognosis. J Neurol Sci 1999;165: 77–83.
[60] Poser S, Ritter G, Bauer HJ, Grosse-Wilde H, et al. HLA-antigens and the prognosis of multiple sclerosis. J Neurol 1981;225:219–21.
[61] Runmarker B, Martinsson T, Wahlstrom J, et al. HLA and prognosis in multiple sclerosis. J Neurol 1994;241:385–90.
[62] Weinshenker BG, Santrach P, Bissonet AS, et al. Major histocompatibility complex class II alleles and the course and outcome of MS: a population-based study. Neurology 1998;51: 742–7.
[63] Barcellos LF, Thomson G, Carrington M, et al. Chromosome 19 single-locus and multilocus haplotype associations with multiple sclerosis. JAMA 1997;1256–71.

[64] Pericak-Vance MA, Rimmler JB, Martin ER, et al. Linkage and association analysis of chromosome 19q13 in multiple sclerosis. Neurogenetics 2001;3:195–201.
[65] Haines JL, Bradford Y, Garcia ME, Reed AD, et al. Multiple susceptibility loci for multiple sclerosis. Hum Mol Genet 2002;11:2251–6.
[66] Schmidt S, Barcellos LF, DeSombre K, et al. Association of polymorphisms in the apolipoprotein E region with susceptibility to and progression of multiple sclerosis. Am J Hum Genet 2002;70:708–17.
[67] Evangelou N, Jackson M, Beeson D, et al. Association of the APOE epsilon4 allele with disease activity in multiple sclerosis. J Neurol Neurosurg Psychiatry 1999;67:203–5.
[68] Oliveri RL, Cittadella R, Sibilia G, et al. APOE and risk of cognitive impairment in multiple sclerosis. Acta Neurol Scand 1999;100:290–5.
[69] Chapman J, Vinokurov S, Achiron A, et al. APOE genotype is a major predictor of long-term progression of disability in MS. Neurology 2001;56:312–6.
[70] Fazekas F, Strasser-Fuchs S, Kollegger H, Schmidt H, et al. Apolipoprotein E epsilon 4 is associated with rapid progression of multiple sclerosis. Neurology 2001;57:853–7.
[71] Ballerini C, Campani D, Rombola G, et al. Association of apolipoprotein E polymorphism to clinical heterogeneity of multiplesclerosis. Neurosci Lett 2000;296:174–6.
[72] Fazekas F, Strasser-Fuchs S, Schmidt H, et al. Apolipoprotein E genotype related differences in brain lesions of multiple sclerosis. J Neurol Neurosurg Psychiatry 2000;69:25–8.
[73] Kuokkanen S, Gschwend M, Rioux JD, et al. Genomewide scan of multiple sclerosis in Finnish multiplex families. Am J Hum Genet 1997;61:1379–87.
[74] Chataway J, Feakes R, Coraddu F, et al. The genetics of multiple sclerosis: principles, background and update results of the UK systematic genome screen. Brain 1998;121: 1869–87.
[75] Saarela J, Schoenberg Fejzo M, Chen D, et al. Fine mapping of a multiple sclerosis locus to 2.5 Mb on chromosome 17q22-q24. Hum Mol Genet 2002;11:2257–67.
[76] Sawcer S, Maranian M, Setakis E, et al. A whole genome screen for linkage disequilibrium in multiple sclerosis confirms disease associations with regions previously linked to susceptibility. Brain 2002;125:1337–47.
[77] Fontaine B, Cournu I, Arnaud I, et al. Chromosome 17q22-q24 and multiple sclerosis genetic susceptibility. American-French Multiple Sclerosis Genetic Group. Genes Immun 1999;1:149–50.
[78] Risch N. Searching for genetic determinants in the new millennium. Nature 2000;405: 847–56.
[79] Gabriel SB, Schaffner SF, Nguyen H, et al. The structure of haplotype blocks in the human genome. Science 2002;296:2225–9.
[80] Daly MJ, Rioux JD, Schaffner SF, et al. High-resolution haplotype structure in the human genome. Nat Genet 2001;29:229–32.
[81] Rioux JD, Daly MJ, Silverberg MS, et al. Genetic variation in the 5q31 cytokine gene cluster confers susceptibility to Crohn's disease. Nat Genet 2001;29:223–8.

ELSEVIER
SAUNDERS

Neurol Clin 23 (2005) 77–105

NEUROLOGIC
CLINICS

The Pathology of Multiple Sclerosis

Claudia F. Lucchinetti, MD[a,*], Joseph Parisi, MD[a], Wolfgang Bruck, MD[b]

[a]Mayo Clinic, 200 First Street, SW, Rochester, MN 55905, USA
[b]Institute of Neuropathology, Robert-Koch-Strasse 40, 37075, Göttingen, Germany

Multiple sclerosis (MS) is a chronic neurologic disease affecting approximately 1 million adults worldwide and 300,000 Americans [1]. Early illustrations by Carswell in 1838 and Cruveilhier in 1841, followed by the detailed clinical and pathologic correlative studies of Charcot in 1868 and 1880, described the pathologic hallmarks of the MS lesion as consisting of focal demyelination, inflammation, scar formation, and varying axonal destruction [2–5]. These lesions are scattered throughout the central nervous system (CNS), with a predilection for the optic nerves, brainstem, spinal cord, cerebellum, and periventricular white matter.

Relapses and progression are the two basic clinical phenomena of prototypic MS [6]. Relapses are considered the clinical expression of acute focal or multifocal inflammatory demyelination disseminated in the CNS, whereas progression reflects the occurrence of chronic demyelination, axonal loss, and gliosis. Early in the disease, remission of symptoms likely is the result of remyelination and resolution of inflammation, but after recurrent attacks, remyelination is limited [7]. Although MS includes inflammatory and demyelinating components, their relative influence on axonal loss is unclear. A combination of inflammatory and noninflammatory factors likely contributes to short- and long-term disability in MS. This review highlights recent advances in experimental neuropathology that have contributed to a better understanding of MS lesion pathogenesis. To develop effective MS therapeutic strategies, it is crucial to appreciate the relationship between inflammation, demyelination, and axonal injury and the relative contribution of each aspect to lesion pathogenesis and clinical disability in MS. The recognition of an inflammatory and a neurodegenerative phase of MS likely

* Corresponding author. Mayo Clinic, Department of Neurology, 200 1st Street, SW, Rochester, MN 55905-0001.

E-mail address: clucchinetti@mayo.edu (C.F. Lucchinetti).

0733-8619/05/$ - see front matter
doi:10.1016/j.ncl.2004.09.002

will require the development of therapies that are specific for different targets, stages, and subtypes of the disease.

The multiple sclerosis lesion

The chronic lesion

Chronic MS is the prototype of the demyelinating diseases and involves predominantly white matter at several CNS sites at different points in time. The demyelinating foci, termed "plaques," are distributed randomly throughout the CNS white matter. Plaques vary in size and number from case to case but are most conspicuous in the periventricular white matter around the angles of the lateral ventricles and at the floor of the fourth ventricle (Fig. 1A, B). The visual system, deep white matter, brainstem, and spinal cord also are commonly involved. The chronic inactive MS plaque is a sharply circumscribed, hypocellular plaque with no evidence of active myelin breakdown. Fibrillary gliosis is prominent and, although axonal density is relatively preserved compared with the extent of axonal loss seen in an

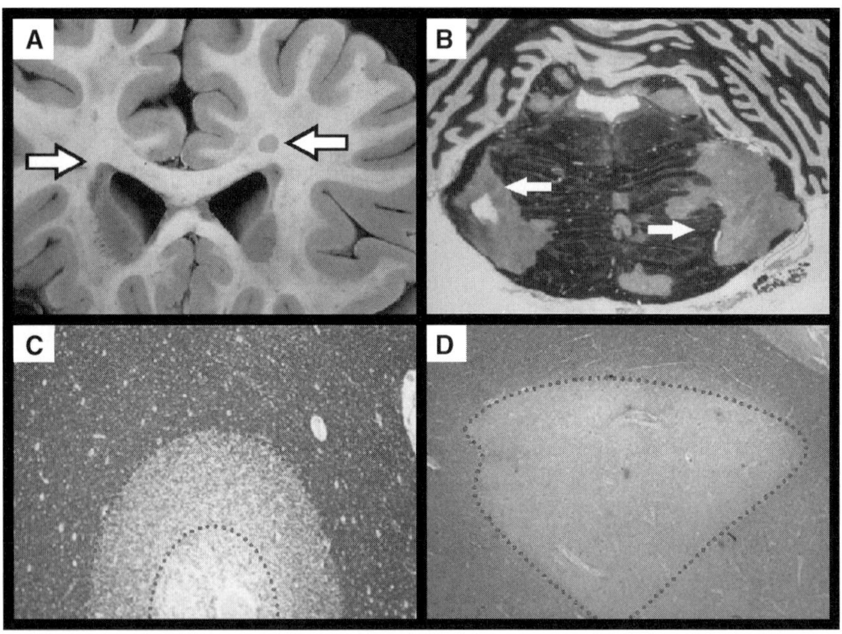

Fig. 1. The chronic MS lesion. (*A*) Macroscopic section through a MS brain with typical periventricular plaques (*arrows*). (*B*) Section of the pons stained for myelin Luxol Fast Blue (LFB)-periodic acid Schiff (PAS) (LFB-PAS). There are numerous demyelinated lesions detectable (*arrows*). (*C, D*) Remyelinated so-called "shadow plaques" are characterized by their reduced staining intensity of myelin. Remyelination either is restricted to the lesion edge (*C*; stained for MBP) or is present throughout the lesion (*D*; LFB-PAS).

infarction, it still may be markedly reduced. Mature oligodendrocytes are markedly diminished or absent from chronic inactive lesions [7] Varying degrees of inflammation may still be present, however, particularly in the perivascular region.

Remyelination in chronic lesions typically is incomplete and restricted largely to the edge of the plaque; however, more extensive remyelination throughout a chronic MS lesion also may be present (see Fig.1C, D). These lesions are referred to as shadow plaques and consist of areas of reduced staining of myelin (myelin pallor) as a result of a decreased ratio between myelin sheath thickness and axonal diameter. Remyelinated lesions may become targets of new demyelinating attacks [8].

Cells consistent with very early stages of oligodendrocyte development have been identified in completely demyelinated plaques devoid of mature oligodendrocytes [9]. Furthermore, a recent study suggests that premyelinating oligodendrocytes may be present in chronic MS lesions, suggesting remyelination at these late states may not be limited by an absence of oligodendrocyte progenitors, rather that damaged axons may not be receptive to remyelination signals [10]. To what extent these cells can be stimulated to divide, repopulate the lesions, and initiate remyelination still must be demonstrated.

The Notch signaling pathway recently has been implicated as a potential mechanism by which remyelination is limited after demyelinating insults to the CNS. During mammalian CNS development, contact-mediated activation of Notch 1 receptors on oligodendrocyte precursors by the ligand Jagged 1 induces Hes5, which inhibits oligodendrocyte maturation [11–13]. In vitro studies show that Jagged 1 signaling inhibits process outgrowth from primary human oligodendrocytes. Jagged 1 is expressed within and around active MS lesions lacking remyelination, whereas lesions with more abundant remyelination lack Jagged 1 expression. Furthermore, Notch 1 and Hes5 localized to immature oligodendrocytes in the same area [12]. Therefore, the Notch pathway may contribute to limited repair in MS and Notch may represent a future therapeutic target.

Remyelination also is evident during the early stages of some MS lesions and may occur simultaneously with ongoing demyelination [13]. During these early stages of myelin sheath formation, inflammation may be prominent within the lesion. The extent of remyelination at these early stages seems to depend on the availability of oligodendrocytes or their progenitor cells in the lesions [14]. Pathologic studies of MS lesions report a varying degree of oligodendrocyte preservation in actively demyelinating lesions [15–17]. A detailed analysis of oligodendrocyte density relative to demyelinating activity in a series of 113 MS cases demonstrated two principal patterns of oligodendrocyte pathology in MS lesions [14]. In the first pattern, oligodendrocytes were variably reduced during active stages of myelin destruction but reappeared within inactive or remyelinating areas (70% of cases examined). The other pattern was characterized by extensive destruction of myelinating cells at active sites of demyelination in the absence of progenitor cell recruitment in inactive plaque areas. In these cases, remyelination was sparse or absent (30% of cases). The profound heterogeneity in extent and topography of oligodendrocyte destruction in active demyelinating lesions suggests that in subsets of patients who have MS, myelin, mature oligodendrocytes, and, possibly, oligodendrocyte progenitors are affected differentially. These observations suggest that different mechanisms of myelin or oligodendrocyte injury may be operating in individual patients who have MS and may influence the likelihood of effective early remyelination within the MS lesion.

The active lesion

Active inflammatory demyelination typically is localized to white matter and characterized by an admixture of lipid-laden macrophages and large reactive astrocytes, accompanied by varying perivascular inflammation

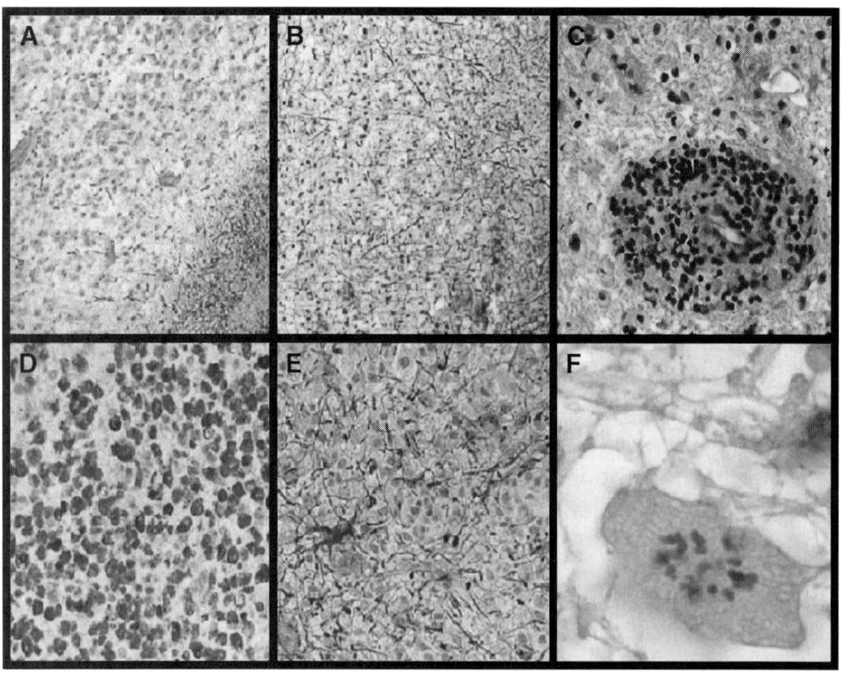

Fig. 2. The active MS lesion. (*A*) Highly cellular lesion with a sharp border. There are numerous macrophages present (LFB-PAS). (*B*) Axons are reduced or lost and form so-called axonal balloons (Bielschowskýs silver impregnation). (*C*) Dense perivascular infiltrate mainly composed of T cells (hematoxylin-eosin). (*D*) The lesion is infiltrated diffusely by high numbers of macrophages removing the myelin debris (Ki-M1P). (*E*) Astrocytes are hypertrophic and form multiple processes glial fibrillary acidic protein (GFAP). (*F*) Hypertrophic astrocyte (Creutzfeld-Peters cell), with granular mitosis.

(Fig. 2A, C–E). The involved areas demonstrate marked pallor of myelin staining with relative preservation of axons, although where damage is most severe, axons also are lost or fragmented and display irregular tortuous and clubbed profiles (see Fig. 2B). Many macrophages become engorged with phagocytosed myelin remnants and debris and assume the appearance of classic gitter cells. These cells are characterized by spherical round nuclei, vacuolated cytoplasm, and discrete cell borders. Intimately intermingled are hypertrophic (reactive) astrocytes with prominent, somewhat polymorphic, nuclei and conspicuous eosinophilic cytoplasm. The so-called "granular mitosis" (also referred to as a Creutzfeld-Peters cell) is an unusual finding in reactive astrocytes in demyelination and other reactive processes. These structures have the appearance of large chromosomes arranged like mitotic figures but represent small fragments of the nucleus (micronuclei) (see Fig. 2F). The presence of these atypical astrocytes suggests the possibility of a glioma; however, reactive astrocytes in active MS lesions are distributed evenly and avoid the tendency to clump together as they do in gliomas.

The criteria for defining an actively demyelinating MS lesion are controversial and often misleading. A stringent definition of demyelinating activity within a plaque can be obtained by studying the structural profile and chemical composition of myelin degradation products within macrophages and examining the sequential expression of inflammatory macrophage activation antigens in the lesions [18]. Minor myelin proteins, such as myelin oligodendrocyte glycoprotein (MOG) or myelin-associated glycoprotein (MAG), are degraded rapidly within macrophages 1 to 2 days after phagocytosis (Fig. 3A). In contrast, major myelin proteins, such as myelin basic protein (MBP) and proteolipid protein (PLP), may persist in macrophages for

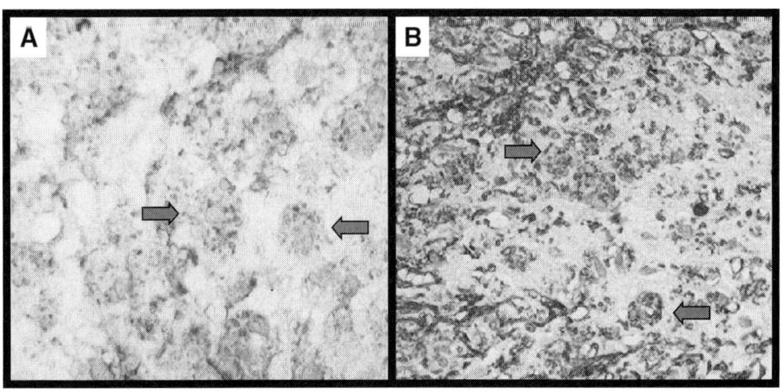

Fig. 3. Definition of demyelinating activity. Detection of myelin proteins in the macrophage cytoplasm allows for definition of different stages of myelin breakdown. Active demyelination is characterized by the presence of minor (eg, MOG; *A*) or major myelin proteins (eg, MBP; *B*) within macrophages.

6 to 10 days (see Fig. 3B). In later stages, the macrophages contain sudanophilic and periodic acid–Schiff (PAS)–positive granular lipids that may persist in the lesion for up to several months.

Normal-appearing white matter damage in multiple sclerosis

Besides the focal demyelinated plaques, a diffuse global injury of the so-called "normal"-appearing white matter (NAWM) is found in the brains of patients who have MS. This is supported by several neuroimaging studies suggesting a diffuse pathology present within the NAWM of patients who have MS. Magnetic resonance spectroscopy (MRS) reveals reduced N-acetyl aspartate (NAA) and elevated creatine levels in the NAWM of primary progressive MS (PPMS) [19–21], and magnetic transfer ratios are reduced in the NAWM of chronic versus relapsing disease [22–24]. Furthermore, brain atrophy in MS is in part independent of T2 lesion load, suggesting that NAWM pathology not only reflects wallerian degeneration of axons traversing macroscopic lesions but also may reflect microscopic or diffuse lesions not detected by MRI [25]. The pathology of the NAWM in MS is characterized by diffuse, mainly $CD8^+$, T-cell infiltrates, gliosis, microglial activation, diffuse axonal injury, and nerve fiber degeneration [26,27]. To what degree these represent reactive changes versus reflecting an inherent abnormality within the white matter of patients who have MS is uncertain.

Gray matter pathology in multiple sclerosis

Although MS generally is considered a disease of the white matter, demyelination also can be found in the deep cerebral nuclei [28] or the cerebral cortex [29]. Cortical MS plaques may be abundant in some patients who have MS. They may appear as subcortical white matter lesions that expand into the adjacent cortex or may occur as cortical perivenous lesions, independent from white matter pathology. In addition, a large number of cortical lesions are band-like demyelinated areas of the upper three to four cortical layers without any topographic relation to cerebral veins [30].

Cortical lesions differ from white matter plaques in several fundamental aspects. They are less inflammatory with a dominant effector cell population of ramified microglia and are not a macrophage phenotype [30]. Although there is a varying extent of axonal injury, the global tissue texture in cortical plaques is preserved better than in white matter lesions, suggesting less global tissue injury. This makes it difficult to appreciate the extent of cortical demyelination on visual inspection of the postmortem brain or with MRI [31].

The presence of apoptotic neurons also has been reported to be increased within the demyelinated cortex [30]. Cortical demyelination may have an impact on neuronal, dendritic, and axonal function, viability, and survival. This may be relevant to the pathogenesis of neurologic and cognitive disability in MS.

Multiple sclerosis pathogenesis

Inflammatory infiltrates in MS lesions consist mainly of T lymphocytes, few B lymphocytes and plasma cells, and extensive macrophage/microglial activation. Activated helper T-cell subsets have distinct cytokine profiles that regulate immune responses. These are divided into two subsets: T_H1 and T_H2 lymphocytes [32]. T_H1 lymphocytes generally produce proinflammatory cytokines, such as interleukin 2 (IL-2), interferon-γ (IFN-γ), and tumor necrosis factor α (TNF-α), whereas T_H2 lymphocytes secrete anti-inflammatory cytokines, such as IL-4, IL-5, IL-6, IL-10, and IL-13.

A limited trafficking of antigen nonspecific T cells occurs across an intact blood-brain barrier (BBB) via the interaction of integrins expressed on the surface of lymphocytes and adhesion molecules present on the endothelial surface of blood vessels. Rolling, adherence, and diapedesis of T lymphocytes are mediated by VCAM/VLA-4 and ICAM/LFA-1 interactions. Genetic and environmental factors (ie, viral infection, bacterial lipopolysaccharides, superantigens, reactive metabolites, and metabolic stress) may facilitate the entry of potentially pathogenic autoreactive T cells and antibodies into the CNS via BBB disruption. In the CNS, local factors upregulate the expression of endothelial adhesion molecules (ICAM-1, VCAM-1, and E-selectin), which further enhances the movement of pathogenic cells into the CNS [33].

Once autoreactive T cells enter the CNS, matrix metalloproteinases (MMPs), especially MMP 9, are believed to contribute to degrading extracellular matrix macromolecules. Beta interferons, which reduce relapse rate and severity, are potent MMP 9 inhibitors [34] and may limit T-cell infiltration and cytokine production [35]. Within the CNS, proinflammatory cytokines activate resident and hematogenous macrophages. Recruitment and attraction of these cells occurs via integrins and chemokines and contribute to tissue injury and demyelination. Selective expression of individual chemokines may influence the cellular composition of inflammatory lesions, because chemokine receptors are associated with either T_H1 or T_H2 responses.

To propagate the inflammatory cascade, T cells, which have entered the CNS, need to be activated by specific antigens. Antigen-specific T-cell activation requires the presentation of antigenic peptides in the context of major histocompatibility complex (MHC) molecules. The trimolecular complex consists of the T-cell receptor, the processed antigen, and the MHC molecule. Perivascular monocytes, microglia, macrophages, parenchymal lymphocytes, and, possibly, astrocytes express MHC antigens in MS. There are two principal types of MHC molecules: class I and class II. These molecules bind peptide antigens as part of the processing they require for presentation to different T lymphocytes. $CD4^+$ lymphocytes recognize antigens in the context of MHC class II molecules, whereas $CD8^+$ lymphocytes recognize antigens in association with MHC class I molecules. This activation is further enhanced by the interaction of costimulatory molecules, such as CD40/CD40 ligand or B7-1 and B7-2/cytotoxic T-lymphocyte antigen-4. The full T-cell activation program is present in MS lesions. MS plaque macrophages express CD40 and B7-2, whereas lymphocytes express mainly CD40L and B7-1 [36]. Once activated, T cells can orchestrate several cellular and humoral responses that could result in tissue injury.

Based on several observations, the inflammatory reaction in MS is believed to reflect a T_H1 autoimmune response. MS pathology has some features similar to experimental autoimmune encephalomyelitis (EAE), an experimental model of T_H1 autoimmunity. There is an upregulation of a variety of T_H1 cytokines, including IL-2, IFN-γ, and TNF-α, which also are found in the CSF of patients who have MS with active disease [37,38]. Autoreactive T cells with a T_H1 cytokine profile have been isolated from the blood and CSF of patients who have MS. There is a pattern of T_H1 chemokine expression in CSF and MS lesions [39]. MS has is linked to specific MHC class II haplotypes [40].

If MS is an autoimmune disease, however, the causative antigen still is unknown, and myelin and nonmyelin candidates are proposed. The evidence supporting a primary and exclusive pathogenic role for T_H1-mediated injury in MS remains indirect and circumstantial. Some therapies that have been beneficial in EAE have yielded ineffective responses or unexpected aggravation of MS [41,42]. A therapeutic approach based on a myelin peptide that induced a T_H-2 shift unexpectedly resulted in severe relapses in an EAE monkey model [43]. Furthermore, most experimental models of EAE result in limited demyelination, in a pattern more closely resembling acute disseminated encephalomyelitis (ADEM). Additional pathogenic factors, therefore, may be required to produce the pathologic hallmark of MS, the demyelinated plaque. These factors may include demyelinating antibodies, cytokines and other soluble mediators, cytotoxic T cells, reactive oxygen and nitrogen species, excitotoxic mechanisms, or primary oligodendrocyte injury [44,45].

Cytotoxic $CD8^+$ T lymphocytes may play an important role in MS lesion pathogenesis. Recent studies demonstrate the ability of $CD8^+$ T cells to mediate demyelinating pathology [46]. $CD8^+$ T cells predominate in many MS lesions and are clonally expanded within MS plaques [47]. $CD8^+$ T cells in the CSF are oligoclonal and support involvement in an antigen-driven pathologic process [48]. MHC class I expression is present on oligodendrocytes, astrocytes, neurons, axons, and endothelial cells in active lesions; therefore, these structures are potential targets for MHC class I–mediated cytotoxic injury [49]. In vitro studies demonstrate $CD8^+$ T cells can lyse neurons, axons, and oligodendrocytes [50,51]. In vivo studies indicate that axonal damage within early active MS lesions correlates with the number of $CD8^+$ T cells [52] Myelin-specific $CD8^+$ T cells even may evoke EAE under certain conditions. Extensive demyelinated lesions are restricted to the brain and are associated with cell death [53,54].

The humoral response also may play an important role in disease pathogenesis. Receptor-mediated phagocytosis is implicated in myelin breakdown [55]. Antibodies against myelin proteins, such as MOG and MBP, are found in the sera and CSF in a subset of patients who have MS [56,57]. In an animal model of MS, demyelination occurs in the presence of antibodies and complement activation [58]. Deposition of antibodies and C9neo along disrupted myelin sheaths, oligodendrocytes, and within macrophages has been demonstrated in MS lesions [59,60]. Anti-MOG antibodies also have been identified within MS lesions [61]. Traditionally, the occurrence of elevated intrathecal immunoglobulin G (IgG) synthesis and oligoclonal bands in the CSF of most patients who have MS is viewed as evidence of a humoral response in MS. In neuromyelitis optica (NMO), however, an inflammatory demyelinating disorder associated with evidence of humorally mediated pathology [62], oligoclonal bands typically are absent [63]. This may reflect a peripheral lymphoid source versus intrathecal synthesis IgG.

The inflammatory response within MS lesions also may be involved in promoting repair. Autoimmune T cells can protect optic nerve neurons after crush injury [64]. Macrophages stimulate remyelination in culture [65], and macrophage depletion actually diminishes remyelination [66]. Furthermore, inflammatory cells within MS lesions synthesize neurotrophic factors, such as brain-derived neurotrophic factor (BDNF) [67]. There likely is, therefore, a delicate balance between pathogenic and reparative factors that determine the final outcome of the MS lesion. Conceivably, the complete blockage of all inflammatory responses in the MS lesion could be counterproductive.

Pathogenic heterogeneity in multiple sclerosis

The limited efficacy of T-cell–directed therapies in MS may be the consequence of a failure to abolish inflammation completely or the inability to intervene more specifically, because neither the trigger of inflammation nor the target autoantigen is known. Alternatively, it may be that MS therapies do not adequately address the potential for pathogenic heterogeneity in this complex disease. The focus of MS research has been on attempts to identify a single cause in hopes of finding a specific therapy effective for all patients. MS is a heterogeneous disease, however, with respect to its clinical, genetic, radiographic, and pathologic features. Furthermore, the observed variability in treatment response to current strategies among patients who have MS is not understood well. In vitro and in vivo studies indicate that inflammatory demyelination can result from various immune and nonimmune mechanisms.

The pathologic analysis of MS lesions reveals a profound heterogeneity between patients with respect to the inflammatory response, patterns of demyelination, oligodendrocyte survival, extent of remyelination, and degree of axonal injury. This variability generally was believed to reflect varying intensity of the same pathogenic process, resulting in different degrees of injury. An examination of several lesions within a given patient, however, when matched for demyelinating activity, demonstrates a striking homogeneity among lesions with respect to pathologic features [60]. MS, therefore, may represent a common name for different pathogenic entities that unify on the special vulnerability of the myelin and oligodendrocyte complex to various immune and toxic mediators [45]. This possibility has important therapeutic implications. If several terminal effector pathways act in parallel within a single patient who has MS, there would be little chance to treat or prevent the disease by interfering with a single mechanism. Alternatively, if a dominant effector pathway operates in a given patient, a specific therapy could be targeted to a specific mechanism.

An understanding of the earliest events in MS lesion pathogenesis requires the analysis of actively demyelinating lesions that show evidence of ongoing myelin degradation. A major restriction of previous MS neuropathologic studies was the result of the limited availability of material from actively demyelinating lesions. Detailed neuropathologic studies of a large number of active MS lesions (n = 82) revealed a profound heterogeneity in immunopathologic patterns of demyelination [60,68]. Although lesion patterns differed between patients, the pattern was identical among all active lesions examined from a given patient. This can be determined only in patients who have MS with available autopsy, serial biopsy, or biopsy/autopsy material.

All active lesions occurred on a background of an inflammatory process, composed mainly of T lymphocytes and macrophages. Despite the similarities in the inflammatory reaction, the lesions segregated into four patterns of demyelination based on plaque geography, extent and pattern of oligodendrocyte pathology, evidence for immunoglobulin deposition and complement activation, and pattern of myelin protein loss (Fig. 4). The four patterns are:

Pattern I: Macrophage-associated demyelination
Pattern II: Antibody/complement-associated demyelination
Pattern III: Distal dying-back oligodendrogliopathy
Pattern IV: Primary oligodendrocyte degeneration

In patterns I and II, macrophages and T cells predominate in well-demarcated plaques that surround small veins and venules; only pattern II lesions demonstrate the local precipitation of immunoglobulin and activated complement in regions of active myelin breakdown. The expression of all the myelin proteins (MBP, PLP, MAG, and MOG) is reduced similarly. Oligodendrocytes are reduced in number at the active edge; however, they reappear within the plaque center and remyelination is extensive. Pattern I (macrophage-associated demyelination) closely resembles myelin destruction in mouse models of autoimmune encephalomyelitis. In these models, mainly toxic products of activated macrophages, such as TNF-α [69] and nitric oxide (NO) [70], mediate destruction of myelin sheaths. Lesions closely similar to pattern II (antibody-associated demyelination) are found in models of EAE induced by sensitization with MOG. In this model,

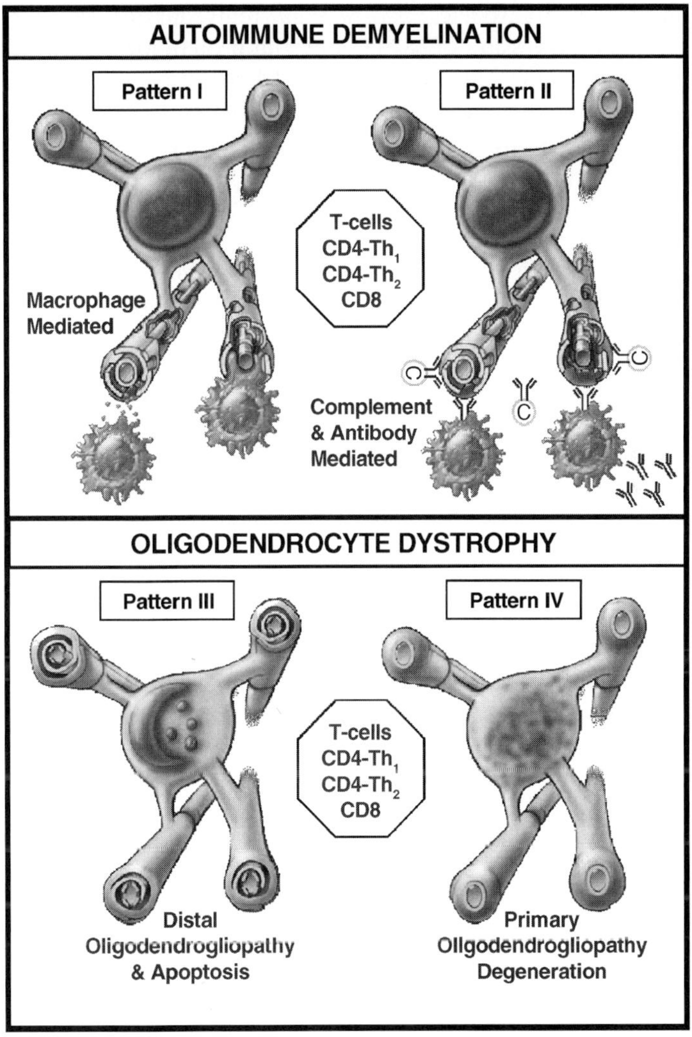

Fig. 4. Immunopathologic patterns of demyelination. Schematic presentation of the four MS subtypes based on the underlying mechanism of myelin/oligodendrocyte destruction.

demyelination is induced by cooperation between encephalitogenic T cells and demyelinating anti-MOG antibodies [71].

Pattern III lesions also contain an inflammatory infiltrate, composed mainly of macrophages, activated microglia, and T cells; however, the lesions are ill defined and typically do not surround vessels. There is no evidence for immunoglobulin or activated complement in these lesions, and there is a selective loss of MAG compared with the other myelin proteins. This pattern is associated with oligodendrocyte apoptosis, a marked reduction in oligodendrocytes, and minimal remyelination. A pronounced reduction in the expression of MAG, a myelin protein localized to the most distal extension of the oligodendrocyte cell body (the periaxonal region), has been described in some MS lesions since the early 1980s [72,73]. This early loss of MAG was believed to reflect a dying-back process in the oligodendrocyte. A similar selective loss of MAG has been described at the periphery of progressive multifocal leukoencephalopathy (PML) lesions, a known viral infection of oligodendrocytes in which the cells are unable to maintain their myelin sheaths [74]. Thus, a pattern of demyelination in which the destruction of MAG precedes one of the major myelin proteins (MBP or PLP) is suggestive of a lesion at the level of the oligodendroglial cell body. MAG loss, therefore, suggests a distal dying-back oligodendrogliopathy, in which the cell body is unable to support the metabolic processes necessary to maintain the distal axon. This pattern is characterized by ultrastructural alterations in the most distal extension of the oligodendroglial processes, the periaxonal region. The morphologic features include a uniform widening of inner myelin lamellae and degeneration of inner glial loops antedating destruction of the myelin sheaths. These pathologic alterations have been described in certain experimental models of toxin and viral-induced demyelination and observed in several stereotactic brain biopsies obtained for diagnostic purposes in cases of early MS [75–77].

The preferential loss of MAG, which is a hallmark of pattern III lesions, also is observed in acute white matter ischemia and in Herpes simplex virus (HSV) and cytomegalovirus (CMV) encephalitis [78]. This pattern of myelin destruction is associated with prominent nuclear expression of hypoxia inducible factor (HIF)–1α, a specific and sensitive marker for hypoxia-like metabolic injury. A profound expression of HIF-1α is shared in acute stroke lesions and pattern III MS lesions, suggesting that a hypoxia-like metabolic injury may contribute to the pathogenesis of inflammatory white matter damage in a subset of patients who have MS and patients who have virus encephalitis [79]. Microarray analysis of normal-appearing white matter from 10 postmortem MS brains revealed upregulation of genes, such as HIF-1α, known to be involved in neuroprotective mechanisms induced by hypoxic preconditioning [80]. Whether or not this upregulation reflects an adaptation of cells to the chronic progressive pathophysiology of MS or, alternatively, represents the activation of neuroprotective mechanisms in response to ischemic preconditioning in a subset of patients remains to be determined.

Pattern IV lesions also contain macrophages and T lymphocytes, but there is no preferential loss of MAG or evidence of immunoglobulin or activated complement deposits within these lesions. Instead, there is evidence of nonapoptotic oligodendroglial death in the adjacent normal-appearing periplaque white matter. The mechanisms responsible for pattern IV lesions (primary oligodendrocyte degeneration), which are the most infrequent in the MS population, and have been restricted to a small group of primary progressive cases, are not clear so far. It is tempting to speculate that in such patients, a genuine metabolic disturbance of oligodendrocytes could render these cells particularly vulnerable to the toxic action of inflammatory mediators. In summary, interindividual, but not intra-individual, heterogeneity with respect to demyelination is a characteristic feature of MS. This may have profound consequences in clinical practice, because distinct patterns may require distinct therapeutic interventions.

Barnett and Prineas recently described extensive oligodendrocyte apoptosis in the absence of inflammation in a pediatric patient who had MS and died 9 months after disease onset and 17 hours after presenting with acute pulmonary edema [81]. The pattern described is similar to the pattern III MS pathology described previously. It is unclear, however, if hypoxic conditions in the setting of the patient's pulmonary edema may have confounded the pathologic observations. The investigators also describe the coexistence of remyelinating lesions and complement activation in other lesions from this and 6 other patients and suggest that all MS lesions begin with this type of pathology. An analysis of multiple active lesions from the authors' pattern III autopsy cases does not reveal evidence for complement activation when using the highly specific monoclonal antibody against C9neo antigen. A subset of pattern III cases with Baló's type of concentric lesions occasionally may demonstrate remyelinating lesions. This is consistent with the observation of remyelination as described by Barnett and Prineas in their pediatric case, which had some features of Baló's concentric sclerosis (BCS) (Stadelmann C, et al, submitted for publication, 2004).

Clinical and paraclinical correlates are needed to differentiate between these pathologic patterns. To date, 210 MS cases have been classified with the following distribution: 19% pattern I, 53% pattern II, 26% pattern III, and 2% pattern IV. All patients who have NMO (Devic's disease) have antibody/complement-associated demyelination but in a distinct pattern (see later discussion). All patients who have Baló's type of concentric lesions have a distal oligodendrogliopathy. Pattern IV has been found only in a small subset of patients who have PPMS [82].

Detailed clinical follow-up of the biopsy cohort (n = 99) fails to reveal any correlation between time of symptom onset, date of biopsy, and pathologic pattern. In addition, the authors have observed a striking correlation between therapeutic response to plasma exchange in patients who have MS with evidence of antibody and complement activation (pattern II pathology, n = 10) on biopsy and no response in pattern I (n = 3) or pattern III (n = 6) cases [83]. The sharp border at the active plaque edge with accumulating macrophages typical of active lesions in patterns I and II MS lesions is associated highly with the presence of ring enhancement on gadolinium-enhanced MRI and hypointense T2 rims, whereas these imaging features are not found in pattern III lesions ($P < 0.001$; 54 cases examined) [84]. These observations support pathogenic heterogeneity in immune effector mechanisms involved in MS lesion formation, which persist over a period of time, rather than a single mechanism dominating the formation of all lesions.

Substrate of irreversible disability in multiple sclerosis

MRI studies reveal that axonal loss in MS lesions correlates with the presence of permanent black holes on T1-weighted MRI [102–105], a reduction in NAA on MRS [106,107], and the extent of atrophy in the spinal cord [108]. Because these imaging parameters correlate with clinical disability, axonal damage likely is responsible for irreversible clinical disability in MS. Although historical neuropathologic descriptions by Charcot in 1880, Marburg in 1906, and Doinikow in 1915 recognized degeneration of axons in MS lesions, they emphasized the primary demyelinating nature of the disease [109]. More recent studies show a high incidence of acute axonal injury in chronic and early MS lesions (Fig. 7A–D) [26,110,111]. The extent of axonal injury varies, ranging from 20% to 90% reduction in axonal density relative to the periplaque white matter. Furthermore, there is interindividual heterogeneity in the extent of acute axonal injury [52].

Whereas the extent of axonal transection in early active lesions correlates with inflammation, the magnitude of axonal loss in chronic lesions suggests mechanisms other than inflammatory demyelination may contribute to axonal damage at later stages. Kornek et al demonstrated that extensive

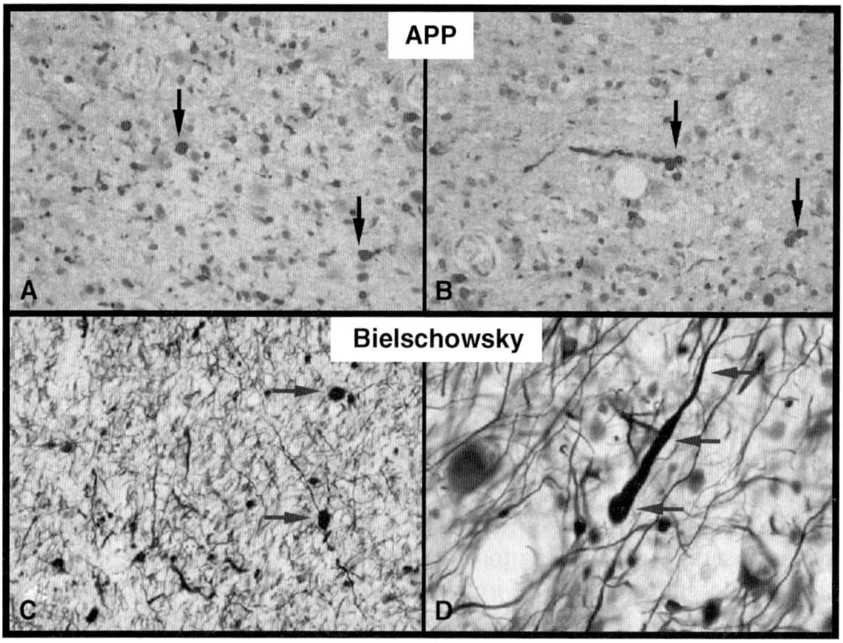

Fig. 7. Axonal damage in MS. *(A, B)* Immunocytochemistry for amyloid precursor protein (APP) showing numerous axons (*arrows*) with disturbances of axonal transport or even transections. (*C, D*) Bielschowsky̌s silver impregnation for axons reveals axonal bulbs (*arrows, C*), a transected axon (*arrows, D*), and a reduced axonal density within the lesions.

acute axonal injury occurs during early stages of demyelination; however, a slow ongoing axonal destruction is present in inactive MS lesions that lack inflammation [26]. Therefore, the mechanisms of axonal destruction in MS may vary depending on the stage of the disease.

Data are limited on the mechanisms of axonal injury (Fig. 8). During the acute stages of the disease, inflammatory mediators likely contribute to axonal injury. An association between the numbers of $CD8^+$ T cells and the extent of axon damage has been reported [52], and experimental studies implicate a CD8-MHC class I–mediated pathway of axon destruction [112]. Furthermore, the attachment of activated CD8 T cells containing cytotoxic granules polarized toward the demyelinated axon suggests direct $CD8^+$ T-cell–mediated cytotoxicity [51]. Macrophages and microglia often are found in close contact with degenerating axons. Toxic inflammatory mediators liberated from these cells, such as proteases, cytokines, and free radicals, including NO, also may lead to axonal injury. At low concentrations, NO induces a functional conduction block. At higher concentrations, NO derivatives may damage axons irreversibly, particularly when they are active electrically [113]. Axon specific antibodies and complement also may be involved in mediating axonal injury. Antiganglioside antibodies were found significantly higher in PPMS than in secondary progressive or

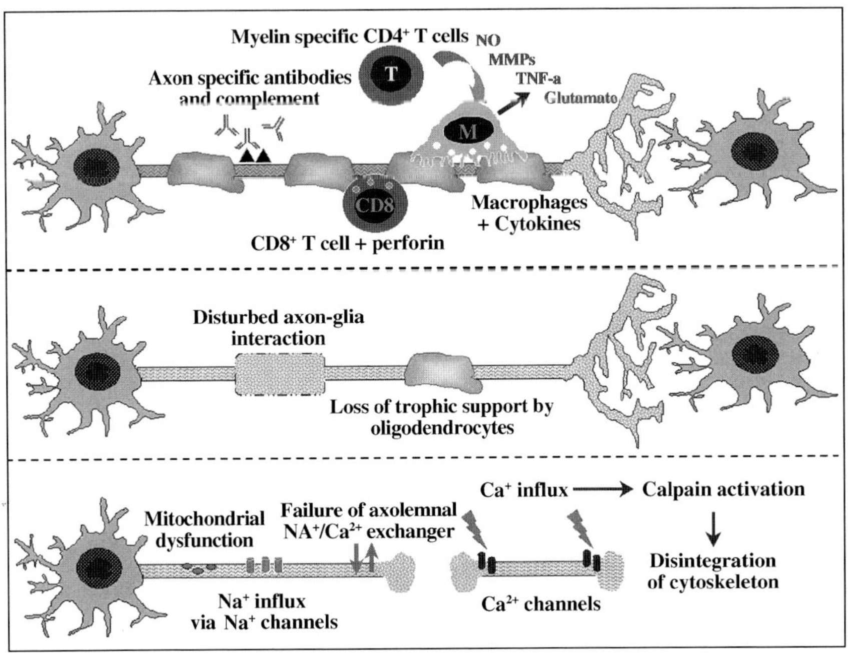

Fig. 8. Mechanisms of axonal destruction. Phases and effector mechanisms of axonal degeneration during active demyelination and in inactive demyelinated lesions. The final pathway of axon destruction is the result of mitochondrial dysfunction, ion influx into the axon, and activation of proteases.

relapsing-remitting MS [114]. Axons exposed to complement after demyelination may activate the complement cascade directly [115].

In contrast, a low-grade axonal degeneration occurs in silent inactive plaques [26]. Although only a few axons are destroyed at a given time point, such lesions may persist in the CNS for years. In addition, repeated demyelination within previously remeylinated lesions may contribute to axonal loss in chronic MS [8]. Chronically demyelinated axons also may degenerate as a result of the lack of trophic support from myelin and oligodendrocytes. Mice lacking certain myelin proteins (MAG and PLP) demonstrate late onset axonal pathology and evidence of an increased incidence of wallerian degeneration [116,117]. Secondary wallerian degeneration also contributes to diffuse axonal loss [118].

Once axonal injury is triggered, a cascade of downstream mechanisms occurs, leading ultimately to axonal disintegration (see Fig. 8) [118]. These mechanisms are similar in a variety of pathologic conditions, including inflammation, ischemia, and trauma. Acute axonal injury leads to a disturbance in axoplasmic membrane permeability and subsequent energy failure, leading to uncontrolled sodium influx into the axoplasm, which reverses the sodium/calcium exchanger and results in excess intraxonal calcium. This activates Ca++-dependent proteases, which degrade cytoskeletal proteins, further impairing axonal transport. Voltage-gated calcium channels (VGCC) accumulate at sites of disturbed axonal transport, leading to further Ca++ influx and eventual dissolution of the axonal cytoskeleton and axonal disintegration. Therapeutic strategies that inhibit different steps in this execution phase of axonal destruction, such as Na+ channel blockers, inhibitors of the Na+-Ca++ exchanger, blockade of VGCC, or inhibition of calcium-dependent proteases, may help limit axonal destruction in MS. Clinical trials are needed with these agents to determine if they slow disease progression.

The relationship between inflammatory demyelination and axonal loss

Although MS includes inflammatory and demyelinating components, their relative influence on axonal loss is unclear. Pathologic studies reveal that myelin and axonal pathology may occur independently. Ongoing axonal injury is present in inactive plaques, and the damage to axons does not seem to depend on the stage of demyelinating activity [52]. Furthermore, acute axonal injury is found in the normal-appearing and periplaque white matter of patients who have MS. Experimental systems reveal that inflammatory demyelination, axonal loss, and neurologic disability can be dissociated. Mice deficient for the MHC class-I light chain (β_2-microglobulin) develop inflammatory demyelination but not early axonal damage or clinical deficit after Theiler's virus infection [112,119]. These data suggest that the mechanisms of inflammatory demyelination and axonal injury may, in part, have separate pathogenic bases.

This apparent dissociation between inflammation, demyelination, and axonal injury is supported by clinical studies. Two observational MS natural history studies have found that once a clinical threshold of irreversible disability is reached, the progression of disability is not affected by relapses, either those before the onset of the progressive phase or those that supervene during this phase [120,121]. The absence of a relationship between relapses and irreversible disability suggests there is dissociation at the biologic level between recurrent acute focal inflammatory demyelination and progressive degeneration of the CNS. This apparent paradox is consistent with the persistence of disability progression in patients who have MS despite infection with HIV [122] or despite suppression of cerebral inflammation after treatment with a potent antileukocyte monoclonal antibody [123]. It also is in keeping with the refractory state of progressive MS to anti-inflammatory therapies. The results of the pivotal North American trial of IFN-β1b in relapsing-remitting disease reveal that although there was suppression of inflammatory disease activity by more than 60% as assessed by MRI, no significant change in progression of neurologic disability was observed after 5 years of follow-up [124]. In another study using IFN-β1b, inflammation was noted to occur less frequently based on MRI measures, yet axonal loss, as measured by atrophy, continued [125]. These findings suggest that therapeutic agents that have a short-term effect on MS relapses may not necessarily delay the development of long-term disability. Therefore, a combination of inflammatory and noninflammatory factors likely contributes to disability in MS.

Summary

The recognition of MS as a heterogeneous disorder with an inflammatory and a neurodegenerative phase requires the development of therapies that address not only the role of other targets in the disease (ie, myelin, oligodendrocyte, and axon) but also the role of different immune effector mechanisms ($CD8^+$ T cells, antibody, complement, and so forth) and the potential need for different therapeutic strategies given at different stages of the disease. Recent genomic and proteomic technologic advances applied to MS neuropathology may help unravel the complexities of the MS lesion. Ultimately, the MS lesion is the target for therapy. A better understanding of the targets and mechanisms involved in lesion pathogenesis hopefully will lead to more effective therapeutic strategies.

References

[1] Anderson DW, Ellenberg JH, Leventhal CM, et al. Revised estimate of the prevalence of multiple sclerosis in the United States. Ann Neurol 1992;31:333–6.

[2] Carswell R. Pathological anatomy: illustrations on elementary forms of disease. London: Logman; 1838.

[3] Cruveilier J. Anatomie pathologique du corps humain. 1841:1829–42.
[4] Charcot J. Lecons sur les maladies du systeme nerveux faites a la salpetriere. Paris: Cert et fils; 1880.
[5] Charcot JM. Histologie de la sclérose en plaques. Gaz Hop Civils Militaires 1868;140–1, 143, 554–5, 557–8, 566.
[6] Lublin FD, Whitaker JN, Eidelman BH, et al. Management of patients receiving interferon beta-1b for multiple sclerosis. Neurol 1996;46:12–8.
[7] Prineas J. The neuropathology of multiple sclerosis. In: Vinken P, Bruyn G, Klawans H, editors. Handbook of clinical neurology. New York: Elsevier Science Publishers; 1985. p. 213–57.
[8] Prineas JW, Barnard RO, Revesz T, et al. Multiple sclerosis. Pathology of recurrent lesions. Brain 1993;116(Pt3):681–93.
[9] Wolswijk G. Chronic stage multiple sclerosis lesions contain a relatively quiescent population of oligodendrocyte precursor cells. J Neurosci 1998;18:601–9.
[10] Chang ATW, Rudick R, Trapp BD. Premyelinating oligodendrocytes in chronic lesions of multiple sclerosis. N Engl J Med 2002;346:165–73.
[11] Kondo T, Raff M. Basic helix-loop-helix proteins and the timing of oligodendrocyte differentiation. Development 2000;127:2989–98.
[12] John G, Shankar S, Shafit-Zagardo B, Massimi A, et al. Multiple sclerosis: re-expression of a developmental pathway that restricts oligodendrocyte maturation. Nat Med 2002;8: 1115–21.
[13] Rodriguez M, Scheithauer B, Kelly P, Forbes G. Ultrastructural analysis of acute demyelinating lesions obtained by stereotaxic biopsy. J Neuropathol Exp Neurol 1989;43: 323.
[14] Lucchinetti CF, Brueck W, Rodriguez M, et al. A quantitative study on the fate of the oligodendrocyte in multiple sclerosis lesions: a study of 113 cases. Brain 1999;122:2279–95.
[15] Raine CS, Scheinberg L, Waltz JM. Multiple sclerosis: oligodendrocyte survival and proliferation in an active established lesion. Lab Invest 1981;45:534–46.
[16] Ozawa K, Suchanek G, Breitschopf H, et al. Patterns of oligodendroglia pathology in multiple sclerosis. Brain 1994;117:1311–22.
[17] Brueck W, Schmied M, Suchanek G, et al. Oligodendrocytes in the early course of multiple sclerosis. Ann Neurol 1994;35:65–73.
[18] Bruck W, Porada P, Poser S, et al. Monocyte/macrophage differentiation in early multiple sclerosis lesions. Ann Neurol 1995;38:788–96.
[19] Davie CA, Barker GJ, Thompson AJ, et al. 1H magnetic resonance spectroscopy of chronic cerebral white matter lesions and normal appearing white matter in multiple sclerosis. J Neurol Neurosurg Psychiatry 1997;63:736–42.
[20] Suhy J, Rooney WD, Goodkin DE. 1H MRSI comparison of white matter and lesions in primary progressive and relapsing-remitting multiple sclerosis. Multiple Sclerosis 2000;6: 148–55.
[21] Filippi M, Campi A, Martinelli V, et al. A brain MRI study of different types of chronic-progressive multiple sclerosis. Acta Neurol Scand 1995;91:231–3.
[22] Leary SM, Silver NC, Stevenson VL, et al. Magnetisation transfer of normal appearing white matter in primary progressive multiple sclerosis. Multiple Sclerosis 1999;1999: 313–6.
[23] Tortorella C, Viti B, Bozzali M. A magnetization trasfer histogram study of normal appearing brain tissue in MS. Neurology 2000;54:186–93.
[24] Dehmeshki J, Silver NC, Leary SM, et al. Magnetisation transfer ratio histogram analysis of primary progressive and other multiple sclerosis subgroups. J Neurol Sci 2001;185: 11–7.
[25] Pelletier J, Suchet L, Witjas T. A longitudinal study of callosal atrophy and interhemispheric dysfunction in relapsing-remitting multiple sclerosis. Arch Neurol 2001;58: 105–11.

[26] Kornek B, Storch MK, Weissert R, et al. Multiple sclerosis and chronic autoimmune encephalomyelitis: a comparative quantitative study of axonal injury in active, inactive, and remyelinated lesions. Am J Pathol 2000;157:267–76.
[27] Evangelou N, Esiri MM, Smith S, et al. Quantitative pathological evidence for axonal loss in normal appearing white matter in multiple sclerosis. Ann Neurol 2000;47:391–5.
[28] Cifelli A, Arridge M, Jezzard P, et al. Thalamic neurodegeneration in multiple sclerosis. Ann Neurol 2002;52:650–3.
[29] Lumsden C. The neuropathology of multiple sclerosis. In: Vinken P, Bruyn G, editors. Handbook of clinical neurology. New York: Elsevier; 1970. p. 217–309.
[30] Peterson JW, Bo L, Mork S, et al. Transected neurites, apoptotic neurons, and reduced inflammation in cortical multiple sclerosis lesions. Ann Neurol 2001;50:389–400.
[31] Kidd D, Barkhof F, McConnell R, et al. Cortical lesions in multiple sclerosis. Brain 1999; 122:17–26.
[32] Romagnani S. The Th 1/Th 2 paradigm. Immunol Today 1997;6:263–6.
[33] Noseworthy JH, Lucchinetti C, Rodriguez M, et al. Multiple sclerosis. N Engl J Med 2000; 343:938–52.
[34] Yong VW, Chabot S, Stuve O, et al. Interferon beta in the treatment of multiple sclerosis: mechanisms of action. Neurology 1998;51:682–9.
[35] Uhm JH, Dooley NP, Stuve O, et al. Migratory behavior of lymphocytes isolated from multiple sclerosis patients: effects of interferon beta-1b therapy. Ann Neurol 3;46: 319–24.
[36] Gerritse K, Laman J, Noelle R, et al. CD40–CD40 ligand interactions in experimental allergic encephalomyelitis and multiple sclerosis. Proc Natl Acad Sci USA 1996;93: 2499–504.
[37] Canella B, Raine CS. The adhesion molecule and cytokine profile of multiple sclerosis lesions. Ann Neurol 1995;37:424–35.
[38] Navikas V, Link H. Review: cytokines and the pathogenesis of multiple sclerosis. J Neurosci Res 1996;45:322–33.
[39] Sorensen T, Tani M, Jensen J, et al. Expression of specific chemokines and chemokine receptors in the central nervous system of multiple sclerosis patients. J Clin Invest 1999;103: 807–15.
[40] Kalman B, Lublin FD. The genetics of multiple sclerosis. A review. Biomed Pharmacother 1999;53:358–70.
[41] Hohlfeld R. Immunotherapy of multiple sclerosis. Consensus and controversies. Nervenarzt 1999;70:297.
[42] Hohlfeld R, Wiendl H. The ups and downs of multiple sclerosis therapeutics. Ann Neurol 2001;49:281–4.
[43] Genain CP, Abel K, Belmar N, et al. Late complications of immune deviation therapy in a nonhuman primate. Science 1996;274:2054–7.
[44] Wingerchuk D, Lucchinetti C, Noseworthy J. Multiple sclerosis: current pathophysiological concepts. Lab Invest 2001;81:263–81.
[45] Noseworthy J, Lucchinetti C, Rodriguez M, et al. Multiple sclerosis. N Engl J Med 2000; 343:938–52.
[46] Haring JS, Pewe LL, Perlman S. Bystander CD8 T cell-mediated demyelination after viral infection of the central nervous system. J Immunol 2002;169:1550–5.
[47] Babbe H, Roers A, Waisman A, et al. Clonal expansion of CD8 T cells dominate the T cell infiltrate in active multiple sclerosis lesions as shown by micromanipulation and single cell polymerase chain reaction. J Exp Med 2000;192:393–404.
[48] Jacobsen M, Cepok S, Quak E, et al. Oligoclonal expansion of memory CD8 + T cells in cerebrospinal fluid from multiple sclerosis patients. Brain 2002;125:538–50.
[49] Hoftberger R, Aboul-Enein F, Brueck W, et al. Expression of major histocompatibility complex class I molecules on the different cell types in multiple sclerosis lesions. Brain Pathol 2004;14:43–50.

[50] Jurewicz A, Biddison WE, Antel JP. MHC class I-restricted lysis of human oligodendrocytes by myelin basic protein peptide-specific CD8 T lymphocytes. J Immunol 1998;160:3056–9.
[51] Neumann H, Medana IM, Bauer J, et al. Cytotoxic T lymphocytes in autoimmune and degenerative CNS diseases. Trends Neurosci 2002;25:313–9.
[52] Bitsch A, Schuchardt J, Bunkowski S, et al. Acute axonal injury in multiple sclerosis. Correlation with demyelination and inflammation. Brain 2000;123(Pt 6):1174–83.
[53] Sun D, Whitaker JN, Huang Z, et al. Myelin antigen-specific CD8 + T cells are encephalitogenic and produce severe disease in C57BL/6 mice. J Immunol 2001;166: 7579–87.
[54] Huseby ES, Liggitt D, Brabb T, et al. A pathogenic role for myelin-specific CD8 + T cells in a model for multiple sclerosis. J Exp Med 2001;194:669–76.
[55] Prineas JW, Graham JS. Multiple sclerosis: capping of surface immunoglobulin G on macrophages engaged in myelin breakdown. Ann Neurol 1981;10:149–58.
[56] Reindl M, Linington C, Brehm U, et al. Antibodies against the myelin oligodendrocyte glycoprotein and the myelin basic protein in multiple sclerosis and other neurological diseases: a comparative study. Brain 1999;122(Pt 11):2047–56.
[57] Berger T, Rubner P, Schautzer F, et al. Antimyelin antibodies as a predictor of clinically definite multiple sclerosis after a first demyelinating event. N Engl J Med 2003;349:139–45.
[58] Mead RJ, Singhrao SK, Neal JW, et al. The membrane attack complex of complement causes severe demyelination associated with acute axonal injury. J Immunol 2002;168:458–65.
[59] Storch MK, Piddlesden S, Haltia M, et al. Multiple sclerosis: in situ evidence for antibody- and complement-mediated demyelination. Ann Neurol 1998;43:465–71.
[60] Lucchinetti CF, Bruck W, Parisi J, et al. Heterogeneity of multiple sclerosis lesions: implications for the pathogenesis of demyelination. Ann Neurol 2000;47:707–17.
[61] Genain CP, Cannella B, Hauser SL, et al. Identification of autoantibodies associated with myelin damage in multiple sclerosis. Nat Med 1999;5:170–5.
[62] Lucchinetti CF, Mandler RN, McGavern D, et al. A role for humoral mechanisms in the pathogenesis of Devic's neuromyelitis optica. Brain 2002;125(Pt 7):1450–61.
[63] Wingerchuk DM, Hogancamp WF, O'Brien PC, et al. The clinical course of neuromyelitis optica (Devic's syndrome). Neurology 1999;53:1107–14.
[64] Moalem G, Leibowitz-Amit R, Yoles E, et al. Autoimmune T cells protect neurons from secondary degeneration after central nervous system axotomy. Nat Med 1999;5:49–55.
[65] Diemel LT, Copelman CA, Cuzner ML. Macrophages in CNS remyelination: friend or foe? Neurochem Res 1998;23:341–7.
[66] Kotter MR, Setzu A, Sim FJ, et al. Macrophage depletion impairs oligodendrocyte remyelination following lysolecithin-induced demyelination. Glia 2001;35:204–12.
[67] Kerschensteiner M, Gallmeier E, Behrens L, et al. Activated human T cells, B cells and monocytes produce brain-derived neurotrophic factor (BDNF) in vitro and in brain lesions: a neuroprotective role for inflammation? J Exp Med 1999;189:865–70.
[68] Lassmann H, Bruck W, Lucchinetti C. Heterogeneity of multiple sclerosis pathogenesis: implications for diagnosis and therapy. Trends Mol Med 2001;7:115–21.
[69] Probert L, Akassoglou K, Pasparakis M, et al. Spontaneous inflammatory demyelinating disease in transgenic mice showing central nervous system-specific expression of tumor necrosis factor alpha. Proc Natl Acad Sci USA 1995;92:11294–8.
[70] Griot C, Vandevelde M, Richard A, et al. Selective degeneration of oligodendrocytes mediated by reactive oxygen species. Free Radical Research Communications 1990;11: 181–93.
[71] Linington C, Bradl M, Lassmann H, et al. Augmentation of demyelination in rat acute allergic encephalomyelitis by circulating mouse monoclonal antibodies directed against a myelin/oligodendrocyte glycoprotein. Am J Pathol 1988;130:443–54.
[72] Itoyama Y, Sternberger NH, Webster HD, et al. Immunocytochemical observations on the distribution of myelin-associated glycoprotein and myelin basic protein in multiple sclerosis lesions. Ann Neurol 1980;7:167–77.

[73] Gendelman HE, Pezeshkpour GH, Pressman NJ, et al. A quantitation of myelin-associated glycoprotein and myelin basic protein loss in different demyelinating diseases. Ann Neurol 1985;18:324–8.

[74] Itoyama Y, Webster HD, Sternberger NH, et al. Distribution of papovavirus, myelin-associated glycoprotein, and myelin basic protein in progressive multifocal leukoencephalopathy lesions. Neurology 1982;11:396–407.

[75] Rodriguez M. Virus-induced demyelination in mice: "dying back" of oligodendrocytes. Mayo Clin Proc 1985;60:433–8.

[76] Rodriguez M, Sheithauer B. Ultrastructure of multiple sclerosis. Ultrastruct Pathol 1994; 18:3–13.

[77] Ludwin S, Johnson E. Evidence of a "dying back" gliopathy in demyelinating disease. Ann Neurol 1981;301–5.

[78] Aboul-Enein F, Rauschka H, Kornek B, et al. Preferential loss of myelin-associated glycoprotein reflects hypoxia-like white matter damage in stroke and inflammatory brain diseases. J Neuropathol Exp Neurol 2003;62:25–33.

[79] Lassmann H. Hypoxia-like tissue injury as a component of multiple sclerosis lesions. J Neurol Sci 2003;206:187–91.

[80] Graumann U, Reynolds R, Steck AJ, et al. Molecular changes in normal appearing white matter in multiple sclerosis are characteristic of neuroprotective mechanisms against hypoxic insult. Brain Pathology 2003;13:554–73.

[81] Barnett MH, Prineas JW. Relapsing and remitting multiple sclerosis: pathology of the newly forming lesion. Ann Neurol 2004;55:458–68.

[82] Lucchinetti CF. Merging of minds and matter. Multiple Sclerosis 2003;9:8.

[83] Keegan M, Konig F, Bitsch A, et al. Multiple sclerosis pathological subtype predicts response to therapeutic plasma exchange. Neurology 2004;62(Suppl 5):7.

[84] Lucchinetti CF, Altintas A, Wegner C, et al. Magnetic resonance imaging correlates of multiple sclerosis pathologic subtypes. Ann Neurol (Suppl 7) 2003;54:67.

[85] Weinshenker BG, Lucchinetti CF. Acute leukoencephalopathies: differential diagnosis and investigation. The Neurologist 1998;4:148–66.

[86] Marburg O. Die sogenannte "akute Multiple Sklerose". J Psychiatric Neurology 1906;27: 211–312.

[87] Wood DD, Bilbao JM, O'Connors P, et al. Acute multiple sclerosis (Marburg type) is associated with developmentally immature myelin basic protein. Ann Neurol 1996;40:18–24.

[88] Courville C. Concentric sclerosis. In: Bruyn PVaG, editor. Handbook of clinical neurology. Amsterdam: Elsevier; 1970. p. 437–51.

[89] Kuroiwa Y. Clinical and epidemiological aspects of multiple sclerosis in Japan. Jpn J Med 1982;21:135–40.

[90] Korte J, Born E, Vos L, et al. Balo concentric sclerosis: MR diagnosis. AJNR Am J Neuroradiol 1994;15:1284–5.

[91] Revel M, Valiente E, Gray F, et al. Concentric MR patterns in multiple sclerosis. Report of two cases. J Neuroradiol 1993;20:252–7.

[92] Chen C, Ro L, Chang C, et al. Serial MRI studies in pathologically verified Balo's concentric sclerosis. J Comput Assist Tomogr 1996;20:732–5.

[93] Garbern J, Spence A, Alvord E. Balo's concentric demyelination diagnosed premortem. Neurology 1986;36:1610–4.

[94] Gharagozloo A, Poe L, Collins G. Antemortem diagnosis of Balo concentric sclerosis: correlative MR imaging and pathologic features. Radiology 1994;191:817–9.

[95] Hanemann C, Kleinschmidt A, Reifenberger G, et al. Balo concentric sclerosis followed by MRI and positron emission tomography. Neuroradiology 1993;35:578–80.

[96] Karaarslan E, Altintas A, Senol U, et al. Balo's concentric sclerosis: clinical and radiologic features of five cases. AJNR Am J Neuroradiol 2001;22:1362–7.

[97] Spiegel M, Kruger H, Hofmann E, et al. MRI study of Balo's concentric sclerosis before and after immunosuppressant therapy. J Neurol;236:487–8.

[98] Wingerchuk DM. Postinfectious encephalomyelitis. Curr Neurol Neurosci Rep 2003;3: 256–64.
[99] Kepes J. Large focal tumor-like demyelinating lesions of the brain: intermediate entity between multiple sclerosis and acute disseminated encephalomyelitis: a study of 31 patients. Ann Neurol 1993;33:18–27.
[100] Masdeu JC, Moreira J, Trasi S, et al. The open ring. A new imaging sign in demyelinating disease. J Neuroimaging 1996;6:104–7.
[101] Lennon VA, Wingerchuk DM, Kryzer TJ, et al. A serum autoantibody marker of neuromyelitis optica. Lancet, in press.
[102] Barnes D, Munro PM, Youl BD, Prineas JW, McDonald WI. The longstanding MS lesion. A quantitative MRI and electron microscopic study. Brain 1991;114:1271–80.
[103] Truyen L, van Waesberghe JH, van Walderveen MA, et al. Accumulation of hypointense lesions ("black holes") on T1 spin-echo MRI correlates with disease progression in multiple sclerosis. Neurology 1996;47:1469–76.
[104] van Walderveen MA, Kamphorst W, Scheltens P, et al. Histopathologic correlate of hypointense lesions on T1-weighted spin-echo MRI in multiple sclerosis. Neurology 1998; 50:1282–8.
[105] van Waesberghe J, Kamphorst W, De Groot C, et al. Axonal loss in multiple sclerosis lesions: magnetic resonance imaging insights into substrates of disability. Ann Neurol 1999; 46:747–54.
[106] Bruck W, Bitsch A, Kolenda H, et al. Inflammatory central nervous system demyelination: correlation of magnetic resonance imaging findings with lesion pathology. Ann Neurol 1997;42:783–93.
[107] Bjartmar C, Kidd G, Mork S, et al. Neurological disability correlates with spinal cord axonal loss and reduced N-acetyl aspartate in chronic multiple sclerosis patients. Ann Neurol 2000;48:893–901.
[108] Losseff N, Wang L, Lai H, et al. Progressive cerebral atrophy in multiple sclerosis. A serial MRI study. Brain 1996;119:2009–19.
[109] Kornek B, Lassmann H. Axonal pathology in multiple sclerosis: a historical note. Brain Pathol 1999;9:651–6.
[110] Ferguson B, Matyszak MK, Esiri MM, et al. Axonal damage in acute multiple sclerosis lesions. Brain 1997;120:393–9.
[111] Trapp BD, Peterson J, Ransohoff RM, et al. Axonal transection in the lesions of multiple sclerosis. N Engl J Med 1998;338:278–85.
[112] Rivera-Quinones C, McGavern D, Schmelzer JD, et al. Absence of neurological deficits following extensive demyelination in a class I-deficient murine model of multiple sclerosis. Nat Med 1998;4:187–93.
[113] Smith KJ, Kapoor R, Hall SM, et al. Electrically active axons degenerate when exposed to nitric oxide. Ann Neurol 2001;49:470–6.
[114] Sadatipour BT, Greer JM, Pender MP. Increased circulating antiganglioside antibodies in primary and secondary progressive multiple sclerosis. Ann Neurol 1998;44:980–3.
[115] Neumann H. Molecular mechanisms of axonal damage in inflammatory central nervous system diseases. Curr Opin Neurol 2003;16:267–73.
[116] Sadahiro S, Yoshikawa H, Yagi N, et al. Morphometric analysis of the myelin-associated oligodendrocytic basic protein-deficient mouse reveals a possible role for myelin-associated oligodendrocytic basic protein in regulating axonal diameter. Neuroscience 2000;98:361–7.
[117] Yoshikawa H. Myelin-associated oligodendrocytic basic protein modulates the arrangement of radial growth of the axon and the radial component of myelin. Med Electron Microsc 2001;34:160–4.
[118] Lassmann H. Axonal injury in multiple sclerosis. J Neurol Neurosurg Psychiatry 2003;74: 695–7.
[119] Murray PD, McGavern DB, Lin X, et al. Perforin-dependent neurologic injury in a viral model of multiple sclerosis. J Neurosci 1998;18:7306–14.

[120] Confavreux C, Vukusic S, Moreau T, et al. Relapses and progression of disability in multiple sclerosis. N Engl J Med 2000;343:1430–8.
[121] Pittock SJ, Mayr WT, McClelland RL, et al. Change in MS-related disability in a population-based cohort—a 10-year follow-up study. Neurology 2004;62:51–9.
[122] Berger JR, Sheremata WA, Resnick L, et al. Multiple sclerosis-like illness occurring with human immunodeficiency virus infection. Neurology 1989;39:324–9.
[123] Coles AJ, Wing MG, Molyneux P, et al. Monoclonal antibody treatment exposes three mechanisms underlying the clinical course of multiple sclerosis. Ann Neurol 1999;46: 296–304.
[124] The IFNB Multiple Sclerosis Study Group and the University of British Columbia MS/ MRI Analysis Group. Interferon b-1b in the treatment of MS: Final outcome of the randomized controlled trial. Neurology 1995;45:1277–85.
[125] Molyneux PD, Kappos L, Polman C, et al. The effect of interferon beta-1b treatment on MRI measures of cerebral atrophy in secondary progressive multiple sclerosis. European Study Group on Interferon Beta-1b in Secondary Progressive Multiple Sclerosis. Brain 2000;123(Pt 11):2256–63.

ELSEVIER
SAUNDERS

Neurol Clin 23 (2005) 107–129

NEUROLOGIC
CLINICS

Neuropathobiology of Multiple Sclerosis

John W. Peterson, PhD, Bruce D. Trapp, PhD*

Department of Neurosciences, The Lerner Research Institute, The Cleveland Clinic Foundation, 9500 Euclid Avenue, Cleveland, OH 44195, USA

Multiple sclerosis (MS) is an inflammatory demyelinating and neurodegenerative disease of the central nervous system (CNS) affecting more than 2 million people worldwide and more than 400,000 individuals in the United States [1,2]. Because of its high prevalence, MS is the leading cause of nontraumatic neurologic disability in young adults in the United States. The majority of patients are female; the female-to-male ratio ranges from 2:1 to 3:1. Tremendous gains have been made in understanding MS during the past several decades, yet the cause of MS remains unknown. Currently, the most accepted hypothesis for MS is that it is an autoimmune disease triggered in genetically susceptible individuals by an unknown environmental agent.

Patients who have MS exhibit four clinical disease courses. The majority (approximately 85%) initially has a relapsing-remitting disease course of MS (RRMS) characterized by clearly defined alternating episodes of neurologic disability and recovery [1,2]. Within 10 years, more than 50%, and by 25 years approximately 90%, of patients who have RRMS exhibit a secondary progressive disease course of MS (SPMS) characterized by steadily increasing permanent neurologic disability [2,3]. Approximately 10% of patients who have MS experience primary progressive MS (PPMS) characterized by a steady decline in neurologic function from disease onset without recovery. The fourth clinical disease course, called progressive relapsing MS (PRMS), is experienced by approximately 5% of patients who have MS and is characterized by steady progressive neurologic decline punctuated by well demarcated acute attacks with or without recovery.

Current therapeutics for patients who have MS predominantly are anti-inflammatory or immunomodulatory. Patients who have RRMS often benefit clinically from the application of anti-inflammatory therapeutics. For patients who have PPMS, PRMS, or SPMS, however, the efficacy of

This work was supported by grant no. NS35058 from the National Institutes of Health.

* Corresponding author.

E-mail address: trappb@ccf.org (B.D. Trapp).

doi:10.1016/j.ncl.2004.09.008

neurologic.theclinics.com

anti-inflammatory therapeutics is of minimal or no clinical benefit in terms of preventing progression of neurologic disability. The identification of the pathophysiologic mechanisms responsible for progression of permanent neurologic disability therefore is of keen interest. In most patients who have MS, the RRMS converts to SPMS, which suggests these disease courses are not distinct etiologically but may be stages of a single biphasic disease course. Elucidation of the mechanisms responsible for the conversion of RRMS to SPMS may provide insight into the mechanisms contributing to progressive neurologic disability in MS.

The pathologic hallmarks of MS lesions include breakdown of the blood-brain barrier (BBB), multifocal inflammation, demyelination, oligodendrocyte loss, reactive gliosis, and axonal degeneration [4]. Although the immune-mediated destruction of CNS myelin and oligodendrocytes is considered the primary pathology of MS, the major cause of permanent neurologic disability is axonal loss [5–7]. Various approaches, including MRI [8–10], magnetic resonance spectroscopy (MRS) [11–13], functional MRI (fMRI) [14–17], and morphologic analysis of MS tissue [18,19], provide evidence for axonal loss as the cause of irreversible neurologic disability in MS.

Neurologic disability in multiple sclerosis

In RRMS, neurologic disability is caused by infiltrating leukocytes, edema from BBB breakdown, and demyelination (Fig. 1). The appearance of neurologic symptoms is rapid, subsiding usually within 4 to 8 weeks. Because demyelination is a slow process, initial symptoms probably result from conduction block caused by inflammation and edema (see Fig. 1B). Relapses often are preceded by increases in the number of immune cells and levels of specific cytokines in cerebrospinal fluid (CSF). Furthermore, gadolinium (Gd)-enhancing MRI lesions correlate with the onset of relapses

→

Fig. 1. (*A*) Pathobiology of neurologic disability in patients who have MS. In normal myelinated axons, action potentials propagate from node to node via saltatory conduction (*arrows*). (*B*) Rapid onset of neurologic symptoms is caused by conduction block as a result of edema from breakdown of the BBB and inflammatory factors from infiltrating leukocytes. Demyelination (*C*) results in loss of saltatory conduction leading to conduction block (*E*). (*D*) Axonal transection also occurs during inflammatory demyelination. Restoration of impulse conduction and neurologic function may occur with remyelination (*F*) or redistribution of Na+ channels along chronically demyelinated axonal segments (*G*). Recent evidence suggests mechanisms compensating for chronic demyelination (*E*) leads to axonal degeneration (*H*). Permanent disability now is associated with axonal transection (*D*), which occurs during inflammatory demyelination (*B*) and degeneration of chronically demyelinated axons (*H*). Axonal loss is clinically silent during RRMS as a result of CNS compensation. (*Adapted from* Trapp BD, Ransohoff RM, Fisher E, et al. Neurodegeneration in multiple sclerosis: relationship to neurological disability. Neuroscientist 1999;5:48–57; with permission.)

in patients who have MS and short disease duration [20–26]. Neurologic symptoms also occur as a result of conduction block caused by demyelination (see Fig. 1C). Demyelination takes place throughout the CNS and often within the same functional systems. Recovery of neurologic function occurs after resolution of inflammation, restoration of the BBB, and early in the disease remyelination.

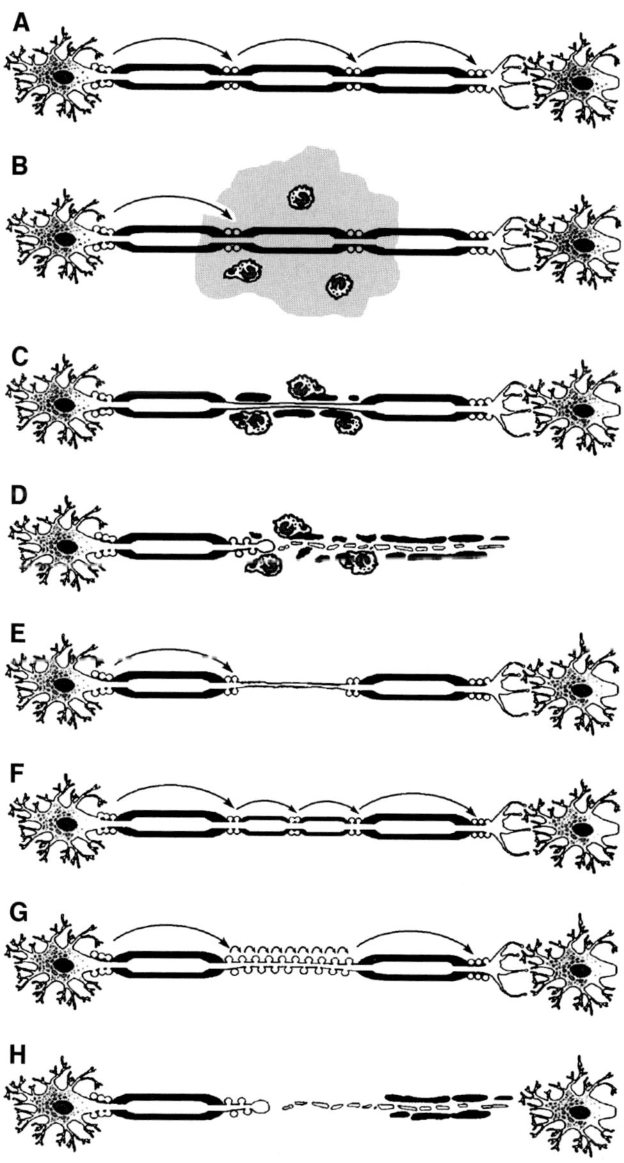

Although inflammatory and demyelinating effects on axonal conduction are sufficient to explain reversible neurologic disability during RRMS, chronic demyelination fails to account adequately for the progressive persistent neurologic disability experienced by patients who have SPMS [27,28]. First, several studies indicate that chronically demyelinated axons redistribute axolemmal ion channels, allowing them to conduct impulses well, although at reduced velocities (see Fig. 1G) [29–31]. Second, inflammatory activity is not prominent and lesion load is stable in many patients who have SPMS. Thus, inflammation, edema, and ongoing demyelination are not expected to make significant contributions to increasing permanent neurologic disability. Other mechanisms must contribute, therefore, to progression of neurologic disability. Several early and more recent studies indicate substantial axonal loss occurs in MS lesions [32,33]. Axonal loss provides a biologic mechanism sufficient to explain irreversible disability in patients who have SPMS.

Axonal loss in multiple sclerosis

Often, axonal injury disrupts axonal transport, resulting in the accumulation of proteins and formation of axonal ovoids. When axons are transected, the proximal axonal segment still connected to the neuronal cell body survives, whereas the distal axonal segment undergoes wallerian degeneration. Anterograde transport from the neuronal perikarya continues leading to the accumulation of organelles, proteins, and a variety of other molecules at the ends of the proximal axonal segments, resulting in the formation of terminal axonal ovoids. Damaged demyelinated axons have been identified in MS by the abnormal accumulation of axonally transported proteins, such as amyloid precursor proteins [18,34], nonphosphorylated neurofilament proteins [19], the pore-forming subunit of N-type calcium channels [35], and metabotropic glutamate receptors [36]. Transected axons were identified and quantified in MS lesions from patients who had disease durations ranging from 2 weeks to 27 years using antibodies to nonphosphorylated neurofilaments (Fig. 2) [19]. Although accumulation of axonal proteins and formation of axonal ovoids suggests axonal transection (see Fig. 2C, E), not all axonal ovoids are the terminal ends of transected axons. En passant axonal ovoids form along intact damaged axons and are identified by the presence of two axonal connections. Whether or not axons with en passant accumulation of axonally transported proteins degenerate or recover normal axonal function is unknown. Analyses of the nonphosphorylated neurofilament-positive ovoids in MS lesions using 3-D reconstruction of confocal microscopy images confirmed that most of the ovoids had only a single axonal connection and, therefore, were transected axons (Fig. 3A). Active lesions contained more than 11,000 terminal ovoids per mm^3, whereas the borders

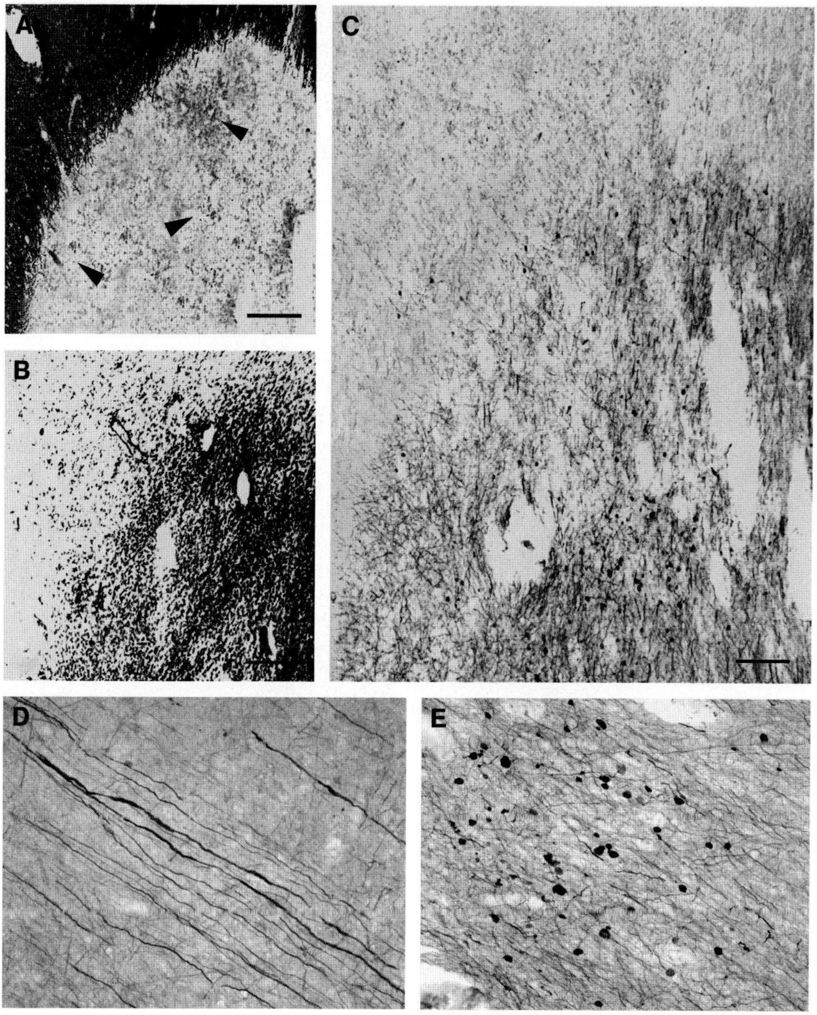

Fig. 2. Abnormal distribution of nonphosphorylated neurofilaments identify demyelinated and damaged axons in MS lesions. An active MS lesion identified by the absence of immunoreactivity to PLP (*A*) and the high density of HLA-DR–positive leukocytes distributed throughout the lesion (*B*). Demyelinated axons and axonal ovoids suggestive of axonal transection were detected in active and chronic active MS lesions (*C, D, E*). Scale bars equal 400 μm in (*A*) and (*B*) and 235 μm in (*C*). (*Adapted from* Trapp BD, Peterson J, Ransohoff RM, et al. Axonal transection in the lesions of multiple sclerosis. N Engl J Med 1998;338:278–85; with permission.)

of chronic active lesions had more than 3000 per mm^3, and the core of chronic active lesions had approximately 900 per mm^3. In comparison, control white matter contained less than one transected axon per mm^3. The identification of significant axonal transection in patients who have short

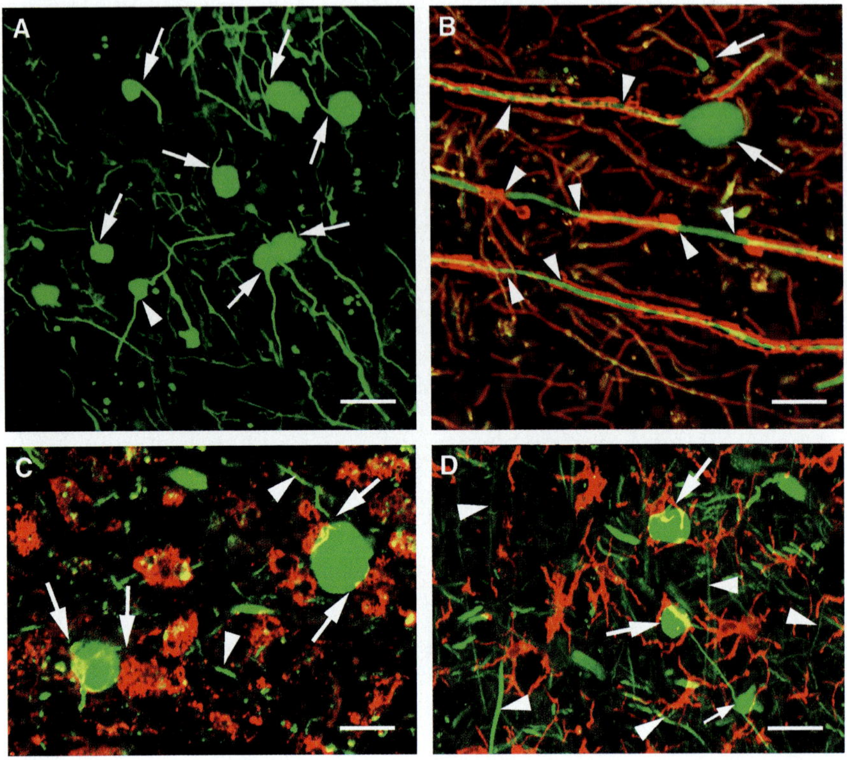

Fig. 3. Confocal analysis of axonal ovoids confirmed transection of axons in MS lesions. (*A*) Most axonal ovoids had single axonal connections indicative of axonal transection (*arrows*), some had two axonal connections (*arrowhead*), indicating the axons had not undergone transection. (*B*) Nonphosphorylated neurofilament-positive axons (green) undergoing demyelination at the border of a chronic active lesion (*arrowheads*; red is myelin basic protein). Two of the axons end in terminal ovoids (*arrows*). Macrophages and microglia associate with transected axons (green) in active MS lesions. (*C*) Macrophages (red) and (*D*) microglia (red) surround terminal axonal swellings (*large arrows*) but do not target normal-appearing axons (*arrowheads*) or swellings in nontransected axons (*small arrow*). Scale bar equals 64 μm in (*A*) and 45 μm in (*B, C, D*). (*Adapted from* Trapp BD, Peterson J, Ransohoff RM, et al. Axonal transection in the lesions of multiple sclerosis. N Engl J Med 1998;338:278–85; with permission.)

disease duration when inflammatory demyelination is predominant helped establish the concept of axonal loss occurring at disease onset in MS (see Fig. 3B).

Immune-mediated axonal loss

Development of neuroprotective therapies is critically dependent on identifying the cellular and molecular mechanisms of axonal transection in MS and understanding the interplay of these mechanisms with disease progression. Elucidating the pathophysiology of axonal injury is complicated, because different or multiple mechanisms of axonal degeneration may occur, depending on the stage of the disease. Positive correlations between inflammatory activity of MS lesions and axonal damage suggest that inflammation modulates axonal pathology in patients who have MS [18,19,35–38]. Even when the disease is subclinical, the link between disease progression and CNS inflammation is correlated [39]. Additionally, axonal damage indicated by the detection of neurofilament proteins in 78% of the CSF samples from patients who have RRMS correlates with clinical disability [40]. MRI provides further support for the dependence of axonal injury on inflammation. For example, progressive brain atrophy is associated with active Gd-enhancing lesions on MRI scans in patients who have RRMS [41]. Correlations between CNS atrophy measured by MRI and clinical disability support atrophy as an indirect indicator of axonal loss [42]. In addition, Gd-enhancing lesions and progressive atrophy can occur without clinical symptoms in patients who have RRMS, indicating the disease can be clinically silent [43–45].

One possible mechanism of axonal degeneration in MS is a specific immunologic attack on the axon. Immune-mediated axonal transection is suggested by the correlation of inflammation with axonal transection. The terminal ovoids of transected axons often are surrounded by macrophages and activated microglia in MS lesions (see Fig. 3C, D) [19]. Neurofilament-positive inclusions sometimes are observed within the macrophages (see Fig. 3C) and microglia (not shown). These observations suggest axons are targeted by macrophages and activated microglia. Whether or not these cells directly attack axons or only remove axonal debris remains to be determined. Direct immunologic targeting of axons is not without precedent. Primary immune-mediated attack against gangliosides on peripheral nervous system axons has been identified as a cause of axonal degeneration in the autoimmune disease, acute motor axonal neuropathy (AMAN), a variant of Guillain-Barré syndrome [46]. The identification of immunoglobulins and the complement activation marker C3d at the nodes of Ranvier indicate antibody binding to an axolemmal molecule [47]. Unlike AMAN, antibodies to axonal components in the CNS are not localized to MS lesions [46,47]. Antibodies to enriched fractions of axolemma are detected, however, in the CSF and serum of patients who have MS [48]. Additionally, because most axons survive the acute demyelinating process, it seems unlikely there is a specific immunologic attack against axons. Recent studies identify cytotoxic $CD8^+$ T cells as mediators of axonal transection in inflammatory lesions in MS tissue [49,50], in experimental autoimmune encephalomyelitis (EAE) mice [51], and in vitro [52,53]. Furthermore, some reports indicate that axonal subpopulations may be targeted by immune-mediated mechanisms [54–56]. Despite the current paucity of direct evidence supporting a specific immunologic attack on axons in MS, the possibility of cell-mediated mechanisms of axon loss should not be ignored.

Axonal loss may take place as a result of nonspecific damage caused by the inflammatory process. Activated immune and glial cells release

increased workload. These preprogrammed neurodegenerative changes dissociate initial inflammatory damage observed early in the disease from progressive tissue degeneration during chronic stages of MS. The observations described previously suggest that oligodendrocytes exert trophic effects on axons at a local level, and disruption of the axonal cytoskeleton plays a role in mediating the pathogenesis of axonal degeneration secondary to demyelination. Furthermore, the effects of chronic demyelination may induce late axonal degeneration in SPMS by initiating deleterious compensatory changes in axons and disrupting axonal transport. Additionally, chronic demyelination results in loss of structural support from myelin for axons. Remyelination is important, therefore, for restoring normal impulse conduction and as a neuroprotective event for preventing axonal degeneration.

Pathology of cortical multiple sclerosis lesions

Demyelination also occurs in the gray matter of patients who have MS [83–87]. Little is known about the impact of cortical pathology on neurologic disability in MS. A recent study detected axonal transection, dendritic transection, and neuronal apoptosis in cortical MS lesions [86]. The incidence of cerebral cortical lesions in MS is described in several studies. Brownell and Hughes report that 26% of the brain lesions in MS involve the gray matter [83]. Approximately 65% of the gray matter lesions are located at the leukocortical junction, affecting the cortex and white matter. The remaining gray matter lesions are located either in the central gray matter (15%) or completely within in the cortex (approximately 19%). Another study of 60 MS brains detected cortical lesions in 93% of the cases, with 59% of the cerebral lesions in the cortex [84]. One brain contained 465 cortical lesions.

Historically, cortical involvement in MS has received little attention, even though it can be extensive in some patients who have MS. There is renewed interest in the involvement of cerebral cortex in MS [88]. The detection of white matter lesions by MRI enables correlations to be made with neurologic symptoms. Patients who have MS, however, often experience neurologic symptoms that do not correlate with the white matter pathology. A recent immunocytochemical study of 110 tissue blocks from 50 MS brains identified and characterized 112 cortical lesions [86]. Based on the distribution of cortical demyelination, three types of cortical lesions were described (Fig. 4). Type I lesions occurred at the leukocortical junction, demyelinating white matter and cortex. Demyelinating lesions, which remained completely within the cortex, were called Type II lesions. Cortical lesions, which extended into the cortex from the pial surface, were called Type III lesions. All three cortical lesion types often were detected in the same MS brains. No single cortical lesion type seems to predominate in individual patients. It is unknown, however, if subgrouping patients who

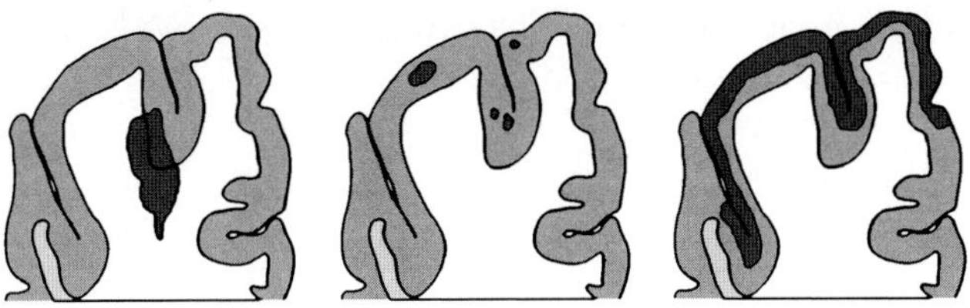

Fig. 4. Three types of cortical lesions were identified in MS. Type I lesions affect subcortical white matter and cortex. Type II lesions are small, circular intracortical lesions, often centered on vessels. Type III lesions extend from the pial surface into the cortex and often involve multiple gyri. Cortex is light gray, white matter is white, and dark gray represents demyelination.

have variable pathogenesis [89] can help identify patients who have particular cortical lesion subtypes. Mechanisms of demyelination and characteristics of the immune response or demyelinating inflammatory environment may be different for each cortical lesion subtype. Another immunocytochemical study prospectively selected the frontal, parietal, and temporal cortices along with cingulate gyrus to analyze the extent of cortical demyelination in postmortem MS brains. Approximately 27% of the cortical area analyzed was demyelinated [87].

There are several reasons why cortical lesions are missed. Cortical myelin is not readily apparent on routine histologic examination of Luxol fast blue staining of postmortem tissue. As described in detail later, cortical lesions are not hypercellular and, therefore, not obvious on hematoxylin-eosin–stained sections. Most important, cortical lesions rarely are detected by routine MRI procedures [85,90]. The dynamics of lesion formation, therefore, are unknown, as is whether or not lesion loads correlate with clinical disabilities or type of disease course.

Decreased inflammation in cortical lesions

The number of inflammatory cells in Type I cortical lesions is significantly less than in white matter lesions [86]. The cortical part of Type I lesions contains 6 times fewer CD68-positive microglia/macrophages and 13 times fewer CD3-positive lymphocytes than the white matter part of the lesions. Reduced inflammatory cells in Type I and Type II cortical lesions compared with white matter lesions has been described [91]. In cortical lesions, perivascular cuffing was rare and, when present, contained few cells [86,91]. Regulation of leukocyte migration in the cortex seems different from that in white matter. One possibility for the lack of cortical leukocytic infiltration may be the differential regulation and expression of cell adhesion molecules by cortical endothelial cells. The molecular regulation of leukocyte trafficking into the brain is elucidated partially [92–95]. Antigen-specific lymphocytes produce proinflammatory cytokines, inducing a cascade of cytokine and chemokine expression by resident astrocytes and microglia [96]. Thus, endothelial cells, astrocytes, and microglia help modulate the inflammatory signals in cortex and in white matter lesions, influencing the inflammatory cell character of the immune response.

The paucity of leukocytes in cortical MS lesions indicates that demyelination can occur without extensive leukocytic infiltration. This suggests that induction of demyelination may not require a large influx of leukocytes and that the trafficking of leukocytes into white matter lesions is related to phagocytosis of myelin debris rather than the destruction of myelin. Type III lesions, which accounted for approximately 50% of the total cortical lesions identified, are the most interesting pattern of demyelination [86]. Many Type III lesions extended from the pial surface to cortical layers three or four, often affecting multiple gyri. This pattern of demyelination suggests that a factor or factors in the CSF may cause demyelination or loss of oligodendrocytes in Type III lesions. There are reports of demyelinating factors in the CSF of patients who have MS [97] or serum from rodents with EAE [98], suggesting that the mechanisms of demyelination may differ in Type III cortical lesions from those in Type I and II cortical lesions.

Neuronal damage in cortical lesions

Transected axons, transected dendrites, and neuronal apoptosis were identified in cortical lesions from patients who had MS whose clinical disease ranged from 2 weeks to 27 years [86]. Substantial neuronal injury occured in cortical lesions despite reduced cortical inflammation. Neurofilament-positive swellings were detected along dendrites and axons, suggesting disruption of normal cellular transport. Confocal analysis identified many of these swellings as the terminal ends of axons and dendrites (Fig. 5A, B). Neuritic (axons and dendrites) transection in cortical lesions correlated with microglial activation numbering 4119/mm^3 in active lesions, 1107/mm^3 in chronic active lesions, and 25/mm^3 in chronic inactive lesions. In comparison, an average of 8 and 1 transected neurites/mm^3 were detected in myelinated cortex from MS and control brains respectively. The correlation between neuritic transection and microglial activation of the lesion suggests that dendrites and demyelinated axons are vulnerable to activated microglia associated with cortical demyelination.

The destruction of dendrites is a previously unidentified pathologic change in MS that can contribute to neurologic disability by decreasing synaptic input into the cortex. The functional deficit induced by axonal transection varies depending on which axons are transected. If transection of efferent axonal inputs occurs close to their targets, they may have the ability to sprout and reinnervate postsynaptic densities. Proximal transection of afferent axonal outputs of cortical neurons (see Fig. 5B), however, results in the irreversible functional loss of the neuron, because reinnerva-

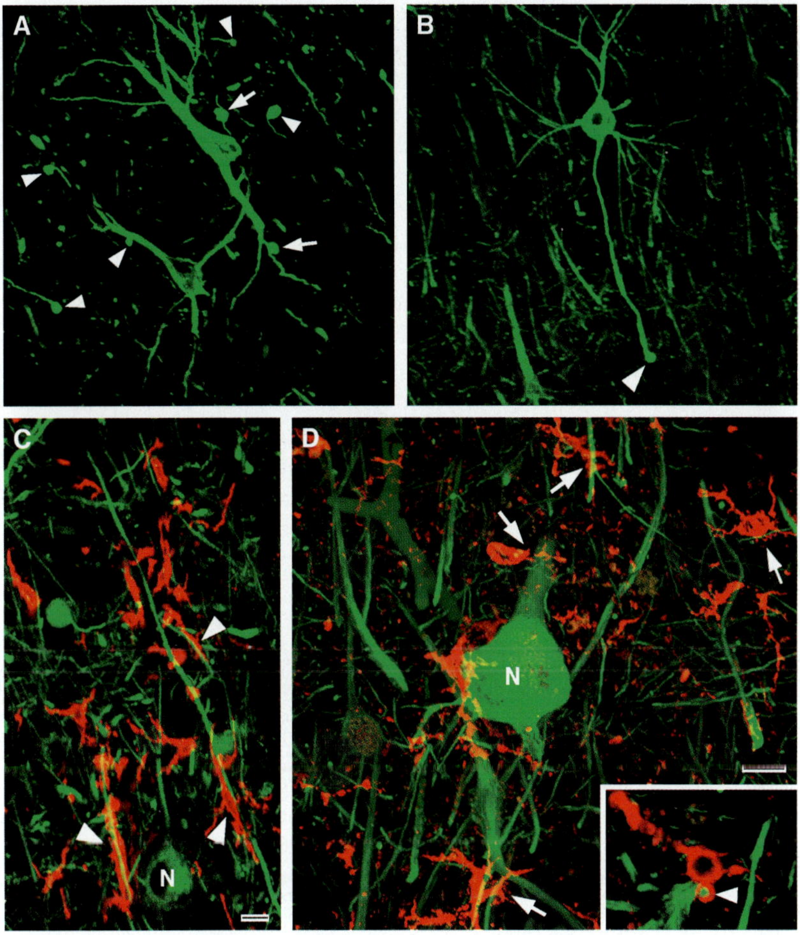

Fig. 5. Neuronal pathology in cortical lesions. (*A, B*) Nonphosphorylated neurofilament-positive ovoids are abundant in cortical lesions (green). Confocal microscopy confirmed most of these ovoids as terminal ends of neurites (*A, arrowheads*) and some as "en passant" swellings (*A, arrows*). Some ovoids close to neuronal perikarya could be identified as axonal (*B, arrowhead*) or dendritic (*A, arrow*). (*C, D*) Microglia (red) target neurons and their processes (green). (*C*) Confocal microscopy-detected ferritin-positive microglia with elongated shapes ensheathing neurites (*arrowheads*). (*D*) More stellate-shaped microglia were identified in close apposition to neuronal perikarya and extending processes to and around neurofilament-positive neurites (*arrows*). (*Inset*) High-magnification image of microglial process (red, *arrowhead*) ensheathing a branch of an apical dendrite (green). N, neuron. (*Adapted from* Peterson JW, Bo L, Mork S, et al. Transected neurites, apoptotic neurons and reduced inflammation in cortical multiple sclerosis lesions. Ann Neurol 2001;50:389–400; with permission.)

tion of the target is not possible. Axonal transection may result in apoptosis or atrophy of the affected neuron depending on the amount of remaining target-derived support [99–102]. The death or atrophy of cortical neurons reduces the trophic support for their afferent neurons and eventually these target-deprived neurons may die or atrophy [100]. Neuronal or axonal damage unrelated to axonal transection also may result in apoptotic neuronal death. A recent study reports that CSF collected during ongoing inflammatory activity from a patient who had PPMS induced apoptosis of neurons in vitro [97], suggesting a diffusible factor in the CSF mediates neuronal damage and death.

If demyelination, deafferentation, or inflammatory mediators secreted by activated microglia causes neuronal apoptosis, then therapeutic intervention may help preserve the neuron and maintain the neuronal circuitry. Detection of substantial neuronal apoptosis in chronic active and chronic inactive lesions suggests that neuronal death may result from chronic insults to neurons, dendrites, or axons in addition to direct immune attack during the demyelinating process [86]. Clearance of apoptotic cells occurs within 24 hours [103,104]. Apoptotic neurons are prevalent in chronic lesions that exist for years. Over time, therefore, neuronal loss by apoptosis is significant.

Microglial targeting of neurons in cortical multiple sclerosis lesions

Microglia are the resident macrophages of the CNS responsible for monitoring pathologic changes [105,106]. In cortical MS lesions, microglia are detected closely associated with neurons [86]. Elongated microglia are oriented perpendicular to the pial surface, closely apposed, and ensheathing apical dendrites and axons in active and chronic active cortical lesions (see Fig. 5C, D). In addition, other highly ramified stellate-shaped microglia often extend processes to neuronal perikarya and ensheathed dendrites or axons (see Fig. 5D). Unlike microglia/macrophages in white matter lesions, which often surround the transected ends of axons [19], microglia in cortical lesions do not seem to target the transected ends of neurites in cortical lesions (see Fig. 5C).

The targeting of neurons by microglia in cortical lesions is suggestive of synaptic stripping [107,108]. It remains to be determined if microglia in cortical lesions actively target synaptic terminals and if the association of microglia with neurons is destructive or protective. It is probable that the microglia target already damaged neurons. For example, activated microglia target damaged neurites and neurons in Alzheimer's disease (AD) [109–111]. Some of the most promising AD therapeutics are anti-inflammatory drugs that target activated microglia [112,113]. Similar anti-inflammatory drugs, which reduce microglial activation in the cerebral cortex, also may benefit patients who have MS.

Contribution of cortical lesions to neurologic disability in multiple sclerosis

The studies described previously implicate cortical lesions as major contributors to disease burden in patients who have MS. Neuronal damage in motor and sensory cortex certainly has an impact on ambulatory decline in patients who have MS. In addition to motor and sensory deficits, 40% to 70% of all individuals diagnosed with MS experience various cognitive deficits [114,115]. Cognitive functions commonly affected include learning, memory, and information processing [114]. A positron emission tomography study demonstrates a correlation between decreased cerebral metabolism and increased MRI lesion load with cognitive dysfunction in MS [116]. Cognitive impairment in patients who have MS has been attributed to subcortical white matter lesions, but often the anatomic location of the subcortical lesions and the identified cognitive deficits do not match. Cortical pathology likely contributes to functional impairment, given the extent and nature of damage to cortical neurons in many MS brains.

Functional consequences

The concept of MS as an inflammatory demyelinating and neurodegenerative disease provides a conceptual framework that explains disease progression and development of permanent neurologic disability in patients who have MS (Fig. 6). The time from clinical disease onset of MS to a score of 4 on the EDSS ranges from 1 to 33 years; however, once patients reach EDSS 4, the time to EDSS 7 is similar among the patients [117]. These observations suggest an initiation of a cascade of neuronal degeneration that occurs once a pathologic threshold is reached. The progression of neurologic disability from EDSS 4 to EDSS 7 occurs by neurodegenerative mechanisms other than inflammatory-mediated axonal transection [2,5,117,118]. The identification of neuronal pathology in MS, specifically the destruction of axons and dendrites along with neuronal apoptosis, provides a pathologic substrate for the progressive disability many patients who have MS experience and suggests early inflammatory activity may initiate a state of preprogrammed neuronal degeneration.

All neurodegenerative diseases have an initial silent stage of neuronal cell loss. The CNS has a remarkable ability to compensate for neuronal damage. For example, it is estimated that 50% to 80% of target neurons in amyotrophic lateral sclerosis and Parkinson's disease, respectively, are lost before neurologic symptoms present clinically [119,120]. In RRMS, lesions outnumber clinical relapses 10 to 1 [21]. Correlations between clinical status and T2 lesion load on MRI scans usually are weak [43,121]. Additionally, clinical features during RRMS are poor predictors of subsequent progression of disability [39]. There is a positive correlation between progressive disability and increasing brain atrophy in individual patients, however, which probably parallels accumulating axonal loss [122]. These data indicate that maintained motor function during early stages of MS may result from adaptive cortical changes, such as the reorganization of functional pathways, which could compensate for axonal damage.

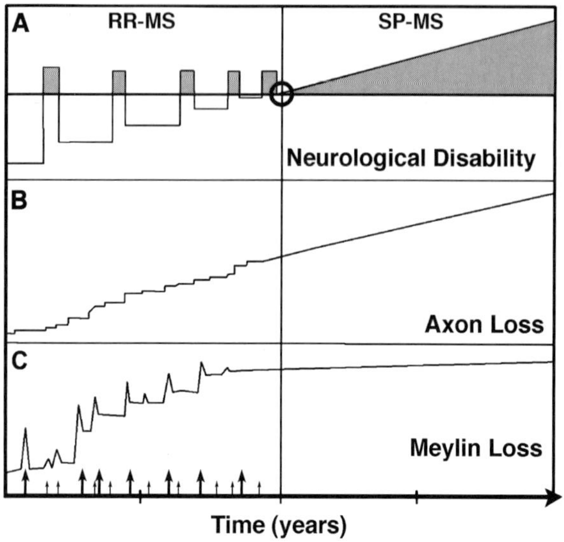

Fig. 6. The most common disease course experienced by patients who have MS is biphasic. (*A*) Initially, patients who have RRMS experience alternating periods of clinical disability punctuated by periods of recovery. When disability (gray) exceeds clinical threshold (*horizontal line*), neurologic symptoms become clinically evident. Clinical diagnosis of SPMS occurs when disability becomes progressive without remission. (*B*) Axon loss begins at disease onset and accumulates with disease duration. Pathologically, the conversion of RRMS to SPMS (*A, circle*) occurs once axon loss surpasses the capacity of the CNS to compensate (*B, vertical line*). (*C*) During RRMS, Gd-enhancing lesions (*arrows*) are prominent, whereas during SPMS, inflammatory activity is negligible. The rate of myelin loss correlates with inflammatory activity with the greatest loss early in the disease during RRMS when inflammation is most active. The amount of demyelination remains relatively stable during SPMS.

The prevention of persistent neurologic disability is the main goal when treating neurologic diseases. Because inflammatory-mediated tissue destruction begins at disease onset and may occur in the absence of clinical symptoms during RRMS, early continuous proactive application of disease-modifying therapy is warranted to prevent and delay accumulating neuronal damage. Thus, inflammation remains a major therapeutic target. Other mechanisms also contribute to neuronal damage during different stages of MS; therefore, clarification of the pathophysiology of neurodegeneration in MS is crucial. In contrast patients who have other neurodegenerative diseases, patients who have MS can be identified early, before the occurrence of extensive neurodegeneration, by the presentation of symptoms mediated by inflammatory demyelination. Neuroprotective therapeutics, therefore, may have a greater probability of clinical efficacy in patients who have MS, because treatment can be initiated before extensive axonal loss. Additionally, patients who have MS may benefit from the combination of neuroprotective therapies and current anti-inflammatory and immunomodulatory treatments. The development of neuroprotective drugs applicable to MS is an urgent goal of MS researchers. Remyelination also would be neuroprotective. Promotion of remyelination restores conduction and oligodendrocyte-derived trophic support and prevents axonal degeneration.

Summary

Neuronal injury is an integral part of MS. Loss of axons, dendrites, and neurons contribute to the irreversible permanent neurologic disability experienced by patients who have MS. Various aspects and potential mechanisms of neuronal injury in MS recently have been described. A multidisciplinary approach and a variety of animal models have increased understanding of the neuropathologic mechanisms involved in the development of permanent neurologic disability. Several lines of evidence indicate that primary inflammatory demyelination underlies early axonal loss during RRMS. Initially this axonal loss clinically is silent. The transition from RRMS to SPMS is hypothesized to occur once a threshold of axonal loss is reached and the compensatory capacity of the CNS is surpassed, resulting in the steady progression of permanent neurologic symptoms.

The concept of MS as an inflammatory neurodegenerative disease has several clinical implications. The development of surrogate markers for axonal loss is needed to monitor neurodegeneration. To prevent and delay disability, early aggressive anti-inflammatory and immunomodulatory treatment should be provided. The development of neuroprotective therapeutics is warranted for MS. Finally, further elucidation of the molecular mechanisms behind axonal injury and their relation to disease stage in MS is essential for the development and refinement of therapeutic strategies.

Acknowledgments

The authors thank Susan De Stefano for assistance with preparation of the manuscript and Dr. Grahame Kidd and Rosalia Yacubova for assistance with the figures.

References

[1] Weinshenker BG. Epidemiology of multiple sclerosis. Neurol Clin 1996;14:291–308.

[2] Noseworthy JH, Lucchinetti C, Rodriguez M, et al. Multiple sclerosis. N Engl J Med 2000; 343:938–52.

[3] Weinshenker BG, Bass B, Rice GP, et al. The natural history of multiple sclerosis: a geographically based study. I. Clinical course and disability. Brain 1989;112:133–46.

[4] Prineas J. Pathology of multiple sclerosis. In: Cook S, editor. Handbook of multiple sclerosis. Basel (Switzerland): Marcel Dekker; 2001. p. 289–324.

[5] Trapp BD, Ransohoff RM, Fisher E, et al. Neurodegeneration in multiple sclerosis: relationship to neurological disability. Neuroscientist 1999;5:48–57.

[6] Bjartmar C, Wujek JR, Trapp BD. Axonal loss in the pathology of MS: consequences for understanding the progressive phase of the disease. J Neurol Sci 2003;206:165–71.
[7] Bruck W, Stadelmann C. Inflammation and degeneration in multiple sclerosis. Neurol Sci 2003;24(Suppl 5):S265–7.
[8] van Waesberghe JH, Kamphorst W, De Groot CJ, et al. Axonal loss in multiple sclerosis lesions: magnetic resonance imaging insights into substrates of disability. Ann Neurol 1999; 46:747–54.
[9] Stevenson VL, Miller DH. Magnetic resonance imaging in the monitoring of disease progression in multiple sclerosis. Mult Scler 1999;5:268–72.
[10] De Stefano N, Guidi L, Stromillo ML, et al. Imaging neuronal and axonal degeneration in multiple sclerosis. Neurol Sci 2003;24(Suppl 5):S283–6.
[11] Narayana PA, Doyle TJ, Lai D, et al. Serial proton magnetic resonance spectroscopic imaging, contrast-enhanced magnetic resonance imaging, and quantitative lesion volumetry in multiple sclerosis. Ann Neurol 1998;43:56–71.
[12] Matthews PM, De Stefano N, Narayanan S, et al. Putting magnetic resonance spectroscopy studies in context: axonal damage and disability in multiple sclerosis. Semin Neurol 1998; 18:327–36.
[13] Arnold DL. Magnetic resonance spectroscopy: imaging axonal damage in MS. J Neuroimmunol 1999;98:2–6.
[14] Reddy H, Narayanan S, Arnoutelis R, et al. Evidence for adaptive functional changes in the cerebral cortex with axonal injury from multiple sclerosis. Brain 2000;123(Pt 11):2314–20.
[15] Pantano P, Iannetti GD, Caramia F, et al. Cortical motor reorganization after a single clinical attack of multiple sclerosis. Brain 2002;125(Pt 7):1607–15.
[16] Rocca MA, Mezzapesa DM, Falini A, et al. Evidence for axonal pathology and adaptive cortical reorganization in patients at presentation with clinically isolated syndromes suggestive of multiple sclerosis. Neuroimage 2003;18:847–55.
[17] Parry AM, Scott RB, Palace J, et al. Potentially adaptive functional changes in cognitive processing for patients with multiple sclerosis and their acute modulation by rivastigmine. Brain 2003;126(Pt 12):2750–60.
[18] Ferguson B, Matyszak MK, Esiri MM, et al. Axonal damage in acute multiple sclerosis lesions. Brain 1997;120:393–9.
[19] Trapp BD, Peterson J, Ransohoff RM, et al. Axonal transection in the lesions of multiple sclerosis. N Engl J Med 1998;338:278–85.
[20] Harris JO, Frank JA, Patronas N, et al. Serial gadolinium-enhanced magnetic resonance imaging scans in patients with early, relapsing-remitting multiple sclerosis: implications for clinical trials and natural history. Ann Neurol 1991;29:548–55.
[21] McFarland HF, Frank JA, Albert PS, et al. Using gadolinium-enhanced magnetic resonance imaging lesions to monitor disease activity in multiple sclerosis. Ann Neurol 1992;32:758–66.
[22] Miller DH, Barkhof F, Nauta JJ. Gadolinium enhancement increases the sensitivity of MRI in detecting disease activity in multiple sclerosis. Brain 1993;116(Pt 5):1077–94.
[23] Koudriavtseva T, Thompson AJ, Fiorelli M, et al. Gadolinium enhanced MRI predicts clinical and MRI disease activity in relapsing-remitting multiple sclerosis. J Neurol Neurosurg Psychiatry 1997;62:285–7.
[24] Weiner HL, Guttmann CR, Khoury SJ, et al. Serial magnetic resonance imaging in multiple sclerosis: correlation with attacks, disability, and disease stage. J Neuroimmunol 2000;104: 164–73.
[25] Khoury SJ, Guttmann CR, Orav EJ, et al. Changes in activated T cells in the blood correlate with disease activity in multiple sclerosis. Arch Neurol 2000;57:1183–9.
[26] Wang HY, Matsui M, Saida T. Immunological disturbances in the central nervous system linked to MRI findings in multiple sclerosis. J Neuroimmunol 2002;125:149–54.
[27] Waxman SG. Demyelinating diseases—new pathological insights, new therapeutic targets. N Engl J Med 1998;338:323–5.

[28] Trapp BD, Ransohoff RM, Fisher E, et al. Neurodegeneration in multiple sclerosis: relationship to neurological disability. Neuroscientist 1999;5:48–57.
[29] Bostock H, Sears TA. The internodal axon membrane: electrical excitability and continuous conduction in segmental demyelination. J Physiol 1978;280:273–301.
[30] Foster RE, Whalen CC, Waxman SG. Reorganization of the axon membrane in demyelinated peripheral nerve fibers: morphological evidence. Science 1980;210:661–3.
[31] Felts PA, Baker TA, Smith KJ. Conduction in segmentally demyelinated mammalian central axons. J Neurosci 1997;17:7267–77.
[32] Kornek B, Lassmann H. Axonal pathology in multiple sclerosis. A historical note. Brain Pathol 1999;9:651–6.
[33] Bjartmar C, Trapp BD. Axonal degeneration and progressive neurologic disability in multiple sclerosis. Neurotox Res 2003;5:157–64.
[34] Gehrmann J, Banati RB, Cuzner ML, et al. Amyloid precursor protein (APP) expression in multiple sclerosis lesions. Glia 1995;15:141–51.
[35] Kornek B, Storch MK, Bauer J, et al. Distribution of a calcium channel subunit in dystrophic axons in multiple sclerosis and experimental autoimmune encephalomyelitis. Brain 2001;124:1114–24.
[36] Geurts JJ, Wolswijk G, Bo L, et al. Altered expression patterns of group I and II metabotropic glutamate receptors in multiple sclerosis. Brain 2003;126(Pt 8):1755–66.
[37] Kornek B, Storch MK, Weissert R, et al. Multiple sclerosis and chronic autoimmune encephalomyelitis: a comparative quantitative study of axonal injury in active, inactive, and remyelinated lesions. Am J Pathol 2000;157:267–76.
[38] Bitsch A, Schuchardt J, Bunkowski S, et al. Acute axonal injury in multiple sclerosis. Correlation with demyelination and inflammation. Brain 2000;123:1174–83.
[39] Rudick RA, Goodman A, Herndon RM, et al. Selecting relapsing remitting multiple sclerosis patients for treatment: the case for early treatment. J Neuroimmunol 1999;98:22–8.
[40] Lycke JN, Karlsson JE, Andersen O, et al. Neurofilament protein in cerebrospinal fluid: a potential marker of activity in multiple sclerosis. J Neurol Neurosurg Psychiatry 1998;64: 402–4.
[41] Zivadinov R, Zorzon M. Is gadolinium enhancement predictive of the development of brain atrophy in multiple sclerosis? A review of the literature. J Neuroimaging 2002;12: 302–9.
[42] Losseff NA, Miller DH. Measures of brain and spinal cord atrophy in multiple sclerosis. J Neurol Neurosurg Psychiatry 1998;64(Suppl 1):S102–5.
[43] Simon JH, Jacobs LD, Campion M, et al. Magnetic resonance studies of intramuscular interferon beta-1a for relapsing multiple sclerosis. The Multiple Sclerosis Collaborative Research Group. Ann Neurol 1998;43:79–87.
[44] Simon JH, Jacobs LD, Campion MK, et al. A longitudinal study of brain atrophy in relapsing multiple sclerosis. The Multiple Sclerosis Collaborative Research Group (MSCRG). Neurology 1999;53:139–48.
[45] Rudick RA, Cohen JA, Weinstock-Guttman B, et al. Management of multiple sclerosis. N Engl J Med 1997;337:1604–11.
[46] Ho TW, McKhann GM, Griffin JW. Human autoimmune neuropathies. Annu Rev Neurosci 1998;21:187–226.
[47] Hafer-Macko C, Hsieh S-T, Li CY, et al. Acute motor axonal neuropathy: an antibody-mediated attack on axolemma. Ann Neurol 1996;40:635–44.
[48] Rawes JA, Calabrese VP, Khan OA, et al. Antibodies to the axolemma-enriched fraction in the cerebrospinal fluid and serum of patients with multiple sclerosis and other neurological diseases. Mult Scler 1997;3:363–9.
[49] Babbe H, Roers A, Waisman A, et al. Clonal expansions of CD8(+) T cells dominate the T cell infiltrate in active multiple sclerosis lesions as shown by micromanipulation and single cell polymerase chain reaction. J Exp Med 2000;192:393–404.

[50] Skulina C, Schmidt S, Dornmair K, et al. Multiple sclerosis: brain-infiltrating CD8 + T cells persist as clonal expansions in the cerebrospinal fluid and blood. Proc Natl Acad Sci USA 2004;101:2428–33.
[51] Huseby ES, Liggitt D, Brabb T. A pathogenic role for myelin-specific CD8(+) T cells in a model for multiple sclerosis. J Exp Med 2001;194:669–76.
[52] Medana I, Martinic MA, Wekerle H. Transection of major histocompatibility complex class I-induced neurites by cytotoxic T lymphocytes. Am J Pathol 2001;159:809–15.
[53] Giuliani F, Goodyer CG, Antel JP, et al. Vulnerability of human neurons to T cell-mediated cytotoxicity. J Immunol 2003;171:368–79.
[54] Ganter P, Prince C, Esiri MM. Spinal cord axonal loss in multiple sclerosis: a post-mortem study. Neuropathol Appl Neurobiol 1999;25:459–67.
[55] Lovas G, Szilagyi N, Majtenyi K, et al. Axonal changes in chronic demyelinated cervical spinal cord plaques. Brain 2000;123:308–17.
[56] Evangelou N, Konz D, Esiri MM, et al. Size-selective neuronal changes in the anterior optic pathways suggest a differential susceptibility to injury in multiple sclerosis. Brain 2001; 124(Pt 9):1813–20.
[57] Hohlfeld R. Biotechnological agents for the immunotherapy of multiple sclerosis. Principles, problems and perspectives [invited review]. Brain 1997;120:865–916.
[58] Piani D, Frei K, Do KQ, et al. Murine brain macrophages induced NMDA receptor mediated neurotoxicity in vitro by secreting glutamate. Neurosci Lett 1991;133: 159–62.
[59] Werner P, Pitt D, Raine CS. Multiple sclerosis: altered glutamate homeostasis in lesions correlates with oligodendrocyte and axonal damage. Ann Neurol 2001;50:169–80.
[60] Bö L, Dawson TM, Wesselingh S, et al. Induction of nitric oxide synthase in demyelinating regions of multiple sclerosis brains. Ann Neurol 1994;36:778–86.
[61] Smith KJ, Lassmann H. The role of nitric oxide in multiple sclerosis. Lancet Neurol 2002;1: 232–41.
[62] Lu F, Selak M, O'Connor J, et al. Oxidative damage to mitochondrial DNA and activity of mitochondrial enzymes in chronic active lesions of multiple sclerosis. J Neurol Sci 2000;177: 95–103.
[63] Rudick RA, Fisher E, Lee JC, et al. Use of the brain parenchymal fraction to measure whole brain atrophy in relapsing-remitting MS. Multiple Sclerosis Collaborative Research Group. Neurology 1999;53:1698–704.
[64] Miller DH, Barkhof F, Frank JA, et al. Measurement of atrophy in multiple sclerosis: pathological basis, methodological aspects and clinical relevance. Brain 2002;125(Pt 8): 1676–95.
[65] De Stefano N, Matthews PM, Fu L, et al. Axonal damage correlates with disability in patients with relapsing-remitting multiple sclerosis. Results of a longitudinal magnetic resonance spectroscopy study. Brain 1998;121:1469–77.
[66] Gonen O, Catalaa I, Babb JS, et al. Total brain N-acetylaspartate: a new measure of disease load in MS. Neurology 2000;54:15–9.
[67] Bjartmar C, Yin X, Trapp BD. Axonal pathology in myelin disorders. J Neurocytol 1999; 28:383–95.
[68] Li C, Tropak MB, Gerial R, et al. Myelination in the absence of myelin-associated glycoprotein. Nature 1994;369:747–50.
[69] Yin X, Crawford TO, Griffin JW, et al. Myelin-associated glycoprotein is a myelin signal that modulates the caliber of myelinated axons. J Neurosci 1998;18:1953–62.
[70] Klugmann M, Schwab MH, Puhlhofer A, et al. Assembly of CNS myelin in the absence of proteolipid protein. Neuron 1997;18:59–70.
[71] Griffiths I, Klugmann M, Anderson T, et al. Axonal swellings and degeneration in mice lacking the major proteolipid of myelin. Science 1998;280:1610–3.
[72] Lappe-Siefke C, Goebbels S, Gravel M, et al. Disruption of Cnp1 uncouples oligodendroglial functions in axonal support and myelination. Nat Genet 2003;33:366–74.

[73] Bjartmar C, Kidd G, Mork S, et al. Neurological disability correlates with spinal cord axonal loss and reduce *N*-acetyl aspartate in chronic multiple sclerosis patients. Ann Neurol 2000;48:893–901.

[74] Garbern JY, Yool DA, Moore GJ, et al. Patients lacking the major CNS myelin protein, proteolipid protein 1, develop length-dependent axonal degeneration in the absence of demyelination and inflammation. Brain 2002;125:551–61.

[75] Scherer S. Axonal pathology in demyelinating diseases. Ann Neurol 1999;45:6–7.

[76] Ames A III. CNS energy metabolism as related to function. Brain Res Brain Res Rev 2000; 34:42–68.

[77] Stys PK, Waxman SG, Ransom BR. Ionic mechanisms of anoxic injury in mammalian CNS white matter: role of Na + channels and Na(+)-Ca2 + exchanger. J Neurosci 1992;12: 430–9.

[78] Leppanen LL, Stys PK. Ion transport and membrane potential in CNS myeliated axons. II: effects of metabolic inhibition. J Neurophysiol 1997;78:2095–107.

[79] Craner MJ, Lo AC, Black JA, et al. Abnormal sodium channel distribution in optic nerve axons in a model of inflammatory demyelination. Brain 2003;126(Pt 7):1552–61.

[80] Craner MJ, Hains BC, Lo AC, et al. Co-localization of sodium channel Nav1.6 and the sodium-calcium exchanger at sites of axonal injury in the spinal cord in EAE. Brain 2004; 127(Pt 2):294–303.

[81] Agrawal SK, Fehlings MG. Mechanisms of secondary injury to spinal cord axons in vitro: role of Na+, Na(+)-K(+)-ATPase, the Na(+)-H + exchanger, and the Na(+)-Ca2+ exchanger. J Neurosci 1996;16:545–52.

[82] Li S, Jiang Q, Stys PK. Important role of reverse Na(+)-Ca(2+) exchange in spinal cord white matter injury at physiological temperature. J Neurophysiol 2000;84: 1116–9.

[83] Brownell B, Hughes JT. Distribution of plaques in the cerebrum in multiple sclerosis. J Neurol Neurosurg Psychiatry 1962;25:315–20.

[84] Lumsden CE. The neuropathology of multiple sclerosis. In: Vinken PJ, Bruyn GW, editors. Handbook of clinical neurology. Amsterdam: Elsevier Science; 1970. p. 217–309.

[85] Kidd D, Barkhof F, McConnell R, et al. Cortical lesions in multiple sclerosis. Brain 1999; 122:17–26.

[86] Peterson JW, Bo L, Mork S, et al. Transected neurites, apoptotic neurons and reduced inflammation in cortical multiple sclerosis lesions. Ann Neurol 2001;50:389–400.

[87] Bo L, Vedeler CA, Nyland HI, et al. Subpial demyelination n the cerebral cortex of multiple sclerosis patients. J Neuropathol Exp Neurol 2003;62:723–32.

[88] Filippi M. Multiple sclerosis: a white matter disease with associated gray matter damage. J Neurol Sci 2001;185:3–4.

[89] Lucchinetti C, Bruck W, Parisi J, et al. Heterogeneity of multiple sclerosis lesions: implications for the pathogenesis of demyelination. Ann Neurol 2000;47:707–17.

[90] Sharma R, Narayana PA, Wolinsky JS. Grey matter abnormalities in multiple sclerosis: proton magnetic resonance spectroscopic imaging. Mult Scler 2001;7:221–6.

[91] Bo L, Vedeler CA, Nyland H, et al. Intracortical multiple sclerosis lesions are not associated with increased lymphocyte infiltration. Mult Scler 2003;9:323–31.

[92] Hickey WF. Migration of hematogenous cells through the blood-brain barrier and the initiation of CNS inflammation. Brain Pathol 1991;1:97–105.

[93] Lassmann H, Zimprich F, Rossler K, et al. Inflammation in the nervous system. Basic mechanisms and immunological concepts. Rev Neurol 1991;147:763–81.

[94] Perry VH, Andersson PB, Gordon S. Macrophages and inflammation in the central nervous system [review]. Trends Neurosci 1993;16:268–73.

[95] von Andrian UH, Mackay CR. T-cell function and migration. Two sides of the same coin. N Engl J Med 2000;343:1020–34.

[96] Lo D, Feng L, Li L, et al. Integrating innate and adaptive immunity in the whole animal. Immunol Rev 1999;169:225–39.

[97] Alcazar A, Regidor I, Masjuan J, et al. Axonal damage induced by cerebrospinal fluid from patients with relapsing-remitting multiple sclerosis. J Neuroimmunol 2000;104:58–67.
[98] Bornstein MB, Appel SH. Tissue culture studies of demyelination. Ann N Y Acad Sci 1965; 122:280–6.
[99] Ginsberg SD, Martin LJ. Axonal transection in adult rat brain induces transsynaptic apoptosis and persistent atrophy of target neurons. J Neurotrauma 2002;19:99–109.
[100] al Abdulla NA, Martin LJ. Projection neurons and interneurons in the lateral geniculate nucleus undergo distinct forms of degeneration ranging from retrograde and transsynaptic apoptosis to transient atrophy after cortical ablation in rat. Neuroscience 2002; 115:7–14.
[101] Hains BC, Black JA, Waxman SG. Primary cortical motor neurons undergo apoptosis after axotomizing spinal cord injury. J Comp Neurol 2003;462:328–41.
[102] Meyer R, Weissert R, Diem R, et al. Acute neuronal apoptosis in a rat model of multiple sclerosis. J Neurosci 2001;21:6214–20.
[103] al Abdulla NA, Portera-Cailliau C, Martin LJ. Occipital cortex ablation in adult rat causes retrograde neuronal death in the lateral geniculate nucleus that resembles apoptosis. Neuroscience 1998;86:191–209.
[104] Olanow CW, Tatton WG. Etiology and pathogenesis of Parkinson's disease. Annu Rev Neurosci 1999;22:123–44.
[105] Streit WJ, Walter SA, Pennell NA. Reactive microgliosis. Prog Neurobiol 1999;57:563–81.
[106] Gonzalez-Scarano F, Baltuch G. Microglia as mediators of inflammatory and degenerative diseases. Annu Rev Neurosci 1999;22:219–40.
[107] Blinzinger K, Kreutzberg G. Displacement of synaptic terminals from regenerating motor neurons by microglial cells. Z Zellforsch Mikrosk Anat 1968;85:145–57.
[108] Graeber MB, Streit WJ, Kreutzberg GW. Axotomy of the rat facial nerve leads to increased CR3 complement receptor expression by activated microglial cells. J Neurosci Res 1988;21: 18–24.
[109] Haga S, Akai K, Ishii T. Demonstration of microglial cells in and around senile (neuritic) plaques in the Alzheimer brain. An immunohistochemical study using a novel monoclonal antibody. Acta Neuropathol 1989;77:569–75.
[110] McGeer PL, Kawamata T, Walker DG, et al. Microglia in degenerative neurological disease. Glia 1992;7:84–92.
[111] Mochizuki A, Peterson JW, Mufson EJ, Trapp BD. Amyloid load and neural elements in Alzheimer's disease and nondemented individuals with high amyloid plaque density. Exp Neurol 1996;142:89–102.
[112] Breitner JC. The role of anti-inflammatory drugs in the prevention and treatment of Alzheimer's disease. Annu Rev Med 1996;47:401–11.
[113] Combs CK, Johnson DE, Karlo JC, et al. Inflammatory mechanisms in Alzheimer's disease: inhibition of beta- amyloid-stimulated proinflammatory responses and neurotoxicity by PPARgamma agonists. J Neurosci 2000;20:558–67.
[114] Rao SM, Leo GJ, Bernardin L, et al. Cognitive dysfunction in multiple sclerosis. I. Frequency, patterns, and prediction. Neurology 1991;41:685–91.
[115] Beatty WW, Paul RH, Wilbanks SL, et al. Identifying multiple sclerosis patients with mild or global cognitive impairment using the Screening Examination for Cognitive Impairment (SEFCI). Neurology 1995;45:718–23.
[116] Blinkenberg M, Rune K, Jensen CV, et al. Cortical cerebral metabolism correlates with MRI lesion load and cognitive dysfunction in MS. Neurology 2000;54:558–64.
[117] Confavreux C, Vukusic S, Moreau T, et al. Relapses and progression of disability in multiple sclerosis. N Engl J Med 2000;343:1430–8.
[118] Bjartmar C, Trapp BD. Axonal and neuronal degeneration in multiple sclerosis: mechanisms and functional consequences. Curr Opin Neurol 2001;14:271–8.
[119] Lloyd KG. CNS compensation to dopamine neuron loss in Parkinson's disease. Adv Exp Med Biol 1977;90:255–66.

[120] Bradley WG. Recent views on amyotrophic lateral sclerosis with emphasis on electrophysiological studies. Muscle Nerve 1987;10:490–502.

[121] Filippi M, Paty DW, Kappos L, et al. Correlations between changes in disability and T2-weighted brain MRI activity in multiple sclerosis: a follow-up study. Neurology 1995; 45:255–60.

[122] Losseff NA, Wang L, Lai HM, et al. Progressive cerebral atrophy in multiple sclerosis. A serial MRI study. Brain 1996;119:2009–19.

ELSEVIER
SAUNDERS

NEUROLOGIC
CLINICS

Neurol Clin 23 (2005) 131–148

Neuroimaging in Multiple Sclerosis

Anthony Traboulsee, MD, FRCPC[a,*],
Guojun Zhao, MD[a], David K.B. Li, MD, FRCPC[b]

[a]*Division of Neurology, Department of Medicine, The University of British Columbia, Vancouver, British Columbia, Canada*
[b]*Department of Radiology, The University of British Columbia, Vancouver, British Columbia, Canada*

MRI is the dominant neuroimaging modality for multiple sclerosis (MS). The revised diagnostic criteria for MS [1] formally incorporate the common MRI abnormalities found in patients who have MS to enable a timely diagnosis in the absence of a second clinical event in the appropriate clinical setting. Once the diagnosis of MS has been established, the long-term significance of the number and extent of MRI abnormalities for individual patients remains unknown. MRI is suited ideally for evaluating the cycle of dynamic changes in vivo, because it provides full coverage of the central nervous system (CNS) in a reasonable time frame and does not have the safety concerns of radiation exposure. Serial MRI studies demonstrate that new MS lesions occur frequently during periods of apparent clinical stability [2–5]. Correlations with clinical disability are only modest, however, as MRI often detects clinically silent disease activity. The suppression of new gadolinium-enhanced T1-weighted (T1) and newly active T2-weighted (T2) lesions on MRI now are standard outcome measures of efficacy for all clinical trials of putative disease-modifying therapies in MS. This article reviews how conventional and advanced MRI techniques provide important biomarkers of MS pathology and are invaluable for monitoring the pathogenesis of MS, including inflammation, degeneration, and repair. It also considers the role of MRI outcomes in clinical trials and in clinical practice.

* Corresponding author. Department of Medicine, The University of British Columbia, S199-2211 Westbrook Mall, Vancouver, BC V6T 2B5, Canada.
E-mail address: trabouls@interchange.ubc.ca (A. Traboulsee).

0733-8619/05/$ - see front matter
doi:10.1016/j.ncl.2004.10.001 *neurologic.theclinics.com*

Imaging principles

MRI quality and acquisition speed have improved dramatically over the past 2 decades (Fig. 1). Today, most clinical MRI scanners have a magnet field strength of 1.5 tesla (T), a 10-fold increase over that of the early 0.15-T machines. Conventional MRI sequences routinely used on a standard clinical scanner commonly include proton density (PD) and T2 spin echo (SE) in addition to fluid-attenuated inversion recovery (FLAIR) for the identification of the hyperintense lesions and gadolinium-enhanced T1 imaging for identifying new lesion activity.

PD, T2, and FLAIR sequences are extremely sensitive in detecting MS lesions (Fig. 2). There are minor advantages and disadvantages with each technique. PD and T2 images are acquired simultaneously (double echo) with conventional SE techniques. Lesion intensity increases with the longer echo time (TE) of the T2 (TE 80–120 milliseconds) compared with PD (TE 15–40 milliseconds) sequences. Faster acquisition sequences (fast or turbo SE) can miss smaller lesions because of the edge blurring associated with the shorter effective TE. Posterior fossa and spinal cord lesions are seen best on T2 images (Fig. 3) [6]. FLAIR is popular for periventricular and juxtacortical lesion identification because of the excellent suppression of cerebrospinal fluid [7].

T1 imaging is less sensitive for detecting lesions, and those that do appear are hypointense black holes, although it is useful when combined with intravenous gadolinium for detecting lesions that have active inflammation. Gadolinium appears bright on MRI and normally is detected only within blood vessels but not in the brain parenchyma, unless there has been a disruption of the blood-brain barrier (Fig. 4). Higher (triple) doses of gadolinium, longer delays between injecting the gadolinium and acquiring

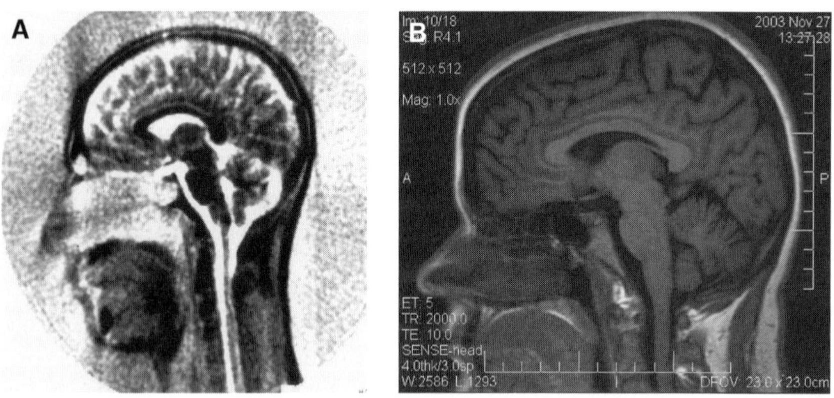

Fig. 1. MR image quality and acquisition speed have improved in the past 2 decades. (*A*) T2-weighted sagittal brain image acquired with a 0.15-T Picker scanner in 1983 at the University of British Columbia. (*B*) T1-weighted sagittal brain image acquired with a 3-T Philips scanner in 2003.

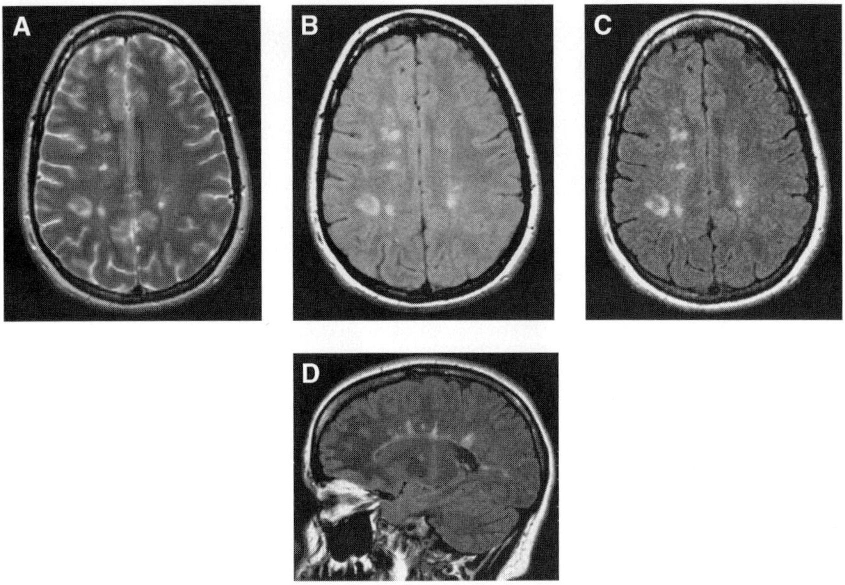

Fig. 2. PD-weighted (*A*), T2-weighted (*B*), and FLAIR (*C*) axial brain images detect MS plaques as hyperintense lesions. T2 images are more sensitive than FLAIR for brainstem and spinal cord lesions. Sagittal FLAIR (*D*) demonstrates lesions in the corpus callosum and the flame-shaped Dawson fingers, which are lesions along subependymal veins. For clinical scans, the Consortium of Multiple Sclerosis Centers MRI working group recommends a slice thickness is 3 mm with no gap and accurate positioning along the subcallosal line.

the postcontrast T1 images, thinner slice, and incorporating a magnetization transfer sequence increase the number of enhancing MS lesions and the intensity of some lesions [8,9].

MRI protocols vary widely across centers making comparison difficult across studies. The clinical MRI protocol recommended by the Consortium of Multiple Sclerosis Centers MRI working group includes sagittal FLAIR, axial FLAIR, and axial PD/T2 using contiguous 3-mm slice thickness with no gap and with accurate repositioning along the subcallosal line [10]. For postcontrast T1 sequences, the recommended dose of gadolinium is 0.1 mmol/kg with a minimum delay of 5 minutes.

Advanced imaging techniques that provide quantitative information about structural changes not readily visible with conventional imaging include magnetization transfer imaging (MTI), quantitative magnetization transfer imaging (qMT), and magnetization transfer ratio (MTR) [11], diffusion-weighted imaging [12], and myelin water imaging [13]. MR spectroscopy (MRS) estimates changes in chemical constituents of lesions and normal-appearing brain tissue (NABT). The ratio of N-acetyl aspartate to creatinine (NAA/Cr) is of particular interest, because NAA is associated primarily with axons and neurons [14]. Functional MRI (fMRI) detects increased blood flow in specific brain regions during the performance of

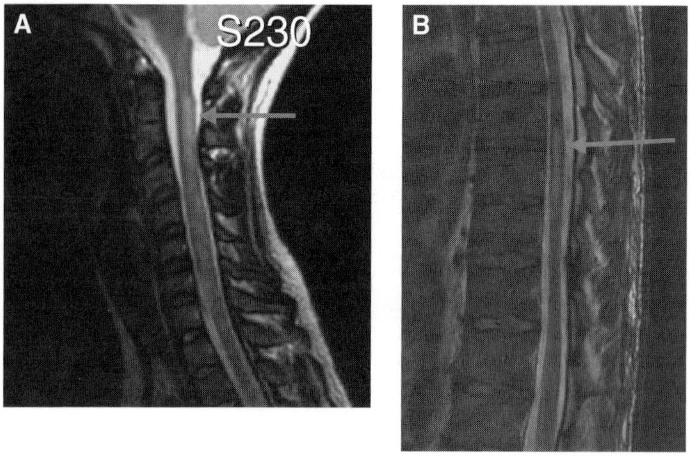

Fig. 3. Sagittal T2-weighted images of MS lesions in the cervical spinal cord.

a simple repetitive task and provides new insight into adaptive mechanisms in response to CNS injury [15]. Most clinical scanners are capable of performing these advanced techniques, and many manufacturers include preprogrammed software packages that perform these functions. These techniques have led to valuable contributions to the understanding of the extent and specificity of MS pathology not readily seen with conventional imaging. Several are being developed for use in clinical trials. Currently,

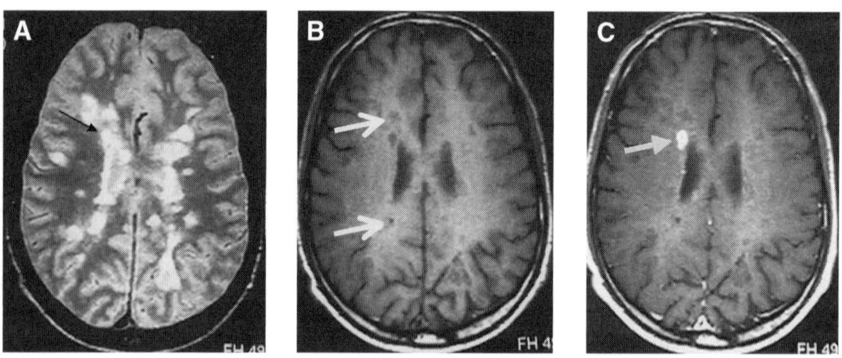

Fig. 4. Axial PD-weighted (*A*) and corresponding Axial T1-weighted brain images before (*B*) and after (*C*) gadolinium injection. T1 images are less sensitive for detecting MS lesions. Gadolinium normally does not appear within the brain parenchyma unless there has been disruption of the blood-brain barrier, such as occurs with acute inflammation in MS. Gadolinium enhancement is transient and usually disappears with 8 weeks. A lesion with persistent gadolinium enhancement beyond 3 months is suspicious for tumor or vascular malformation. T1 hypointense lesions (black holes) that do not enhance include resolving edema (subacute black holes) and severely damaged lesions (chronic black holes). The recommended dose of gadolinium is 0.1 mmol/kg with a minimum delay of 5 minutes.

however, they add little to the diagnostic work-up or ongoing management of individual patients.

Biomarkers of inflammation

The classic MRI appearance of MS is multiple white matter lesions with periventricular predominance on PD/T2 and FLAIR sequences (see Fig. 2). These lesions correlate well with the typical plaques of MS seen on postmortem studies [16]. MS lesions vary in age and in degree of inflammation, gliosis, and axonal loss, despite a similar MRI appearance with T2 imaging. MS lesions are more hydrophilic as a result of loss of myelin lipid and increased water content. They appear as bright T2 lesions because of the longer T2 relaxation times and may appear dark on T1 sequences because of prolonged T1 relaxation times.

MRI is sensitive in detecting most lesions. The sensitivity for smaller lesions can be increased with high field imaging (ie, 3 T and greater) [17]. T2 lesions are not specific, however, for plaque age, degree of myelin loss, amount of inflammation and edema, or the degree of axonal loss [18]. The short T2 relaxation times for lipids make them effectively invisible on conventional MRI. Therefore, the lipid loss resulting from myelin sheath breakdown in demyelination does not contribute directly to the abnormalities seen on MRI. Other pathologies, therefore, such as infarctions, infection, tumors, and inflammation, can produce similar MRI signal changes.

The most common location of MS lesions on MRI is the periventricular region. It is unusual not to see any lesions in this region and it tends to have the heaviest lesion burden within the brain. Lesions often are seen in the corpus callosum, in the temporal lobes, in the brainstem and cerebellum, or at the gray-white matter junction (juxtacortical). Dawson fingers are seen best on sagittal images and refer to the oval, elongated lesions in the corona radiata and the centrum semiovale. These lesions are oriented along subependymal veins that are perpendicular to the walls of the ventricles, representing perivenular inflammation that is a unique pathologic feature of MS (see Fig. 2) [19]. The sagittal image also is useful for demonstrating lesions within the corpus callosum. Approximately 17% of patients who have relapsing-remitting MS (RRMS) have dirty-appearing white matter (DWM); it especially is common adjacent to the occipital horn. These large, diffuse lesions have poorly defined boundaries and extend over several contiguous slices [20]. MTI studies indicate that the degree of tissue abnormalities within DWM seems to be intermediate between NABT and lesions [21]. Occasionally, lesions develop within this region.

A fat suppression technique is required to detect lesions within the optic nerve; thus, the overall incidence of optic nerve lesions is unknown. In one small study, this technique was able to detect optic nerve involvement in 76% of patients; only 4 of the 25 patients had a history of optic neuritis [22].

It is unusual to see the combination of brain and spinal cord lesions in any disease except MS. Spinal cord lesions can be found in 50% to 90% of patients who have MS and are seen most commonly in the cervical cord (see Fig. 3) [23]. These lesions tend to involve in the posterior and lateral regions, occupy less than half the area of the cord on axial images [24], and rarely extend beyond two vertebral segments [25]. Many patients have multiple spinal cord lesions [25].

New disease activity on MRI includes gadolinium-enhancing T1 lesions and new or enlarging T2 lesions, indicating new inflammation. Gadolinium enhancement (see Fig. 4) is transient and can precede new T2 lesions by hours or days [26]. Approximately 30% to 40% of active patients who have RRMS have evidence of gadolinium activity at the time of enrollment in a therapeutic trial [27]. The majority (90%) of patients who have active RRMS have new MRI activity when imaging is performed monthly, and gadolinium detects approximately 88% of that new activity. For 12% of active lesions, however, this is detected only as a new T2 lesion or enlarging pre-existing lesion [28]. A biopsy study of 40 patients correlates these contrast- or gadolinium-enhancing lesions with histopathologic evidence of breakdown of the blood-brain barrier and proinflammatory T-cells infiltrating the brain parenchyma [29]. The enhancement often is more solid and homogeneous with fresh lesions, particularly when they are small. It may appear ring-like, with lesions that are larger and several weeks old. Enhancement usually lasts 4 weeks, with a gradual decline during the following 2 to 4 weeks [30]. In contrast to tumors or vascular lesions, it is unusual for a MS lesion to have gadolinium enhancement beyond 3 months. Gadolinium enhancement is sensitive to steroids and other anti-inflammatory treatments. The majority of new T2 lesions enhance with gadolinium, and pre-existing T2 lesions also can enhance, indicating new activity. In general, newly enhancing lesions are seen twice as often as new T2 activity (new or enlarging T2 lesions) (Fig. 5).

New and enlarging T2 lesions also represent new disease activity as a result of inflammation. The lesions increase in size during the acute phase, mostly because of the edema associated with inflammatory infiltrates, expanding the extracellular space around the lesions. Within 4 weeks, the lesions reach their maximum size [5]. The process is self-limiting, and the lesions slowly decrease in size over the next 6 to 8 weeks as edema resolves and remyelination occurs. Most new T2 lesions leave a smaller residual T2 lesion [31]. Thus, the size of an acute T2 lesion may overestimate the extent of the damage because of the reversible edema associated with the new inflammation compared with a similarly sized stable, chronic T2 lesion. Approximately 90% of patients who have active RRMS demonstrate new T2 activity with annual or biannual imaging [27]. There is enormous variability among individuals, some showing no new lesions and others having up to 75 or more new lesions [32]. On average, patients who have MS develop 4 new T2 lesions per year [33].

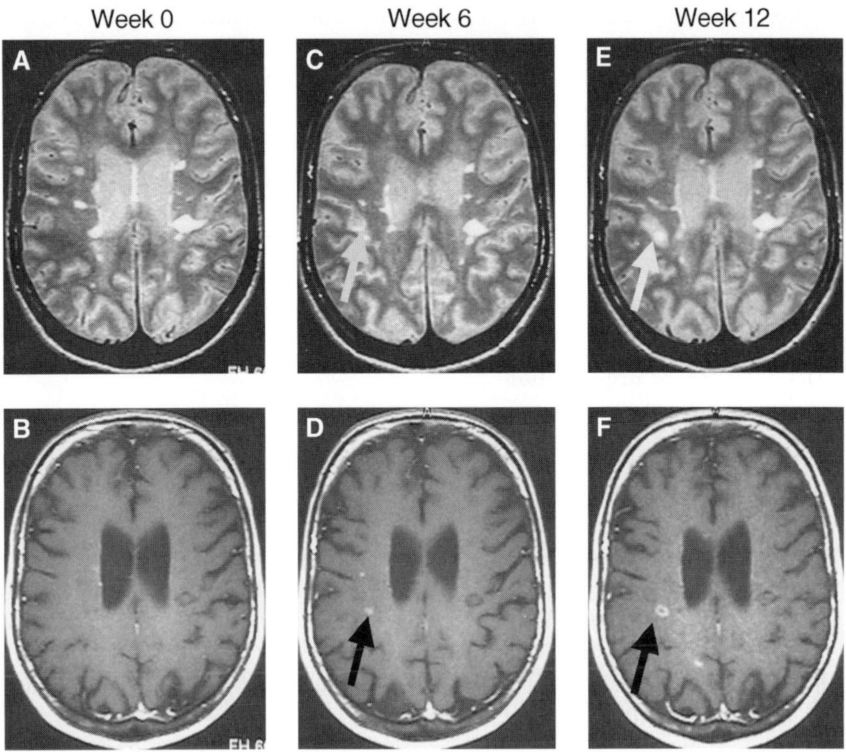

Fig. 5. Biomarkers of inflammation include gadolinium-enhancing lesions and new and enlarging T2 lesions. 3 sets of images collected serially 6 weeks apart. Top row are PD weighted axial images (*A,C,E*) and bottom row are corresponding post gadolinium T1 weighted images (*B,D,F*). 2 new gadolinium enhancing lesions are seen at week 6, one of which is still enhancing at week 12 (black arrow). Gadolinium enhancement can accompany a new T2 lesion (red arrow) or occur in pre-existing T2 lesions. T2 lesions can also enlarge as a marker of new inflammation (yellow arrow). For interpretation of the references to color in this figure legend, the reader is referred to the web version of the article.

Reactivation of pre-existing T2 lesions is common and can be detected with re-enhancement with gadolinium, enlargement on T2 imaging, or both. Eventually, adjacent lesions fuse and several small lesions may end up forming a large confluent lesion [34]. The net accumulation of new and enlarging lesions increases the total T2 volume or burden of disease (T2 BOD) by 5% to 10% annually [35], although some patients may experience a net decrease because of the resolving edema associated with large lesions.

Conventional MRI does not necessarily detect all new inflammatory activity. Cortical plaques also are common and, currently, not easily detected with conventional MRI techniques [36]. These lesions have a similar signal intensity as the gray matter and often are missed with conventional MRI [37]. FLAIR sequences currently are preferred for the detection of cortical lesions [38]. The tight junctions responsible for the maintenance of the blood-brain barrier integrity are impaired in the normal-appearing white matter (NAWM) and provide a route for subtle leakage of inflammatory cells [39]. There also are subtle changes that develop in the NAWM months before the development of a new gadolinium-enhancing or T2 lesion that can be detected with MTI [40,41]. Functional imaging techniques capable of labeling specific cell receptors or cell types can detect microglial proliferation within active lesions using positron emission tomography [42,43], and the migration of magnetic labeled T cells can be tracked with conventional MRI [44]. These techniques may provide additional sensitivity and specificity for detecting and quantifying inflammation occurring within lesions and in the NABT.

MRI measures of degeneration

The damage induced by inflammation in MS is not restricted to the myelin sheath. Axonal loss is a common finding in postmortem studies within acute and chronic MS lesions and also throughout the NAWM [45]. The pathologic basis of progressive and irreversible disability in MS most likely is the result of the extent of axonal damage [46].

On the accompanying unenhanced T1 image, some T2 lesions appear hypointense or as so-called T1 "black holes" (see Fig. 4). A proportion of these black holes are acute lesions that enhance when gadolinium is given and almost half of these resolve slowly over months [47]. Thus, chronic black holes can be defined as T2 lesions that are nonenhancing and hypointense T1 lesions, that persist for a minimum of 6 months after their first appearance, and that have a signal intensity on T1 images less than or equal to that of gray matter. The chronic T1 hypointense black holes are associated with a lower concentration of NAA using MRS. This correlates pathologically

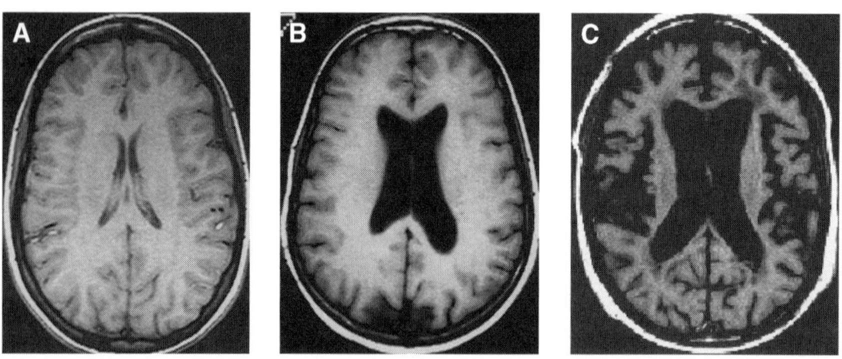

Fig. 6. Cerebral atrophy is common and progressive in MS. It can be detected at the time of a single attack of demyelination. It represents the final common pathway of global degeneration due to axonal loss, myelin loss, and gliosis. (*A*) Axial T1 weighted image at the level of the lateral ventricles in a normal 42 year old volunteer. (*B*) (*C*) Images from the same level for 2 MS patients demonstrating moderate (*B*) to severe (*C*) atrophy with enlargement of the lateral ventricles, widening of sulci, and loss of brain parenchyma.

with greater tissue destruction and axonal loss [48] compared with chronic, stable T2 lesions without a corresponding T1 black hole. Furthermore, these lesions may have a better correlation with clinical disability because of their greater pathologic specificity for severe axonal loss [49].

Brain and spinal cord atrophy was recognized post mortem in patients who had MS before the widely available neuroimaging techniques (Fig. 6). It is likely that atrophy is the result of axonal loss, in addition to myelin loss, and shrinkage resulting from gliosis. Global brain atrophy, therefore, is another important measure of the neurodegenerative component of MS [50]. Atrophy is more common and severe in secondary progressive MS (SPMS) [51]. It should be appreciated that atrophy can be detected even after a single attack of demyelination in patients who have only a small number of T2 lesions [52]. These early patients also have abnormalities throughout the NAWM, including decreased MTR values [53], and may have decreased NAA/Cr compared with healthy age-matched control patients [54], suggesting that significant tissue loss and irreversible axonal loss occur early in the disease course. Cerebral and spinal cord atrophy in MS are progressive and changes can be detected after 1 year. The annual rate of cerebral atrophy is approximately 0.6% to 0.8%, which is 2 to 3 times the rate in the normal population [55–57]. This equates to a loss of approximately 20 mL of brain tissue per year and an annual increase in ventricle size of 1.6 mL, which is 5 times the rate of control patients [58].

In general, correlations between global atrophy measures and disability have been modest [50], even though it is believed to be the common final pathway of neurodegeneration in MS. The Kurtzke EDSS measures correlate better with cervical cord atrophy ($r = -0.7$) [59], reflecting the inherent bias of this clinical scale for mobility-related disability. At a mildly impaired expanded disability status scale (EDSS) of 3, the average cord area was reduced by 12%, whereas at a severe level of disability (EDSS of 8), the average cord area was reduced by 35%.

Brain volume changes are complex and may be affected by inflammation, edema, and hydration; the use of high-dose intravenous steroids for an acute clinical relapse temporarily can decrease brain volumes [60]. The degree of brain atrophy can be explained only partly by the severity of other MRI abnormalities, individually or combined, including total T2 BOD, T1 black holes, and gadolinium-enhanced lesional activity [61–63], possibly indicating that the pathologic mechanisms leading to progressive tissue loss and atrophy are partially independent of the mechanisms underlying lesion formation.

Pathologically, the damage inflicted by MS is not restricted to plaques; low levels of inflammatory infiltrates, gliosis, and axonal loss can be seen in nonlesional brain tissue. On conventional MRI, however, that damage is not readily apparent in the NAWM and normal-appearing gray matter (NAGM) except as generalized atrophy. MTI can detect global decreases in MTR histogram values throughout the NAWM [64] and NAGM [65], indicating a loss of complex tissues, including myelin. These NAWM MTR abnormalities are more severe with advanced disease, as seen in populations that have SPMS. MRS, despite its limited resolution, also has been used to detect significant decreases in NAA/Cr ratios in NAWM. These abnormalities, representing axonal loss, also are progressive [66].

Repair mechanisms and functional adaptation

The gadolinium enhancement associated with new lesion activity is a transient event, reflecting a self-limiting inflammatory process with restoration of the blood-brain barrier. There is resolution of edema in the acute inflammatory lesion, evidenced by the decrease in the size of the T2 lesion and the disappearing acute and subacute T1 black holes. In new lesions that have a significant decrease of NAA, there may be a partial recovery of that signal, suggesting that a component of NAA loss represents axonal dysfunction rather than axonal transection. Similar recovery also has been seen with MTR measures, probably reflecting remyelination and resolution of edema. Myelin water imaging is a potential tool for monitoring remyelination in the recovering lesion [67].

The lack of a strong correlation between the extent of MRI abnormalities and clinical disability may be explained in part by adaptive mechanisms within the CNS. fMRI detects increased blood flow to an area of cortex associated with repetitive motor or cognitive tasks. Several groups have found that patients who have MS activate larger areas of cortex than age-matched control patients for simple tasks, such as finger tapping. The extent of the increase in fMRI activity correlates well with the degree of axonal loss, as measured by NAA [68]. Furthermore, these adaptive changes can be detected early in the disease course, after a single attack of demyelination [69]. Patients who have MS and who have low levels of fMRI activation performed poorly in a series of cognitive tests compared with patients who were able to activate large areas of cortex [70]. This suggests that not only are these adaptive mechanisms critical for maintaining function but also there may be a limited threshold beyond which recruitment is no longer possible.

Role of MRI outcomes in clinical trials

Clinical trials rely on objective outcome measures that reflect some aspect of the disease and that change within a short period of time. Over the past decade, MRI measures have become established as important outcomes in all phases of clinical drug development and for the final approval of these therapies. MRI can measure many aspects of the pathogenesis of MS, including inflammation and degeneration. These measures serve as valuable biomarkers of MS pathology. A limitation, however, is that the MRI outcomes are only weak predictors of future clinical outcome for individual patients and, appropriately, remain as secondary outcomes of efficacy for phase III studies.

Early studies focused on the inflammatory aspects of the disease, including clinical relapses and new MRI activity (gadolinium-enhancing lesions and enlarging T2 and new T2 lesions). In the RRMS studies, the high-dose, high-frequency interferon-β treatment suppressed more than 80% of new MRI activity and prevented any significant accumulation of annual T2 burden [28,71–73]. The reduction in clinical relapses was only a modest 33%, however, with perhaps an even lesser impact on preventing progression of disability in the short-term follow-up. In several of the SPMS clinical trials, the significant benefit seen in MRI outcomes was accompanied by a disappointing lack of clinical benefit in terms of preventing progressive disability [74]. Other SPMS studies have demonstrated that suppressing new lesions on MRI does not necessarily prevent progressive cerebral atrophy, which may be a useful outcome measure for future studies in this population [75].

Standard and exploratory MRI measures can be quantified easily and blinded for analysis at a central MRI reading center. The common MRI measures used in clinical trials include gadolinium-enhancing lesions, T2 lesions, T1 hypointense lesion volume, and brain volumes. These have been standardized for multicenter studies using clinical MRI scanners that vary in field strength, by manufacturer, and in software and local expertise. Exploratory MRI measures, such as MRS, which measures whole brain or single voxel NAA/Cr, and MTI, are more difficult to standardize and use in multicenter studies. These advanced techniques rely on local expertise and are sensitive to scanner software changes that occur often during a 2-year clinical trial.

Many putative therapies for treating MS are studied initially for their impact on suppressing the MRI measures of inflammation (gadolinium-enhancing lesions and active T2 lesions) as a proof of concept before committing to larger, more expensive phase III studies of clinical efficacy. This can be achieved within 6 months or possibly a shorter period of time with small sample sizes. To detect significant changes in neurodegenerative measures, however, such as brain and spinal cord atrophy, MTR histograms of NABT, and MRS of NAWM, a study would require a longer duration (1 to 3 years depending on the measure) with a larger population. Furthermore, demonstrating that brain or spinal cord atrophy does not occur with any therapy alone is insufficient and also would require validation against a clinical meaningful outcome, such as preventing the progression of disability.

Role of MRI in monitoring individual patients

The MRI measures of the greatest practical use for monitoring individual patients remain gadolinium-enhancing lesions, new T2 lesions, and estimates of total lesion burden in the brain and spinal cord. These features are helpful, although not required, for establishing the diagnosis of MS. For patients who have had a single attack of demyelination and go on to have definite MS, the baseline number, volume of lesions, and rate of increase of total lesion volume over 5 years have some prognostic value for future disability [76]. A normal early scan seems to predict a more benign course. With regard to clinical outcome, there is enormous variability among individuals, regardless of their early MRI findings.

In general, MRI measures rarely are used for prognosis in MS because of the poor correlation with clinical outcome measures and the poor predictive value of short-term studies. For patients who have established MS, the predictive value of new MRI lesions for short-term clinical outcomes, such as relapses and disability, remains poor [77]. A meta-analysis by Filippi et al [78] of 281 patients who had MS found a significant, but weak, correlation between the development of new or enlarging T2 lesions over 2 to 3 years and worsening EDSS. It is possible that with a longer follow-up, these correlations could improve.

There are several explanations for the poor correlation with clinical scales of disability. One advantage of MRI is detecting lesions in the absence of clinical symptoms. The factors that determine neurologic expression are a combination of location, intensity, and nature of pathology in the active lesion. Most new MRI lesions are clinically silent and patients who have RRMS have 5 to 10 silent MRI attacks for every clinical relapse they experience [79,80]. A small lesion in the spinal cord has a greater clinical impact than a similar lesion in the cerebrum. The severity of the pathologic process in that lesion affects the severity of the symptoms expressed and may explain the stronger correlation between chronic black holes and EDSS. Lesions that occur in the frontal or temporal lobes and atrophy of the corpus callosum correlate well with cognitive dysfunction that is not reflected by the EDSS [81–83]. Patients who have MS for more than 15 years and a low EDSS (<3.5) may not necessarily have benign disease since they could have significant cognitive dysfunction. The capacity of the CNS to adapt to injury also has an impact on the correlation between MRI measures and clinical function.

Individual MRI measures correlate only modestly with disability. To improve the correlation and predictive value of MRI with clinical outcomes, MRI measures of inflammation and neurodegeneration can be combined [84]. The improvement in correlations with EDSS, however, still remains modest when MRI outcomes, including T2 burden, atrophy, and NABT MTR, are combined [64]. In part, this reflects the limited nature of clinical scales, such as the EDSS, which does not quantify all aspects of clinical dysfunction. It also reflects the fact that many T2 lesions and NABT abnormalities are clinically silent and do not contribute directly to the disability, whereas functional reorganization minimizes the impact that lesions have on clinical disability.

Applying the results obtained from group or population outcomes from clinical trials to treatment decisions for individual patients remains unproven. Most, but not all, new MRI activity can be suppressed with some treatments, especially high-dose, high-frequency interferons. Of patients who took high-dose interferon, however, 69% still had evidence of new T2 activity when scanned biannually for 2 years, albeit considerably less activity than that seen in the placebo group [28]. A small percentage of patients who took placebo did not have any new lesions, and a significant proportion did not have any significant increase in overall T2 burden after 2 years. A stable MRI does not necessarily indicate a clinical stable patient, nor does an active MRI predict a poor short-term clinical outcome. The individual variation in the response to treatment, with a similar spread in responses in those who took placebo and in those who were treated, makes it difficult to use MRI for monitoring treatment response outside of clinical trials.

Most clinicians agree that MRI is biomarker for the pathology of MS. Thus, new MRI activity reflects active inflammation, and the accumulation of T2 burden, chronic black holes, and progressive brain and spinal cord atrophy reflect worsening degeneration irrespective of the clinical status. Validation with long-term, meaningful clinical outcomes still is required before any of these MRI measures can be used and applied in the management of individual patients and selection of treatments. Some of this information will come from several important long-term follow-up studies of patients who were enrolled in the early pivotal studies. Some of these early studies were conducted before gadolinium was available, however, and there have been dramatic technologic improvements that may make it difficult to quantify the degree of brain atrophy accurately. Nonetheless, they will provide valuable insight into the prognostic value of early MRI findings in a well-defined population of patients.

Summary

MRI is a safe and invaluable technique for monitoring and understanding the pathology of MS in vivo from the earliest stage of the disease. In the past 2 decades, it has been discovered that a considerable amount of new disease activity occurs in the absence of clinical symptoms in patients who otherwise would be classified as in remission. Advanced techniques and pathologic correlations have improved the understanding of the extent of disease in otherwise NABT and demonstrated that irreversible axonal loss and atrophy can occur early in the disease course. This may be an important outcome for new therapies. A variety of conventional and advanced MRI techniques provides unique and complementary insight into the central mechanisms underlying MS pathogenesis, including inflammation, degeneration, repair, and adaptation. Some, but not all, MRI techniques are standardized easily with routine clinical MRI scanners and can be used in multicenter therapeutic trials. The limited clinical correlation reflects, in part, the unique sensitivity of MRI in detecting clinically silent disease. Applying the results obtained from group or population outcomes from clinical trials to making treatment decisions for individual patients remains unproved. The poor correlation between clinical status and MRI measures and the yet-to-be-proved long-term prognostic value of MRI limit its use for monitoring treatment response in individual patients. The next decade will bring continued technologic advances in the development of MRI scanners, advanced image processing tools, and a better understanding of the development and treatment of MS.

References

[1] McDonald WI, Compston A, Edan G, et al. Recommended diagnostic criteria for multiple sclerosis: guidelines from the International Panel on the diagnosis of multiple sclerosis. Ann Neurol 2001;50:121–7.

[2] Harris JO, Frank JA, Patronas N, et al. Serial gadolinium-enhanced magnetic resonance imaging scans in patients with early, relapsing-remitting multiple sclerosis: implications for clinical trials and natural history. Ann Neurol 1991;29:548–55.

[3] Isaac C, Li DKB, Genton M, et al. Multiple sclerosis: a serial study using MRI in relapsing patients. Neurol 1988;38:1511–5.

[4] McFarland HF, Frank JA, Albert PS, et al. Using gadolinium-enhanced magnetic resonance imaging lesions to monitor disease activity in multiple sclerosis. Ann Neurol 1992;32:758–66.

[5] Willoughby EW, Grochowski E, Li DKB, et al. Serial magnetic resonance scanning in multiple sclerosis: a second prospective study in relapsing patients. Ann Neurol 1989;25: 43–9.

[6] Gawne-Cain ML, O'Riordan JI, Thompson AJ, et al. Multiple sclerosis lesion detection in the brain: a comparison of fast fluid-attenuated inversion recovery and conventional T2-weighted dual spin echo. Neurology 1997;49:364–70.

[7] Rydberg JN, Riederer SJ, Rydberg CH, et al. Contrast optimization of fluid-attenuated inversion recovery (FLAIR) imaging. Magn Reson Med 1995;34:868–77.

[8] Filippi M, Yousry T, Campi A, et al. Comparison of triple dose versus standard dose gadolinium-DTPA for detection of MRI enhancing lesions in patients with MS. Neurology 1996;46:379–84.

[9] Silver NC, Good CD, Barker GJ, et al. Sensitivity of contrast enhanced MRI in multiple sclerosis. Effects of gadolinium dose, magnetization transfer contrast and delayed imaging. Brain 1997;120(Pt 7):1149–61.

[10] Consortium of Multiple Sclerosis Centers. Available at: http://www.mscare.org/. Accessed November, 2004.

[11] Ostuni JL, Richert ND, Lewis BK, et al. Characterization of differences between multiple sclerosis and normal brain: a global magnetization transfer application. AJNR Am J Neuroradiol 1999;20:501–7.

[12] Ciccarelli O, Werring DJ, Wheeler-Kingshott CAM, et al. Investigation of MS normal-appearing brain using diffusion tensor MRI with clinical correlations. Neurology 2001;56: 926–33.

[13] Whittall KP, MacKay AL, Li DK, et al. Normal-appearing white matter in multiple sclerosis has heterogeneous, diffusely prolonged T(2). Magn Reson Med 2002;47:403–8.

[14] De Stefano N, Narayanan S, Francis SJ, et al. Diffuse axonal and tissue injury in patients with multiple sclerosis with low cerebral lesion load and no disability. Arch Neurol 2002;59: 1565–71.

[15] Cifelli A, Matthews PM. Cerebral plasticity in multiple sclerosis: insights from fMRI. Mult Scler 2002;8:193–9.

[16] Stewart WA, Hall LD, Berry K, et al. Magnetic resonance imaging (MRI) in multiple sclerosis (MS): pathological correlation studies in eight cases. Neurology 1986;36(Suppl 1):320.

[17] Keiper MD, Grossman RI, Hirsch JA, et al. MR identification of white matter abnormalities in multiple sclerosis: a comparison between 1.5 T and 4 T. AJNR Am J Neuroradiol 1998;19: 1489–93.
[18] Barnes D, Munro PM, Youl BD, et al. The longstanding MS lesion. A quantitative MRI and electron microscopic study. Brain 1991;114:1271–80.
[19] Horowitz AL, Kaplan RD, Grewe G, et al. The ovoid lesion: a new MR observation in patients with multiple sclerosis. AJNR Am J Neuroradiol 1989;10:303–5.
[20] Zhao GJ, Li DK, Wang XY, et al. MRI of dirty-appearing white matter in MS. Neurology 2000;54:A121.
[21] Ge Y, Grossman RI, Babb JS, et al. Dirty-appearing white matter in multiple sclerosis: volumetric MR imaging and magnetization transfer ratio histogram analysis. AJNR Am J Neuroradiol 2003;24:1935–40.
[22] Davies MB, Williams R, Haq N, et al. MRI of optic nerve and postchiasmal visual pathways and visual evoked potentials in secondary progressive multiple sclerosis. Neuroradiology 1998;40:765–70.
[23] Bot JC, Barkhof F, Lycklama a Nijeholt G, et al. Differentiation of multiple sclerosis from other inflammatory disorders and cerebrovascular disease: value of spinal MR imaging. Radiology 2002;223:46–56.
[24] Thielen KR, Miller GM. Multiple sclerosis of the spinal cord: magnetic resonance appearance. J Comput Assist Tomogr 1996;20:434–8.
[25] Tartaglino LM, Friedman DP, Flanders AE, et al. Multiple sclerosis in the spinal cord: MR appearance and correlation with clinical parameters. Radiology 1995;195:725–32.
[26] Miller DH, Rudge P, Johnson G, et al. Serial gadolinium enhanced magnetic resonance imaging in multiple sclerosis. Brain 1988;111:927–39.
[27] Miller DH, Khan OA, Sheremata WA, et al. A controlled trial of natalizumab for relapsing multiple sclerosis. N Engl J Med 2003;348:15–23.
[28] Li DK, Paty DW. Magnetic resonance imaging results of the PRISMS trial: a randomized, double-blind, placebo-controlled study of interferon-beta1a in relapsing-remitting multiple sclerosis. Prevention of Relapses and Disability by Interferon-beta1a Subcutaneously in Multiple Sclerosis. Ann Neurol 1999;46:197–206.
[29] Nesbit GM, Forbes GS, Scheithauer BW, et al. Multiple sclerosis: histopathologic and MR and/or CT correlation in 37 cases at biopsy and three cases at autopsy. Radiology 1991;180: 467–74.
[30] Kermode AG, Tofts PS, Thompson AJ, et al. Heterogeneity of blood-brain barrier changes in multiple sclerosis: an MRI study with gadolinium-DTPA enhancement. Neurology 1990; 40:229–35.
[31] Koopmans RA, Li DKB, Oger JJF, et al. The lesion of multiple sclerosis: Imaging of acute and chronic stages. Neurology 1989;39:959–63.
[32] The Once Weekly Interferon for MS Study Group. Evidence of interferon beta-1a dose response in relapsing-remitting MS: the OWIMS Study. Neurology 1999;53: 679–86.
[33] Paty DW. Magnetic resonance imaging in the assessment of disease activity in multiple sclerosis. Can J Neurol Sci 1988;15:266–72.
[34] Koopmans RA, Li DKB, Grochowski E, Cutler PJ, Paty DW. Benign versus chronic progressive multiple sclerosis: magnetic resonance imaging features. Ann Neurol 1989;25: 74–81.
[35] Paty DW, Li DK, Oger JJ, et al. Magnetic resonance imaging in the evaluation of clinical trials in multiple sclerosis. Ann Neurol 1994;36(Suppl):S95–6.
[36] Peterson JW, Bö L, Mörk S, et al. Transected neurites, apoptotic neurons, and reduced inflammation in cortical multiple sclerosis lesions. Ann Neurol 2001;50:389–400.
[37] Kidd D, Barkhof F, McConnell R, et al. Cortical lesions in multiple sclerosis. Brain 1999; 122:17–26.

[38] Boggild MD, Williams R, Haq N, Hawkins CP. Cortical plaques visualised by fluid-attenuated inversion recovery imaging in relapsing multiple sclerosis. Neuroradiology 1996; 38(Suppl 1):S10–3.
[39] Plumb J, McQuaid S, Mirakhur M, et al. Abnormal endothelial tight junctions in active lesions and normal-appearing white matter in multiple sclerosis. Brain Pathol 2002;12: 154–69.
[40] Filippi M, Rocca MA, Martino G, et al. Magnetization transfer changes in the normal appearing white matter precede the appearance of enhancing lesions in patients with multiple sclerosis. Ann Neurol 1998;43:809–14.
[41] Pike GB, De Stefano N, Narayanan S, et al. Multiple sclerosis: magnetization transfer MR imaging of white matter before lesion appearance on T2-weighted images. Radiology 2000; 215:824–30.
[42] Banati RB, Newcombe J, Gunn RN, et al. The peripheral benzodiazepine binding site in the brain in multiple sclerosis: quantitative in vivo imaging of microglia as a measure of disease activity. Brain 2000;123:2321–37.
[43] Debruyne JC, Versijpt J, Van Laere KJ, et al. PET visualization of microglia in multiple sclerosis patients using [11C]PK11195. Eur J Neurol 2003;10:257–64.
[44] Anderson SA, Shukaliak-Quandt J, Jordan EK, et al. Magnetic resonance imaging of labeled T-cells in a mouse model of multiple sclerosis. Ann Neurol 2004;55:654–9.
[45] Trapp BD, Peterson J, Ransohoff RM, et al. Axonal transection in the lesions of multiple sclerosis. N Engl J Med 1998;338:278–85.
[46] McDonald WI, Ron MA. Multiple sclerosis: the disease and its manifestations. Philos Trans R Soc Lond B Biol Sci 1999;354:1615–22.
[47] Bagnato F, Jeffries N, Richert ND, et al. Evolution of T1 black holes in patients with multiple sclerosis imaged monthly for 4 years. Brain 2003;126:1782–9.
[48] van Walderveen MA, Barkhof F, Pouwels PJ, et al. Neuronal damage in T1-hypointense multiple sclerosis lesions demonstrated in vivo using proton magnetic resonance spectroscopy. Ann Neurol 1999;46:79–87.
[49] Truyen L, van Waesberghe JH, van Walderveen MA, et al. Accumulation of hypointense lesions ("black holes") on T1 spin-echo MRI correlates with disease progression in multiple sclerosis. Neurology 1996;47:1469–76.
[50] Miller DH, Barkhof F, Frank JA, et al. Measurement of atrophy in multiple sclerosis: pathological basis, methodological aspects and clinical relevance. Brain 2002;125: 1676–95.
[51] van Walderveen MA, Barkhof F, Tas MW, et al. Patterns of brain magnetic resonance abnormalities on T2-weighted spin echo images in clinical subgroups of multiple sclerosis: a large cross-sectional study. Eur Neurol 1998;40:91–8.
[52] Brex PA, Jenkins R, Fox NC, et al. Detection of ventricular enlargement in patients at the earliest clinical stage of MS. Neurology 2000;54:1689–91.
[53] Traboulsee A, Dehmeshki J, Brex PA, et al. Normal-appearing brain tissue MTR histograms in clinically isolated syndromes suggestive of MS. Neurology 2002;59:126–8.
[54] Tourbah A, Stievenart JL, Abanou A, et al. Normal-appearing white matter in optic neuritis and multiple sclerosis: a comparative proton spectroscopy study. Neuroradiology 1999;41: 738–43.
[55] Fox NC, Jenkins R, Leary SM, et al. Progressive cerebral atrophy in MS: a serial study using registered, volumetric MRI. Neurology 2000;54:807–12.
[56] Rudick RA, Fisher E, Lee JC, et al. Use of the brain parenchymal fraction to measure whole brain atrophy in relapsing-remitting MS. Multiple Sclerosis Collaborative Research Group. Neurology 1999;53:1698–704.
[57] Rovaris M, Comi G, Rocca MA, et al. Short-term brain volume change in relapsing-remitting multiple sclerosis: Effect of glatiramer acetate and implications. Brain 2001;124: 1803–12.

[58] Ge Y, Grossman RI, Udupa JK, et al. Brain atrophy in relapsing-remitting multiple sclerosis and secondary progressive multiple sclerosis: longitudinal quantitative analysis. Radiology 2000;214:665–70.
[59] Losseff NA, Webb SL, O'Riordan JI, et al. Spinal cord atrophy and disability in multiple sclerosis. A new reproducible and sensitive MRI method with potential to monitor disease progression. Brain 1996;119:701–8.
[60] Hoogervorst EL, Polman CH, Barkhof F. Cerebral volume changes in multiple sclerosis patients treated with high-dose intravenous methylprednisolone. Mult Scler 2002;8:415–9.
[61] Losseff NA, Wang L, Lai HM, et al. Progressive cerebral atrophy in multiple sclerosis. A serial MRI study. Brain 1996;119:2009–19.
[62] Paolillo A, Pozzilli C, Gasperini C, et al. Brain atrophy in relapsing-remitting multiple sclerosis: relationship with 'black holes', disease duration and clinical disability. J Neurol Sci 2000;174:85–91.
[63] Zivadinov R, Zorzon M. Is gadolinium enhancement predictive of the development of brain atrophy in multiple sclerosis? A review of the literature. J Neuroimaging 2002;12:302–9.
[64] Traboulsee A, Dehmeshki J, Peters KR, et al. Disability in multiple sclerosis is related to normal appearing brain tissue MTR histogram abnormalities. Mult Scler 2003;9:566–73.
[65] Ge Y, Grossman RI, Udupa JK, et al. Magnetization transfer ratio histogram analysis of normal-appearing gray matter and normal-appearing white matter in multiple sclerosis. J Comput Assist Tomogr 2002;26:62–8.
[66] De Stefano N, Matthews PM, Fu L, et al. Axonal damage correlates with disability in patients with relapsing-remitting multiple sclerosis. Results of a longitudinal magnetic resonance spectroscopy study. Brain 1998;121:1469–77.
[67] MacKay A, Whittall K, Adler J, et al. In vivo visualization of myelin water in brain by magnetic resonance. Magn Reson Med 1994;31:673–7.
[68] Reddy H, Narayanan S, Arnoutelis R, et al. Evidence for adaptive functional changes in the cerebral cortex with axonal injury from multiple sclerosis. Brain 2000;123(Pt 11): 2314–20.
[69] Filippi M, Rocca MA, Mezzapesa DM, et al. Simple and complex movement-associated functional MRI changes in patients at presentation with clinically isolated syndromes suggestive of multiple sclerosis. Hum Brain Mapp 2004;21:108–17.
[70] Mainero C, Caramia F, Pozzilli C, et al. fMRI evidence of brain reorganization during attention and memory tasks in multiple sclerosis. Neuroimage 2004;21:858–67.
[71] Anonymous. Randomised double-blind placebo-controlled study of interferon beta-1a in relapsing/remitting multiple sclerosis. PRISMS (Prevention of Relapses and Disability by Interferon beta-1a Subcutaneously in Multiple Sclerosis) Study Group. Lancet 1998;352: 1498–504.
[72] Paty DW, Li DKB. Interferon beta-1b is effective in relapsing-remitting multiple sclerosis. II. MRI analysis results of a multicenter, randomized, double-blind, placebo-controlled trial. UBC MS/MRI Study Group and the IFNB Multiple Sclerosis Study Group. Neurology 1993;43:662–7.
[73] The IFNB Multiple Sclerosis Study Group. Interferon beta-1b is effective in relapsing-remitting multiple sclerosis. I. Clinical results of a multicenter, randomized, double-blind, placebo-controlled trial. Neurology 1993;43:655–61.
[74] SPECTRIMS Study Group. Randomized controlled trial of interferon-beta-1a in secondary progressive MS: clinical results. Neurology 2001;56:1496–504.
[75] Molyneux PD, Kappos L, Polman C, et al. The effect of interferon beta-1b treatment on MRI measures of cerebral atrophy in secondary progressive multiple sclerosis. European Study Group on Interferon beta-1b in secondary progressive multiple sclerosis. Brain 2000; 123(Pt 11):2256–63.
[76] Brex PA, Ciccarelli O, O'Riordan JI, et al. A longitudinal study of abnormalities on MRI and disability from multiple sclerosis. N Engl J Med 2002;346:158–64.

[77] Kappos L, Moeri D, Radue EW, et al. Predictive value of gadolinium-enhanced magnetic resonance imaging for relapse rate and changes in disability or impairment in multiple sclerosis: a meta-analysis. Gadolinium MRI Meta-analysis Group. Lancet 1999;353:964–9.
[78] Filippi M, Paty DW, Kappos L, et al. Correlations between changes in disability and T2-weighted brain MRI activity in multiple sclerosis: a follow-up study. Neurology 1995;45: 255–60.
[79] Smith ME, Stone LA, Albert PS, et al. Clinical worsening in multiple sclerosis is associated with increased frequency and area of gadopentetate dimeglumine-enhancing magnetic resonance imaging lesions. Ann Neurol 1993;33:480–9.
[80] Thorpe JW, Kidd D, Moseley IF, et al. Serial gadolinium-enhanced MRI of the brain and spinal cord in early relapsing-remitting multiple sclerosis. Neurology 1996;46:373–8.
[81] Damian MS, Schilling G, Bachmann G, et al. White matter lesions and cognitive deficits: relevance of lesion pattern? Acta Neurol Scand 1994;90:430–6.
[82] Edwards SG, Liu C, Blumhardt LD. Cognitive correlates of supratentorial atrophy on MRI in multiple sclerosis. Acta Neurol Scand 2001;104:214–23.
[83] Pozzilli C, Fieschi C, Perani D, et al. Relationship between corpus callosum atrophy and cerebral metabolic asymmetries in multiple sclerosis. J Neurol Sci 1992;112:51–7.
[84] Wolinsky JS, Narayana PA, Noseworthy JH, et al. Linomide in relapsing and secondary progressive MS: part II: MRI results. MRI Analysis Center of the University of Texas-Houston, Health Science Center, and the North American Linomide Investigators. Neurology 2000;54:1734–41.

ELSEVIER
SAUNDERS

Neurol Clin 23 (2005) 149–175

NEUROLOGIC
CLINICS

Immunology of Multiple Sclerosis

Amit Bar-Or, MD, FRCPC[a,b,c,*]

[a]*Montreal Neurological Institute, McGill University, Quebec, Montreal, Canada*
[b]*Microbiology and Immunology, McGill University, Quebec, Montreal, Canada*
[c]*Montreal Neurological Hospital, McGill University Hospital Center, Quebec, Montreal, Canada*

Involvement of the immune system in multiple sclerosis (MS) is multifaceted and only partially understood. The approval of several immune-modulating therapies that have a favorable impact on the disease course has fueled an interest in further elucidating disease mechanisms in an effort to develop treatments that are more effective and easier to tolerate. This is reflected in an exponential growth of the MS literature (Fig. 1). Publications related to the immunology of MS represent a major contribution to this rapid growth. A more complete understanding of the MS process, however, requires consideration not only of immune system responses but also of a complex neurobiology and the intricacies of immune-neural interaction. These include dynamics at the level of the blood-brain barrier (BBB), principles of normal central nervous system (CNS) homeostasis, the impact of immune mediators on neural responses and on the CNS reparative process, and the effects of the CNS responses on the biology of the invading inflammatory cells. A detailed review of such a broad literature is beyond the scope of this article. The goal here is to focus on aspects of the immune response that seem relevant to the pathophysiology of MS and, in particular, to the rational application and development of current and future immune therapies.

A rich body of research has emerged over the years from studies of animal models of MS, such as experimental autoimmune encephalomyelitis

The author is supported by the Canadian Institutes of Health Research, the Multiple Sclerosis Society of Canada (MSSC), the Wadsworth Foundation, and the Immune Tolerance Network. He is recipient of the Don Paty Career Scientist Award of the MSSC and the FRSQ Chercheur Boursier-Clinicien.

Dedicated to Dad–To his name true. For his own children and for children everywhere.

* Neuroimmunology Unit, Montreal Neurological Institute, 3801 University Street, Room #111, Montreal, Quebec H3A 2B4, Canada.

E-mail address: amit.bar-or@mcgill.ca

doi:10.1016/j.ncl.2004.11.001

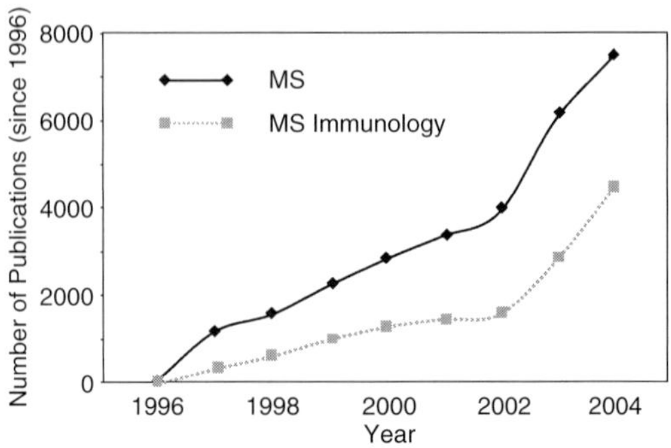

Fig. 1. Growth of literature in MS and in MS immunology. Number of new publications since 1996 in the overall field of MS (*diamonds and solid line*) and in the area of MS immunology (*squares and broken line*). Publications in the area of MS immunology make an important contribution to the recent surge in the overall MS literature.

(EAE) and Theiler's virus encephalomyelitis. Although these important studies continue to provide fundamental insights into principles of immune-CNS interaction and into more general themes of autoimmunity, immune regulation, and neurobiology, this article focuses on studies of humans-in particular patients who have MS. This article considers how well MS meets the definition and requirements of an autoimmune disease. A simplified model of MS immunopathophysiology is presented to illustrate the basic principles by which peripheral immune mediators are believed to interact with the BBB and have an impact on the CNS compartment. This model serves to identify the putative sites of action of currently approved and future MS therapies. A parallel theme considered in this article relates to understanding the immune mechanisms that underlie different clinical features of MS, such as relapses, remissions, and progression of disability. Overall, this article examines the understanding of presumed immune contributions to MS and should provide a useful background for more detailed discussions of specific therapeutic strategies.

Autoimmunity and autoimmune disease

In addition to playing a role in the body's response to tissue injury, a major function of the normal immune system involves immune surveillance, designed to ward off potentially malignant cells and infectious pathogens. To accomplish the latter, the immune system must identify anything that is foreign, which means it must have the fundamental capacity to distinguish between foreign antigens and self-antigens. The main cells in the immune system responsible for recognizing specific antigens are the T cells and B cells. These are cells of the adaptive immune response that can develop memory to particular targets after initial exposure and then are able to respond more efficiently to the same target in the future. The normal immune repertoire includes T cells and B cells that have the potential to react to self-antigens. These self, or autoreactive, cells normally are kept in check as part of the state of tolerance to self-antigens. This is referred to as the normal state of autoimmunity and likely serves important homeostatic functions.

When the normal state of autoimmunity becomes dysregulated and tolerance to particular self-antigens is broken, misguided immune responses can cause damage by targeting a person's own tissue. This is referred to as autoimmune disease [1]. The challenge of restoring self-tolerance is a fundamental therapeutic goal in the field of autoimmune disease. Why some individuals develop autoimmune diseases and why there is selectivity toward particular target organs remain unclear. The prevailing belief is that these diseases manifest when immune dysregulation is triggered by environmental exposures (such as one or more common viruses) in genetically susceptible hosts (likely reflecting involvement of several risk-conferring and protective genes, each contributing relatively little to the overall susceptibility).

Is multiple sclerosis initiated as an autoimmune disease?

MS often is referred to as an autoimmune disease because of the abnormal presence of immune mediators at sites of injury within the CNS. The immune system responds to all forms of tissue injury, however, and the mere presence of immune mediators at these sites does not necessarily mean that the immune system is responsible for triggering the initial injury. To establish that a disease has an autoimmune etiology, several criteria must be met. It must be shown that (1) immune mediators are present at the site of pathology in patients who have the illness; (2) these immune mediators are not present in persons or tissues who do not have the disease; (3) the putative immune mediators can be used to transfer the disease passively; and (4) removal of these mediators has therapeutic effects. In contrast to myasthenia gravis, which fulfills all of these criteria, the case for MS is less clear-cut.

There are at least two ways in which a dysregulated immune response may be involved in CNS injury during the MS disease process. The prevailing view (Fig. 2A), based in large part on animal models such as EAE, is that primary dysregulation of peripheral immune responses leads to a CNS-directed autoimmune disease and inflammatory tissue injury. The initial inflammatory injury of the CNS sets the stage for subsequent waves of inflammation, some of which are seen clinically as relapses or as newly evolving gadolinium-enhancing or T2 hyperintense lesions on MRI. The CNS inflammation also triggers a more degenerative process that is an important substrate for chronic progression of disability. This degenerative process may contribute to, and be directly exacerbated by, waves of

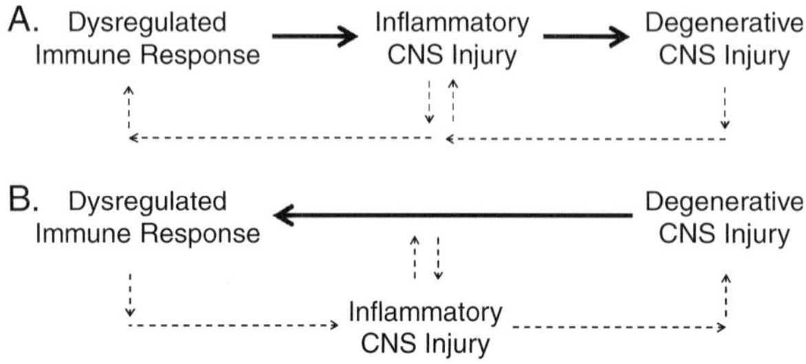

Fig. 2. Two views of disease initiation in MS. (*A*) The model of primary autoimmune disease suggests that dysregulated peripheral immune activation is the initiating event, resulting in inflammatory CNS tissue injury. The CNS then may be subject to additional waves of immune attack and to a partially independent process of degeneration. (*B*) An alternative model is based on a primary CNS abnormality that triggers an immune response with subsequent inflammatory CNS injury. The immune response may contribute to further damage directly and exacerbate the primary CNS degenerative process.

inflammation from the periphery but also could proceed relatively independently of peripheral immune activation, especially as evident later in the disease course. An alternate view (Fig. 2B) invokes a primary CNS degenerative process that could trigger a secondary immune response. Failure to regulate such an immune response could result in superimposed CNS-directed inflammatory injury, which would exacerbate the CNS degenerative process. Support for this latter model comes from imaging studies in which diffuse compromise to normal-appearing white matter (extending beyond the multifocal T2 hyperintense MRI lesions) is reported in patients at the time of their first clinical episode of MS [2,3] and from pathology studies suggesting that an oligodendrogliopathy may be an early event in the MS disease process [4]. As an extension to such a model, it is intriguing to speculate that patients who have the primary progressive form of MS may experience a primary CNS degenerative process which, for some, reason does not trigger clinically evident waves of superimposed inflammatory assault.

Whether immune dysregulation is a primary initiating event or a secondary response in MS, the presence of activated immune cells and mediators at the site of CNS pathology and observations that manipulating immune responses in patients can aggravate or diminish disease activity support the argument that immune responses are not merely epiphenomena of CNS tissue injury but, rather, play an important role in the pathophysiology of MS. The following sections consider how immune responses are believed to contribute to MS relapses, remissions, and disease progression.

Peripheral immune activation—the presumed trigger of multiple sclerosis relapses

In general, triggering immune-mediated tissue injury can be considered in the context of a simplified three-compartment model: (1) the immune system (including thymus, bone marrow, spleen, lymph nodes, and blood); (2) a target organ; and (3) the barrier that separates them. In the case of MS, the immune system is separated from the CNS target by the BBB (Fig. 3). According to this model, a key event in the triggering of an MS relapse is the activation outside the target organ (see Fig. 3, step 1) of T cells that can recognize antigens in the CNS. Through a sequence of subsequent events, these activated immune cells then undergo adhesion to the endothelial barrier (step 2), attraction (step 3), and active invasion (step 3) into the target organ where they may become reactivated (step 5) and subsequently participate in the disease process (step 6). The differentiation state of the invading cells determines if they contribute to injury or, possibly, counter the injury process. This model is used as a framework to discuss how abnormalities at each of these steps may contribute to the MS process and how targeting one or more of these steps may be of therapeutic benefit.

The principle that triggering an autoreactive immune response in the periphery can translate into an attack of inflammatory CNS disease in humans first was considered after Pasteur's introduction of neural tissue–containing vaccine as a therapy for rabies, resulting in episodes of acute disseminated encephalomyelitis, referred to as postvaccination acute disseminated encephalomyelitis [5]. This provided the basis for the development of the commonly used EAE model of MS, in which peripheral immunization with myelin components (including myelin basic protein [MBP], myelin oligodendrocyte glycoprotein [MOG], and proteolipid

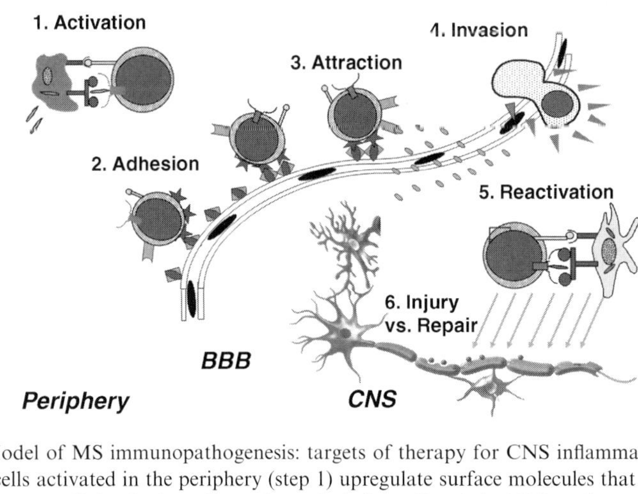

Fig. 3. Model of MS immunopathogenesis: targets of therapy for CNS inflammatory disease. Immune cells activated in the periphery (step 1) upregulate surface molecules that enable them to adhere more efficiently (step 2) to the endothelial cells of the BBB and respond to local chemokine gradients (step 3). Active secretion of matrix proteases (step 4) facilitates immune-cell invasion into the CNS where they may become reactivated (step 5) and have an impact on the biology of CNS elements (step 6). *Adapted from* Bar-Or A, Oliveira EM, Anderson DE, et al. Molecular pathogenesis of multiple sclerosis. J Neuroimmunol 1999;100:252–9.

protein [PLP]) induces inflammatory CNS demyelination [6–8]. Notably, EAE also can be induced in naive animals by means of adoptive transfer of activated (but not resting) myelin reactive CD4+ T cells from animals that have established EAE [9]. The particular strain of animal, the specific antigen selection, and the immunization regimen can result in distinct phenotypes of EAE that have a characteristic anatomic predilection, such as the spinal cord or optic nerve, or characteristic clinical patterns, including relapsing and chronic disease forms [8]. Additional models of induction of immune-mediated CNS demyelination include those in which a viral infection, such as Theiler's, results in the activation of autoreactive T cells directed against the CNS [10,11]. Generation of such cells develops presumably in response to CNS antigens released as a consequence of the injury to neural cell caused by the virus [12]. Collectively, these animal models establish that activation of peripheral T cells that recognize CNS antigens can result in a CNS inflammatory disease.

Analogous to EAE, initiation of MS (or at least an MS relapse) is believed triggered by peripheral activation of autoaggressive CNS-directed T cells. A brief review of T-cell activation and differentiation thus is warranted. T cells recognize antigens that bind with sufficient strength (affinity and avidity) to their T-cell receptor (TCR). For this recognition to occur, the appropriate antigen fragment must be presented to the TCR within the pocket of the major histocompatibility complex (MHC) expressed on the surface of antigen presenting cells (APC). Examples of APC include dendritic cells, monocyte/macrophage, CNS microglial cells, and B cells. Successful binding of the TCR by the antigen-MHC complex delivers a stimulatory signal to the T cell. Although the TCR signal is generally required for a T cell to be activated, this signal alone usually is not sufficient for full activation. Additional signals, collectively referred to as costimulatory signals, also are required and may be delivered by APC that express costimulatory molecules on their surface. A T cell that is stimulated via its TCR in the absence of costimulation may become anergic, which means it no longer is capable of reacting to its antigen. In contrast, a fully activated T cell can proliferate and release a range of cytokines and other effector molecules that may have a direct impact on the target organ, or act through modulation of the functions of other immune cells. APC become activated and upregulate their surface expression of costimulatory molecules when they are exposed to cues in their local environment, such as infectious particles (for example, through Toll-like receptors [TLR]), tissue injury, or various other inflammatory mediators [13]. Several families of costimulatory molecules and their receptors have been identified and likely play key roles in regulating immune responses in health and disease states. One important costimulatory pathway is represented by the engagement of CD28 or CTLA-4 on T cells by the CD80 (B7.1) or CD86 (B7.2) costimulatory molecules. Engagement of CD28 by B7 molecules induces a stimulatory signal, whereas the same B7 molecules engaging

CTLA-4 mediate an inhibitory signal. The integration of signals mediated by the TCR and by the profile of costimulatory molecules expressed in a particular microenvironment determines if a T cell becomes activated and may also influence the effector functions of the T cell [14,15]. Modulating T-cell responses by targeting the B7 costimulatory pathway and more recently described costimulatory molecules and their ligands [16–19] provides an attractive therapeutic approach for immune-mediated diseases, including MS.

As part of the normal immune response, T cells can differentiate into subsets that are distinguished based on the profile of cytokines they secrete [20,21]. This is part of the normal immune system's way of generating effector T cells that can respond in different ways, depending on the circumstance. How T cells differentiate is critically dependent on their microenvironment during initial activation. In addition to the overall strength of activating signals, including the profile of costimulation, cytokines represent important contextual cues that can drive T-cell differentiation. In particular, cytokines released by APC can critically define T-cell responses. For example, the presence of cytokines, such as interleukin (IL)-12 or IL-23, can preferentially generate T cells that subsequently secrete interferon (IFN)-γ, and tumor necrosis factor α (TNF-α) [22]. These T cells are effective as part of the normal antiviral response and are referred to arbitrarily as T helper cells type 1 (Th1) [23]. In contrast, T cells that initially become activated in the absence of IL-12, but in the presence of IL-4, subsequently produce cytokines, including IL-4, IL-5, IL-13, and possibly IL-10. These are referred to as Th2 cells and play an important effector role against parasitic infections. When the normal balance between the body's Th1 and Th2 responses is not regulated properly, disease states can occur, examples of which include too much of a Th2 response that may contribute to asthma or atopic conditions and too much of a Th1 response that is implicated in certain autoimmune disease states. In the EAE model, adoptive transfer of CNS-autoreactive Th1 T cells typically induces disease, whereas transfer of Th2 cells that recognize the same CNS antigens usually does not induce disease. Moreover, the Th2 cells may protect the animal from getting Th1-mediated disease. Based on these observations, it is suggested that, in MS, CNS-directed Th1 responses may be proinflammatory and cause damage, whereas Th2 responses may be anti-inflammatory and protective [24–27]. Additional subsets of T cells that play important roles in immune regulation have been described [28] (discussed later). It should be stressed that the Th1/Th2 paradigm does not capture the true complexity of immune regulation and should not be taken as dogma. For example, in the EAE model, driving Th2 responses too far can result in a CNS inflammatory disease caused by the Th2 cells [29,30]. Nonetheless, the appreciation that T cells can adopt distinct effector profiles and that dysregulation among different subsets of T cells may contribute to pathologic states is relevant.

What is the evidence that T cells reactive to particular CNS antigens are involved in the MS disease process? No single antigen has been identified as the major CNS target in MS. It is likely that the predominant target during MS attacks is different across individuals and, indeed, may change within the same patient over the course of the illness, in a process termed epitope spread. Although several T cell targets are likely [31–36], many studies have focused on T-cell reactivity to MBP, in part because it is easier to isolate human MBP for in vitro studies, compared with the less water-soluble PLP, or with MOG, which is present in small amounts. Consistent with the concept of normal autoimmunity, described previously, it is well established that all individuals (including those who do not have MS) have circulating T cells that can react to CNS antigens, including MBP [37–39]. Thus, the mere presence of these CNS-reactive T cells is not enough to cause the illness. There is evidence that compared with normal individuals, MBP-reactive T cells from patients who are in a higher state of activation [40,41], require fewer costimulatory signals to become reactivated [42,43] and preferentially belong to the memory, rather than the naive, T-cell pool [44–46]. There is also some support of the contention that in patients who have MS, the MBP-reactive T cells are more likely to produce proinflammatory (Th1) than anti-inflammatory mediators [47,48]. Most studies of CNS autoreactivity tend to focus on the CD4 helper T-cell subset, in part because of technical difficulties in maintaining CD8 cytotoxic T cells in culture. Accumulating evidence, however, points to an important contribution of CD8 T cells to MS pathophysiology. Pathologic evaluation reveals a prominence of CD8 over CD4 T-cell responses within MS lesions [49,50] and molecular studies describe specific CD8 (rather than CD4) T cells expanding and persisting long-term within the CNS compartment of patients [49,51]. A high prevalence of CNS autoreactive CD8 T cells is confirmed in the circulation of patients who have MS compared with control patients [52–54]. The roles of natural killer (NK) cells, NK T cells and γ/δ T cells in MS also are under investigation.

The most direct evidence to date that peripheral activation of CNS autoreactive T cells may have an impact on the MS disease process has emerged from careful immune monitoring of patients treated with an altered peptide ligand (APL) of MBP. Initial studies in EAE identified that administration of a particular APL of an encephalitogenic epitope of MBP led to a Th2 shift in MBP reactivity and improved clinical outcomes [55,56]. The same APL subsequently was introduced into early-phase clinical trials of MS. A phase II study using low doses of the APL injected subcutaneously seemed to induce Th2 responses to MBP in patients and suggested possible benefit on MRI outcomes [57]. A phase I study of the same APL administered at a higher dose was halted, however, when several patients experienced increased MRI activity, with or without clinical correlates [58]. In these individuals, elegant immune monitoring identified a strong induction of MBP-reactive CD4 T cells in the periphery and in the cerebrospinal fluid (CSF). These MBP-reactive T cells were notable for their production of high levels of the Th1 cytokine, IFN-γ. Based on the EAE and MS studies noted previously, MS therapeutics often are considered in terms of their capacity to inhibit the activation of CNS autoreactive Th1 cells or promote Th2 responses to CNS targets. It must be stressed that the relationship between Th1 and Th2 responses (loosely designated as proinflammatory and anti-inflammatory, respectively) and tissue damage or protection in MS remains only partially understood, as recent studies suggest that Th1 responses may not always be detrimental [59,60]. Indeed, cells of the immune system are not all bad or all good. The challenge is to define which immune responses are pathogenic and when, so that the most effective therapies can be developed. Nonetheless, a paradigm that continues to be pursued in trials of experimental therapeutics of MS is that the ability to induce immune deviation from Th1 to Th2 responses is a desirable attribute of the therapy.

Where and how might CNS-reactive T cells become activated in patients who have MS? T cell sensitization could occur either within the CNS or in regional draining lymph nodes. Support for the former is derived from observations that lymphocyte trafficking is ongoing in the CNS even under physiologic conditions [61–64] and that perivascular and parenchymal microglia have the capacity to serve as competent antigen-presenting cells [27,65]. The profile of costimulatory molecules on APC may be relevant. The expression of CD80 (B7.1) may be upregulated selectively in MS plaques [66,67], and CD80, but not CD86, was found to be upregulated on immune cells in peripheral blood and CSF of patients who had MS compared with control patients [68]. In EAE, blockade of CD80 signaling was shown to inhibit the induction phase of the disease [69–71]. The CSF and meninges of patients may contain structures that resemble germinal centers, where chronically activated B cells or plasma cells are seen to express high levels of costimulatory molecules and may function as efficient APC to T cells [72].

Another (not mutually exclusive) possibility is that CNS autoreactive cells encounter fragments of the CNS self-antigens that are released or carried by APC into cervical lymph nodes, now known to drain from the brain/CNS [73–75]. T cells reactive to the CNS might also become activated in the periphery when they encounter fragments of nonself-antigens (foreign) that are sufficiently similar to the self-antigen that they activate the self-reactive cells. In support of this mechanism, termed molecular mimicry, are observations that some human MBP-reactive T cells can be activated by epitopes derived from common viruses, such as herpes simplex, Epstein-Barr, or influenza, when presented by the same MHC molecules [76,77]. Extending this concept further is the principle of structural equivalence, wherein different MHC molecules loaded with distinct peptides can create complexes of sufficiently similar structure that they are recognized by the same CNS-reactive T cell in patients who have MS [78].

Interaction of immune cells with the blood-brain barrier: adhesion, attraction, and invasion

Peripheral activation induces immune cells to express several families of molecules that facilitate their migration into the target organ (see Fig. 3) through a tightly regulated sequence of overlapping events [79,80]. Upregulation of selectin and integrin adhesion molecules that interact with ligands expressed on the endothelial cells of the BBB contribute to the immune cell rolling and tethering/arresting, respectively (step 2). Chemokines secreted by activated immune cells, endothelial cells, or injured tissue can promote integrin activation and contribute to further cellular arrest [81]. Chemokines also drive the migration of cells expressing the corresponding chemokine receptors toward the source of the chemical gradient (step 3). Production of enzymes (step 4), such as the matrix metalloproteinases (MMP), results in breakdown of the basement membrane and facilitates tissue infiltration [82]. Evidence from EAE and MS studies implicating these molecular steps in disease pathogenesis identifies potential therapeutic targets for MS (discussed later).

Selective expression of adhesion molecules in multiple sclerosis

Elevated levels of the adhesion molecules, including intercellular adhesion molecule 1 (ICAM-1) and vascular cell adhesion molecule 1 (VCAM-1), have been observed on endothelial cells of MS lesions and these levels have been shown to correlate with the extent of leukocyte infiltration [80,83–85]. The ligands for ICAM-1 and VCAM-1 (LFA-1 and VLA-4, respectively) have been identified on the perivascular inflammatory cells within MS lesions [86]. In EAE, myelin autoreactive T cells fail to cross the BBB in VLA-4–deficient animals [87,88], and treatment of wild type animals with monoclonal antibody directed against VLA-4 results in diminished infiltration of the CNS by inflammatory cells with a concomitant diminution in disease severity [89,90]. These observations provide the foundation for therapeutic targeting of cell migration in patients who have MS. Expression of adhesion molecules, such as VCAM-1 and LFA-1, is also seen on glial cells in MS lesions [91], and this may point to additional roles for these molecules in antigen presentation and possibly T-cell costimulation [86,92,93]

Selective expression of chemokine receptors and chemokines in multiple sclerosis

The interaction of chemokine receptors with their corresponding chemokines represents a fundamental mechanism by which the complex movement of immune cells throughout the body is orchestrated. These interactions are also involved in the trafficking of immune cells into the CNS of patients who have MS (see Fig. 2, step 3). Studies show that (1) the majority of cells in the CSF of patients who have MS are memory T cells that express CCR7, consistent with a central memory phenotype of cells that participate in immune surveillance; (2) essentially all T cells within MS lesions do not express CCR7, consistent with the effector memory phenotype; and (3) cells expressing surface markers of maturing dendritic cells (MHC Class II, CD68, CD86, and the chemokine receptor CCR7) are abundant within CNS lesions and in the CSF of patients who have MS [75]. These observations are consistent with a model in which the afferent limb of the CNS immune response involves, at least in part, dendritic cells, which undergo maturation upon antigenic capture within the CNS lesions. The maturing dendritic cells then migrate via the CSF into deep cervical lymph nodes. There, they may present CNS antigens to T cells, which turn into central memory (CCR7+) cells. These central memory T cells then participate in the efferent limb of CNS immune responses by entering the CSF and differentiating into effector memory (CCR7−) T cells upon restimulation by antigen within the CNS compartment. The effector memory T cells are retained within the MS lesions, where they contribute to the disease process [75].

Certain chemokines seem to recruit T cells and monocytes/dendritic cells selectively into the inflamed CNS and are associated with EAE disease activity [94]. In MS lesions, Regulated on Activation Normal T cell Expressed and Secreted (RANTES) (CCL5) that is chemotactic for lymphocytes and monocytes expressing CCR5 is expressed by activated perivascular T cells, predominantly at the edge of active plaques [95]. Astrocytes express MCP-1 (CCL2), a chemokine that attracts monocytes expressing CCR2 [96]. Compared with CSF from neurologic controls, MS CSF was shown to contain elevated levels of CCL5 and IP-10 (CXCL10) chemotactic for activated T cells expressing the chemokine receptor CXCR3 [97]. An increased frequency of CD4+ and CD8+ T cells from the CSF of patients who have MS expressed CXCR3. Immunohistochemistry confirmed an increased perivascular expression of CXCR3 and CCR5 on immune cells in MS lesions. Thus, the data suggest that the CCL2/CCR2, CXCL10/CXCR3, and CCL5/CCR5 pathways may have selective roles in MS pathogenesis. It has been suggested that certain chemokines and chemokine receptors are preferentially involved in trafficking of proinflammatory Th1 T-cell populations [95,97–100], although this may not always be the case for individual T cells [101].

Selective expression of matrix metalloproteinases in multiple sclerosis

The transmigration of immune cells across the BBB and into the extracellular matrix is based on the capacity of activated immune cells to secrete matrix proteases. The best-known family is called the MMP (see Fig. 2, step 4), comprising tightly regulated proteolytic enzymes that have been ascribed many roles in normal tissue development, remodeling, and immune responses. Dysregulation of MMP and the related family of ADAM molecules may contribute to abnormal tissue invasion by neoplastic or immune cells [82,102–104]. MMP and A Disintegrin And Metalloprotease (ADAMs) may be secreted or expressed on the surface of cells, typically as proenzymes requiring proteolytic cleavage for their own activation and undergoing downregulation by tissue inhibitors of metalloproteinases [105]. The MMP can be expressed by activated immune cells and glial cells (eg, astrocytes and microglia) [106–108]. Their potential contribution to the MS disease process may include (1) disruption of basement membrane of the BBB and the tissue matrix [105], thereby facilitating parenchymal infiltration of immune cells [106]; (2) proteolytic cleavage of membrane-bound proinflammatory cytokines, such as TNF-α [109,110]; and (3) direct damage to CNS elements [111]. MMP also may be relevant during repair and regeneration within the CNS [82]. In patients who have MS, increased activity of several CSF proteolytic enzymes has been reported, compared with normal individuals [112,113]. For example, gelatinase B (MMP-9) levels are increased in serum and CSF of patients who have MS during acute relapse, and the elevated levels correlate with the degree of BBB disruption, as evidenced by the number of gadolinium-enhancing lesion on MRI [114,115]. Comparisons across normal human immune-cell subsets (T cells, B cells, and monocytes) reveal distinct profiles of MMP, ADAM, and TIMP molecule expression [116,117]. Monocytes express a broader range and seem to produce higher amounts of different proteolytic enzymes compared with T cells and B cells [116], which is consistent with the observation that invading monocytes/macrophages are a major contributor to the MS inflammatory lesions.

The multistep molecular machinery discussed previously (adhesion molecules, chemokines, and matrix proteases) forms the basis for how normal immune cells migrate across different endothelial barriers, including the BBB, as part of the process of physiologic immune surveillance and during desired adaptive immune responses [61–64]. Ongoing studies in EAE and MS aim to elucidate how dysregulation of these families of molecules may contribute to pathophysiology and how distinct steps of cell trafficking may be targeted therapeutically, while minimizing the impact on normal immune functions.

B-cell and antibody responses in multiple sclerosis

Like T cells, B cells are able to recognize particular antigens, which they do through their B-cell receptor (BCR). After activation, typically involving BCR engagement by antigen followed by costimulatory signals from T cells (T cell 'help'), B cells can proliferate and differentiate into memory B cells or into plasma cells that produce immunoglobulin (antibody). Involvement of B cells in MS generally has been considered in terms of the possible activation of CNS autoreactive B cells, leading to production of CNS-directed autoantibodies. Molecular studies confirm that MS lesions and CSF contain B cells that probably expanded in response to antigenic encounter within the CNS compartment. The frequently elevated levels of CSF immunoglobulin in MS and common manifestation of an oligoclonal-banding pattern have long been appreciated. Pathologic studies of MS lesions reveal tissue deposition of immunoglobulin and complement and the presence of immunoglobulin bound to myelin fragments within phagocytic macrophage [118,119], suggesting that complement-mediated injury and antibody-dependent cytotoxicity (ADCC), respectively, may contribute to the MS disease process [120,121]. In spite of these studies, the antigenic targets of CNS B cells and antibodies in MS have not been elucidated. Measurements of antimyelin antibodies in MS point to a possible role for them as markers of disease activity [122,123]. Such antibodies seem to be of relatively low affinity, however, and their contribution to pathology is not established [124]. CNS-directed antibodies may, in fact, be beneficial by functioning to remove debris, including growth inhibitory molecules [125], and possibly supporting remyelination [126,127]. B cells also may have roles that extend beyond their potential to become antibody-producing cells. For example, certain B cell subsets can function as effective APC [128]. It has been postulated that chronically activated autoreactive B cells [129] and B cells within germinal center–like structures within the CNS may contribute to the propagation of MS disease activity through activation of T cells [72,130,131]. Recent studies suggest that human B cells may contribute actively to the regulation of immune responses through secretion of effector cytokines [132,133] and that abnormalities in this function may be relevant to autoimmune diseases, including MS [132,134]. Targeting B-cell responses, therefore, may be of therapeutic relevance in subsets of patients who have MS. The molecular interactions that seem to underlie human B-cell entry into the CNS (involving adhesion molecules, chemokines, and MMP) partially overlap but are not identical to those employed by T cells [116,117]. This is important when considering the impact of T-cell–directed therapies on B-cell physiology and how to optimally approach the development of B-cell–directed therapies.

Immune reactivation and effector mechanisms within the central nervous system

Once within the CNS compartment, the infiltrating immune cells may become reactivated (see Fig. 2, step 5). This could occur through antigen presentation by resident microglia or by invading monocytes/macrophage and dendritic cells [135–138]. The inflammatory milieu of locally released cytokines, chemokines, and MMP can induce bystander activation of APC and of primed T cells and B cells, even in the absence of their particular antigen. Local damage results in exposure of additional myelin components that may become primary targets of subsequent waves of infiltrating cells, leading to epitope spread and possibly contributing to clinical relapses [139].

There are many likely mechanisms by which active immune responses can have an impact on the biology of myelin, oligodendrocytes, and neural elements within the CNS of patients who have MS (step 6 and Tables 1 and 2). Antigen-specific injury may be mediated by CD4 and CD8 T cells. CNS autoreactive antibodies may contribute through complement fixation or ADCC. Nonspecific cytotoxicity mediated by CD4 [140] and CD8 [141] T cells also have been demonstrated in vitro. Several nonspecific soluble (humoral) immune mediators are believed to participate in CNS tissue injury in MS, including proinflammatory cytokines, nitric oxide, oxygen radicals, matrix proteases, glutamate, and proapoptotic signals [27,46,59, 142].

Immune mechanisms of recovery from acute attacks

Immune and nonimmune mechanisms contribute to recovery from an MS relapse. Nonimmune mechanisms are discussed elsewhere and may include early redistribution of sodium channels on demyelinated nerve segments [143], remyelination [144], axonal regeneration, and reorganization of networks [145]. Immune mechanisms contributing to recovery include resolution of the processes that actively mediate injury and promotion of immune responses that suppress injury or promote protection and repair. Resolution of active inflammation requires clearance of infiltrating immune cells, which occurs when these cells emigrate out of the CNS or when they undergo apoptosis in situ. Such resolution serves to limit ongoing injury and enables reversal of acute edema. Thus, local expression of proinflammatory cytokines and proretention chemokines, and the balance between proapoptotic and antiapoptotic molecules, influence whether or not activated immune cells persist within MS lesions and have an impact on recovery [59].

Table 1
Possible immune-mediated mechanisms of central nervous system injury

Cytotoxicity mediated by immune cells, including:

1. Antigen-specific CNS-reactive CD8 T cells and CD4 T cells
2. Non–antigen-specific CD8 and CD4 T cells (bystander injury)
3. Macrophage; reactive microglia
4. NK cells; NK T cells; γ/δ T cells
5. Failure to downregulate the immune response (prolonged retention or limited apoptosis of proinflammatory cells)
6. Apoptotic signals (leading to death of CNS cells)

Injury by soluble (humoral) immune mediators, including:

1. Antigen-specific CNS-reactive antibodies: injury through complement fixation or ADCC
2. Proinflammatory cytokines (including Th1 cytokines, osteopontin, TNF-α, and IL-1β)
3. Nitric oxide and reactive oxygen species
4. Leukotrienes, plasminogen activators
5. MMP
6. Glutamate-mediated cytotoxicity

Table 2
Possible immune-mediated mechanisms of recovery and central nervous system protection and repair

Mediators that could serve to decrease proinflammatory responses, including:
1. Anti-inflammatory cytokines (including Th2 cytokines, IL-10, and TGF-β)
2. Anti-inflammatory antigen-presenting cells
3. Regulatory/suppressive T-cell subsets (Tr1, Th2, Th3, CD4+CD25hi; CD8 HLA-E)
4. Proapoptotic signals (leading to death of proinflammatory immune cells)
5. TIMP

Mechanisms that could promote CNS protection and repair, including:
1. Release of neurotrophic factors (BDNF, NGF, and others)
2. Clearance of inhibitory myelin molecules (Nogo, MAG) by macrophage/microglia
3. Cytokines promoting CNS progenitor cells (eg, TNF-α acting via TNF-R2) and remyelination (IL-1β)
4. Protective autoimmunity
5. Promyelinating antibodies
6. Some prostaglandins, lipoxins, antithrombin

Although it was believed that activated immune cells in the CNS were invariably detrimental, several lines of evidence now point to potential beneficial roles of CNS inflammation (see Table 2). Th2 cytokines are known to inhibit Th1 differentiation and it is possible that activated Th2 cells within the CNS could limit proinflammatory Th1 responses through bystander suppression. Modulation of infiltrating monocyte/macrophage and resident microglia toward a Type-2 APC phenotype could promote anti-inflammatory Th2 responses within the CNS [138]. Overly aggressive shifts toward Th2 responses may be detrimental [29,30], however, and Th1 responses have been implicated as beneficial in the context of CNS inflammation under certain conditions, pointing to a possible role for protective autoimmunity [146].

Other distinct cell subsets, acting via cell-cell contact or release of soluble anti-inflammatory factors, may mediate immune regulatory functions [147–149]. In this context, the roles of particular CD4 T cells (such as $CD25^{hi}$ regulatory cells, IL-10–producing Tr1 cells, or transforming growth factor [TGF]-β–producing Th3 cells) [150–152] and CD8 T cells (such as HLA-E–restricted CD8 suppressors) [153,154] in MS are of considerable interest.

In addition to the provision of downregulatory or anti-inflammatory signals, further mechanisms by which immune responses may be beneficial in the CNS of patients who have MS include active contributions to survival and repair through release of neurotrophic factors [155,156], cytokines (TNF-α) that may induce proliferation of oligodendrocyte progenitor cells [157], and myelin-directed antibodies that actually may support remyelination [125,126,158,159]. Immune responses also may make a passive contribution to a more permissive CNS environment through the removal of molecules that otherwise inhibit axonal regeneration, such as Nogo and

Myelin Associated Glycoprotein (MAG) [160]. Certain immune mediators (such as IL-1β, TNF-α, and apoptotic molecules) may have detrimental and beneficial effects during CNS inflammation (see Tables 1 and 2). For example, IL-1β can contribute to CNS injury by promoting the action of MMP and by exacerbating glutamate cytotoxicity but also is required for the production of Ciliary Neurotrophic Factor (CNTF) [161] and is able to promote remyelination by inducing insulin-like growth factor 1 [162]. Similarly, TNF-α is considered a Th1 proinflammatory cytokine that may be directly cytotoxic when acting via TNFR1 but can be supportive of remyelination when acting via TNFR2. This poses particular therapeutic challenges and may explain why anti–TNF-α therapies (which work well for patients who have rheumatoid arthritis) have been unsuccessful and, indeed, detrimental in MS.

Immune mechanisms of disease progression

Persistence and progression of neurologic disability in MS is attributed to failure of remyelination and irreversible axonal injury. A more complete understanding of MS pathophysiology requires detailed consideration of the neurobiology of the disease and the complexities of neuroimmune interactions (discussed elsewhere). The contribution of inflammatory mechanisms to such disease evolution remains to be defined fully. Failure of the resolution phase of acute relapses as a result of persistence of pro-retention and pro-survival cues (see Table 1) may play a role in prolonging the injurious impact of infiltrating immune cells. Chronic activation of resident CNS glial cells, such as microglia and astrocytes, may provide the basis for the generation or maintenance of progressive pathologic responses, even in the absence of acute waves of infiltrating inflammatory cells from the periphery. The activated cells residing within the CNS could be sources of potential effector molecules that contribute to smoldering tissue injury. They may become activated through TLR or by scavenging the CNS debris itself. There is speculation that germinal center–like structures develop within the CNS, providing the nidus for chronic activation [72,130,131].

Loss of oligodendrocytes in the latter phases of disease could reflect an increased vulnerability of these cells after an earlier sublethal inflammatory compromise [163]. For example, chronic exposure of oligodendrocytes to inflammatory mediators can upregulate intracellular p53 leading to surface upregulation of death receptors, which then make cells more susceptible to apoptosis mediated by Fas-ligand and TNF Related Apoptosis-inducing Ligand (TRAIL). It is speculated that the relative lack of remyelination in chronic lesions may reflect drop-out of progenitor cells that were targets of earlier immune-mediated injury [164]. Axons, in turn, rely on trophic support from oligodendrocytes and, in their absence, become more vulnerable to insults that otherwise have a lesser impact. It thus is likely that a combination of otherwise sublethal injuries (some of which may be immune mediated) contribute to the chronic loss of CNS elements, consistent with a multi-hit model [27]. It also is likely that the mechanisms described previously contribute to CNS tissue injury from the earliest stages of the disease. In EAE, there is considerable overlap between acute and chronic disease patterns, suggesting that overlapping pathogenic mechanisms exist across monophasic, recurrent, and chronic phenotypes in humans. Whether or not the mechanisms underlying chronic progression in patients who have the primary progressive form of MS are identical to those that account for the more common secondary progression form of disease remains speculative.

A framework for considering the putative modes of action of therapies for multiple sclerosis

Studies of the mode of action of immunosuppressive and immunomodulating therapies in patients who have MS continue to improve our understanding of the immunopathology of the disease. Developing and incorporating immune assays into well-designed trials of experimental therapies for MS is paramount. Such mechanistic studies not only provide proof of biologic concept and insights into the in vivo mode of action of the therapy in question but also provide critical windows into the disease itself. Combining clinical, imaging, and biologic outcome measures enables more comprehensive prospective monitoring of patients in trials and the development and validation of biomarkers of disease activity, treatment response, and prognosis. The simplified model discussed previously (see Fig. 3) identifies potential targets for intervention in MS. In general terms, treatments that can prevent CNS-reactive cells from becoming abnormally activated or from entering their target, treatments that can shift the immune response from a proinflammatory to an anti-inflammatory profile, and treatments that can promote CNS protection and repair are considered beneficial in MS. Therapies can thus be considered in terms of their potential to (1) inhibit costimulation and peripheral immune activation of proinflammatory cells or promote the same for anti-inflammatory cells (step 1); (2) modulate CNS infiltration through inhibition or promotion of selected molecules involved in adhesion (step 2), attraction (step 3), or transmigration (step 4); (3) have an impact on immune reactivation within the CNS or the capacity to suppress or regulate immune effector profiles (step 5); and (4) contribute to local tissue protection and repair (step 6).

For example, converging studies suggest that the IFN-β medications share the same therapeutic mechanisms of action in MS, which could include: (1) suppressing activation of T cells, possibly by inhibiting the upregulation of costimulatory molecules [68]; (2) inducing the production of the immune suppressive cytokine IL-10 [165]; and (3) limiting the ability of inflammatory cells from entering the CNS by inhibiting immune cell expression of adhesion molecules [166] and suppressing production of

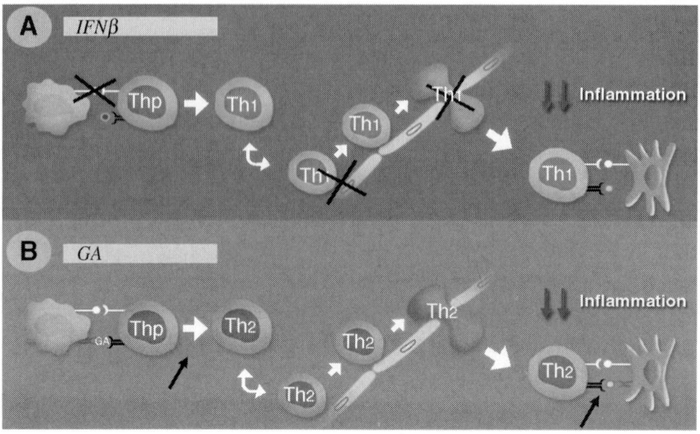

Fig. 4. Therapeutic mechanisms of action of IFN-β and GA in MS. (*A*) IFN-β medications likely mediate their therapeutic effect in MS by interfering with T-cell activation and by inhibiting expression of adhesion molecules and MMP. This results in decreased adhesion and transmigration of activated immune cells into the CNS and decreased inflammation and damage. (*B*) GA likely mediates its therapeutic effect in MS by modulating the response profile of activated immune cells that then migrate into the CNS. There, these cells are believed to counter the local inflammation and decrease damage.

matrix proteases (Fig. 4) [167–169]. In contrast, studies of the therapeutic mode of action of glatiramer acetate in MS initially considered its capacity to inhibit the activation of myelin-directed T cells [170], subsequently focusing on its ability to promote the generation of anti-inflammatory T cells [171–179] and type-2 (anti-inflammatory) APC [138] that migrate into the CNS, where they may counter inflammatory responses and possibly contribute to protection of CNS elements through the release of neurotrophic factors [180,181]. More detailed discussion of the currently used immunomodulators and immunosuppressants and future therapies of MS can be found in the articles elsewhere in this issue.

Acknowledgments

The author wishes to thank Dr. Tina Trollmo for her helpful comments and Arlene Berg for assistance in preparing the manuscript.

References

[1] Ermann J, Fathman CG. Autoimmune diseases: genes, bugs and failed regulation. Nat Immunol 2001;2:759–61.

[2] Filippi M, Bozzali M, Rovaris M, et al. Evidence for widespread axonal damage at the earliest clinical stage of multiple sclerosis. Brain 2003;126(Pt 2):433–7.

[3] De Stefano N, Narayanan S, Francis GS, et al. Evidence of axonal damage in the early stages of multiple sclerosis and its relevance to disability. Arch Neurol 2001;58:65–70.
[4] Barnett MH, Prineas JW. Relapsing and remitting multiple sclerosis: pathology of the newly forming lesion. Ann Neurol 2004;55:458–68.
[5] Stuart G, Krikorian KS. The neuro-paralytic accidents of anti-rabies treatment. Ann Trop Med Parasitol 1928;22:327–77.
[6] Rivers TM, Schwentker FF. Encephalomyelitis accompanied by myelin destruction experimentally produced in monkeys. J Exp Med 1935;61:689–702.
[7] Kabat EA, Wolf A, Bezer AE. The rapid production of acute disseminated encephalomyelitis in rhesus monkeys by injection of heterologous and homologous brain tissue with adjuvants. J Exp Med 1947;85:117–30.
[8] Wekerle H, Kojima K, Lannes-Vieira J, et al. Animal models. Ann Neurol 1994;36(Suppl): S47–53.
[9] Paterson PY. Transfer of allergic encephalomyelitis in rats by means of lymph node cells. J Exp Med 1960;111:119–36.
[10] Miller SD, Vanderlugt CL, Begolka WS, et al. Persistent infection with Theiler's virus leads to CNS autoimmunity via epitope spreading. Nat Med 1997;3:1133–6.
[11] Miller SD, McRae BL, Vanderlugt CL, et al. Evolution of the T-cell repertoire during the course of experimental immune-mediated demyelinating diseases. Immunol Rev 1995;144: 225–44.
[12] Miller SD, Katz-Levy Y, Neville KL, et al. Virus-induced autoimmunity: epitope spreading to myelin autoepitopes in Theiler's virus infection of the central nervous system. Adv Virus Res 2001;56:199–217.
[13] Cook DN, Pisetsky DS, Schwartz DA. Toll-like receptors in the pathogenesis of human disease. Nat Immunol 2004;5:975–9.
[14] Anderson DE, Bieganowska KD, Bar-Or A, et al. Paradoxical inhibition of T-cell function in response to CTLA-4 blockade; heterogeneity within the human T-cell population. Nat Med 2000;6:211–4.
[15] Vijayakrishnan L, Slavik JM, Illes Z, et al. An autoimmune disease-associated CTLA-4 splice variant lacking the B7 binding domain signals negatively in T cells. Immunity 2004; 20:563–75.
[16] Chitnis T, Khoury SJ. Role of costimulatory pathways in the pathogenesis of multiple sclerosis and experimental autoimmune encephalomyelitis. J Allergy Clin Immunol 2003; 112:837–50.
[17] Dong C, Juedes AE, Temann UA, et al. ICOS co-stimulatory receptor is essential for T-cell activation and function. Nature 2001;409:97–101.
[18] Okazaki T, Iwai Y, Honjo T. New regulatory co-receptors: inducible co-stimulator and PD-1. Curr Opin Immunol 2002;14:779–82.
[19] Salama AD, Chitnis T, Imitola J, et al. Critical role of the programmed death-1 (PD-1) pathway in regulation of experimental autoimmune encephalomyelitis. J Exp Med 2003; 198:71–8.
[20] Abbas AK, Murphy KM, Sher A. Functional diversity of helper T lymphocytes. Nature 1996;383:787–93.
[21] O'Garra A. Cytokines induce the development of functionally heterogeneous T helper cell subsets. Immunity 1998;8:275–83.
[22] Murphy CA, Langrish CL, Chen Y, et al. Divergent pro- and antiinflammatory roles for IL-23 and IL-12 in joint autoimmune inflammation. J Exp Med 2003;198:1951–7.
[23] Mosmann TR, Coffman RL. Heterogeneity of cytokine secretion patterns and functions of helper T cells. Adv Immunol 1989;46:111–47.
[24] Hohlfeld R, Wekerle H. Immunological update on multiple sclerosis. Curr Opin Neurol 2001;14:299–304.
[25] Hemmer B, Archelos JJ, Hartung HP. New concepts in the immunopathogenesis of multiple sclerosis. Nat Rev Neurosci 2002;3:291–301.

[26] Steinman L, Martin R, Bernard C, et al. Multiple sclerosis: deeper understanding of its pathogenesis reveals new targets for therapy. Annu Rev Neurosci 2002;25:491–505.
[27] Antel JP, Bar-Or A. Multiple sclerosis: therapy. In: Lazzarini R, editor. Myelin biology and disorders. New York: Elsevier Academic Press; 2004. p. 791–806.
[28] Antel J, Owens T. Multiple sclerosis and immune regulatory cells. Brain 2004;127(Pt 9): 1915–6.
[29] Genain CP, Abel K, Belmar N, et al. Late complications of immune deviation therapy in a nonhuman primate. Science 1996;274:2054–7.
[30] Pedotti R, Mitchell D, Wedemeyer J, et al. An unexpected version of horror autotoxicus: anaphylactic shock to a self-peptide. Nat Immunol 2001;2:216–22.
[31] Ota K, Matsui M, Milford EL, et al. T-cell recognition of an immunodominant myelin basic protein epitope in multiple sclerosis. Nature 1990;346:183–7.
[32] Sun JB, Olsson T, Wang WZ, et al. Autoreactive T and B cells responding to myelin proteolipid protein in multiple sclerosis and controls. Eur J Immunol 1991;21:1461–8.
[33] Markovic-Plese S, Fukaura H, Zhang J, et al. T cell recognition of immunodominant and cryptic proteolipid protein epitopes in humans. J Immunol 1995;155:982–92.
[34] Kerlero de Rosbo N, Hoffman M, Mendel I, et al. Predominance of the autoimmune response to myelin oligodendrocyte glycoprotein (MOG) in multiple sclerosis: reactivity to the extracellular domain of MOG is directed against three main regions. Eur J Immunol 1997;27:3059–69.
[35] Allegretta M, Nicklas JA, Sriram S, et al. T cells responsive to myelin basic protein in patients with multiple sclerosis. Science 1990;247:718–21.
[36] Pender MP, Csurhes PA, Wolfe NP, et al. Increased circulating T cell reactivity to GM3 and GQ1b gangliosides in primary progressive multiple sclerosis. J Clin Neurosci 2003;10: 63–6.
[37] Martin R, Jaraquemada D, Flerlage M, et al. Fine specificity and HLA restriction of myelin basic protein-specific cytotoxic T cell lines from multiple sclerosis patients and healthy individuals. J Immunol 1990;14:540–8.
[38] Pender MP, Csurhes PA, Greer JM, et al. Surges of increased T cell reactivity to an encephalitogenic region of myelin proteolipid protein occur more often in patients with multiple sclerosis than in healthy subjects. J Immunol 2000;165:5322–31.
[39] Pette M, Fujita K, Kitze B, et al. Myelin basic protein-specific T lymphocyte lines from MS patients and healthy individuals. Neurology 1990;40:1770–6.
[40] Zhang J, Markovic-Plese S, Lacet B, et al. Increased frequency of interleukin 2-responsive T cells specific for myelin basic protein and proteolipid protein in peripheral blood and cerebrospinal fluid of patients with multiple sclerosis. J Exp Med 1994;179:973–84.
[41] Bielekova B, Sung MH, Kadom N, et al. Expansion and functional relevance of high-avidity myelin-specific CD4 + T cells in multiple sclerosis. J Immunol 2004;172: 3893–904.
[42] Scholz C, Patton KT, Anderson DE, et al. Expansion of autoreactive T cells in multiple sclerosis is independent of exogenous B7 costimulation. J Immunol 1998;160:1532–8.
[43] Lovett-Racke AE, Trotter JL, Lauber J, et al. Decreased dependence of myelin basic protein-reactive T cells on CD28-mediated costimulation in multiple sclerosis patients. A marker of activated/memory T cells. J Clin Invest 1998;101:725–30.
[44] Burns J, Bartholomew B, Lobo S. Isolation of myelin basic protein-specific T cells predominantly from the memory T-cell compartment in multiple sclerosis. Ann Neurol 1999;45:33–9.
[45] Bielekova B, Muraro PA, Golestaneh L, et al. Preferential expansion of autoreactive T lymphocytes from the memory T-cell pool by IL-7. J Neuroimmunol 1999;100:115–23.
[46] Bar-Or A, O'Connor K, Hafler DA. Multiple sclerosis. In: Austen KF, Frank MM, Atkinson JP, Cantor H, editors. Samter's immunologic diseases. 6th edition. Philadelphia: Lippincott Williams & Wilkins; 2001. p. 711–37.

[47] Becher B, Giacomini PS, Pelletier D, et al. Interferon-gamma secretion by peripheral blood T-cell subsets in multiple sclerosis: correlation with disease phase and interferon-beta therapy. Ann Neurol 1999;45:247–50.

[48] Biddison WE, Cruikshank WW, Center DM, et al. CD8 + peptide-specific T cells can chemoattract CD4 + myelin peptide-specific T cells: importance of IFN-inducible protein 10. J Immunol 1998;160:444–8.

[49] Babbe H, Roers A, Waisman A, et al. Clonal expansions of CD8(+) T cells dominate the T cell infiltrate in active multiple sclerosis lesions as shown by micromanipulation and single cell polymerase chain reaction. J Exp Med 2000;192:393–404.

[50] Hoftberger R, Aboul-Enein F, Brueck W, et al. Expression of major histocompatibility complex class I molecules on the different cell types in multiple sclerosis lesions. Brain Pathol 2004;14:43–50.

[51] Skulina C, Schmidt S, Dornmair K, et al. Multiple sclerosis: brain-infiltrating CD8 + T cells persist as clonal expansions in the cerebrospinal fluid and blood. Proc Natl Acad Sci USA 2004;101:2428–33.

[52] Tsuchida T, Parker KC, Turner RV, et al. Autoreactive CD8 + T-cell responses to human myelin protein-derived peptides. Proc Natl Acad Sci USA 1994;91:10859–63.

[53] Buckle GJ, Hollsberg P, Hafler DA. Activated CD8 + T cells in secondary progressive MS secrete lymphotoxin. Neurology 2003;60:702–5.

[54] Crawford MP, Yan SX, Ortega SB, et al. High prevalence of autoreactive, neuroantigen-specific CD8 + T cells in multiple sclerosis revealed by novel flow cytometric assay. Blood 2004;103:4222–31.

[55] Karin N, Mitchell DJ, Brocke S, et al. Reversal of experimental autoimmune encephalomyelitis by a soluble peptide variant of a myelin basic protein epitope: T cell receptor antagonism and reduction of interferon gamma and tumor necrosis factor alpha production. J Exp Med 1994;180:2227–37.

[56] Young DA, Lowe LD, Booth SS, et al. IL-4, IL-10, IL-13, and TGF-beta from an altered peptide ligand-specific Th2 cell clone down-regulate adoptive transfer of experimental autoimmune encephalomyelitis. J Immunol 2000;164:3563–72.

[57] Kappos L, Comi G, Panitch H, et al. Induction of a non-encephalitogenic type 2 T helper-cell autoimmune response in multiple sclerosis after administration of an altered peptide ligand in a placebo-controlled, randomized phase II trial. The Altered Peptide Ligand in Relapsing MS Study Group. Nat Med 2000;6:1176–82.

[58] Bielekova B, Goodwin B, Richert N, et al. Encephalitogenic potential of the myelin basic protein peptide (amino acids 83–99) in multiple sclerosis: results of a phase II clinical trial with an altered peptide ligand. Nat Med 2000;6:1167–75.

[59] Martino G, Adorini L, Rieckmann P, et al. Inflammation in multiple sclerosis: the good, the bad, and the complex. Lancet Neurol 2002;1:499–509.

[60] Moalem G, Leibowitz-Amit R, Yoles E, et al. Autoimmune T cells protect neurons from secondary degeneration after central nervous system axotomy. Nat Med 1999;5: 49–55.

[61] Wekerle H, Linington C, Lassmann H, et al. Cellular immune reactivity within the CNS. Trends Neurosci 1986;9:271–7.

[62] Hickey WF, Hsu BL, Kimura H. T-lymphocyte entry into the central nervous system. J Neurosci Res 1991;28:254–60.

[63] Kivisäkk P, Mahad DJ, Callahan MK, et al. Human cerebrospinal fluid central memory CD4 + T cells: evidence for trafficking through choroid plexus and meninges via P-selectin. Proc Natl Acad Sci USA 2003;100:8389–94.

[64] Hickey WF. Migration of hematogenous cells through the blood-brain barrier and the initiation of CNS inflammation. Brain Pathol 1991;1:97–105.

[65] Wekerle H. Antigen presentation by CNS glia. In: Kettenmann H, Ranson B, editors. Neuroglia. Oxford (England): Oxford University Press; 1994.

[66] Williams K, Ulvestad E, Antel JP. B7/BB-1 antigen expression on adult human microglia studied in vitro and in situ. Eur J Immunol 1994;24:3031–7.

[67] Windhagen A, Newcombe J, Dangond F, et al. Expression of costimulatory molecules B7–1(CD80), B7–2 (CD86), and interleukin 12 cytokine in multiple sclerosis lesions. J Exp Med 1995;182:1985–96.

[68] Genc K, Dona DL, Reder AT. Increased CD80(+) B cells in active multiple sclerosis and reversal by interferon beta-1b therapy. J Clin Invest 1997;99:2664–71.

[69] Kuchroo VK, Das MP, Brown JA, et al. B7–1 and B7–2 costimulatory molecules activate differentially the Th1/Th2 developmental pathways: application to autoimmune disease therapy. Cell 1995;80:707–18.

[70] Racke MK, Scott DE, Quigley L, et al. Distinct roles for B7–1 (CD-80) and B7–2 (CD-86) in the initiation of experimental allergic encephalomyelitis. J Clin Invest 1995;96: 2195–203.

[71] Miller SD, Vanderlugt CL, Lenschow DJ, et al. Blockade of CD28/B7–1 interaction prevents epitope spreading and clinical relapses of murine EAE. Immunity 1995;3:739–45.

[72] Corcione A, Casazza S, Ferretti E, et al. Recapitulation of B cell differentiation in the central nervous system of patients with multiple sclerosis. Proc Natl Acad Sci USA 2004; 101:11064–9.

[73] Cserr HF, Harling-Berg CJ, et al. Drainage of brain extracellular fluid into blood and deep cervical lymph and its immunological significance. Brain Pathol 1992;2:269–76.

[74] de Vos AF, van Meurs M, Brok HP, et al. Transfer of central nervous system autoantigens and presentation in secondary lymphoid organs. J Immunol 2002;169:5415–23.

[75] Kivisäkk P, Mahad DJ, Callahan MK, et al. Expression of CCR7 in multiple sclerosis: implications for CNS immunity. Ann Neurol 2004;55:627–38.

[76] Wucherpfennig KW, Strominger JL. Molecular mimicry in T cell-mediated autoimmunity: viral peptides activate human T cell clones specific for myelin basic protein. Cell 1999;80: 695–705.

[77] Wucherpfennig KW. Infectious triggers for inflammatory neurological diseases. Nat Med 2002;8:455–7.

[78] Lang HL, Jacobsen H, Ikemizu S, et al. A functional and structural basis for TCR cross-reactivity in multiple sclerosis. Nat Immunol 2002;3:940–3.

[79] Springer TA. Traffic signals for lymphocyte recirculation and leukocyte emigration: the multistep paradigm. Cell 1994;76:301–14.

[80] Ransohoff RM. Mechanisms of inflammation in MS tissue: adhesion molecules and chemokines. J Neuroimmunol 1999;98:57–68.

[81] Campbell JJ, Hedrick J, Zlotnik A, et al. Chemokines and the arrest of lymphocytes rolling under flow conditions. Science 1998;279:381–4.

[82] Yong VW, Power C, Forsyth P, et al. Metalloproteinases in biology and pathology of the nervous system. Nat Rev Neurosci 2001;2:502–11.

[83] Sobel RA, Mitchell ME, Fondren G. Intercellular adhesion molecule-1 (ICAM-1) in cellular immune reactions in the human central nervous system. Am J Pathol 1990;136: 1309–16.

[84] Washington R, Burton J, Todd RF 3rd, et al. Expression of immunologically relevant endothelial cell activation antigens on isolated central nervous system microvessels from patients with multiple sclerosis. Ann Neurol 1994;35:89–97.

[85] Cannella B, Raine CS. The adhesion molecule and cytokine profile of multiple sclerosis lesions. Ann Neurol 1995;37:424–35.

[86] Bo L, Peterson JW, Mork S, et al. Distribution of immunoglobulin superfamily members ICAM-1, -2, -3, and the beta 2 integrin LFA-1 in multiple sclerosis lesions. J Neuropathol Exp Neurol 1996;55:1060–72.

[87] Baron JL, Madri JA, Ruddle NH, et al. Surface expression of alpha 4 integrin by CD4 T cells is required for their entry into brain parenchyma. J Exp Med 1993;177:57–68.

[88] Kuchroo VK, Martin CA, Greer JM, et al. Cytokines and adhesion molecules contribute to the ability of myelin proteolipid protein-specific T cell clones to mediate experimental allergic encephalomyelitis. J Immunol 1993;151:4371–82.
[89] Yednock TA, Cannon C, Fritz LC, et al. Prevention of experimental autoimmune encephalomyelitis by antibodies against alpha 4 beta 1 integrin. Nature 1992;356: 63–6.
[90] Soilu-Hanninen M, Roytta M, Salmi A, et al. Therapy with antibody against leukocyte integrin VLA-4 (CD49d) is effective and safe in virus-facilitated experimental allergic encephalomyelitis. J Neuroimmunol 1997;72:95–105.
[91] Brosnan CF, Cannella B, Battistini L. Cytokine localization in multiple sclerosis lesions: correlation with adhesion molecule expression and reactive nitrogen species. Neurology 1995;45(6 Suppl 6):S16–21.
[92] Damle NK, Klussman K, Leytze G, et al. Costimulation with integrin ligands intercellular adhesion molecule-1 or vascular cell adhesion molecule-1 augments activation-induced death of antigen-specific CD4 + T lymphocytes. J Immunol 1993;151:2368–79.
[93] Moingeon P, Chang HC, Wallner BP, et al. CD2-mediated adhesion facilitates T lymphocyte antigen recognition function. Nature 1989;339:312–4.
[94] Karpus WJ, Ransohoff RM. Chemokine regulation of experimental autoimmune encephalomyelitis: temporal and spatial expression patterns govern disease pathogenesis. J Immunol 1998;161:2667–71.
[95] Hvas J, McLean C, Justesen J, et al. Perivascular T cells express the pro-inflammatory chemokine RANTES mRNA in multiple sclerosis lesions. Scand J Immunol 1997;46: 195–203.
[96] Van Der Voorn P, Tekstra J, Beelen RH, et al. Expression of MCP-1 by reactive astrocytes in demyelinating multiple sclerosis lesions. Am J Pathol 1999;154:45–51.
[97] Sorensen TL, Tani M, Jensen J, et al. Expression of specific chemokines and chemokine receptors in the central nervous system of multiple sclerosis patients. J Clin Invest 1999;103: 807–15.
[98] Siveke JT, Hamann A. T helper 1 and T helper 2 cells respond differentially to chemokines. J Immunol 1998;160:550–4.
[99] Balashov KE, Rottman JB, Weiner HL, et al. CCR5(+) and CXCR3(+) T cells are increased in multiple sclerosis and their ligands MIP-1alpha and IP-10 are expressed in demyelinating brain lesions. Proc Natl Acad Sci USA 1999;96:6873–8.
[100] Misu T, Onodera H, Fujihara K, et al. Chemokine receptor expression on T cells in blood and cerebrospinal fluid at relapse and remission of multiple sclerosis: imbalance of Th1/Th2-associated chemokine signaling. J Neuroimmunol 2001;114:207–12.
[101] Nanki T, Lipsky PE. Lack of correlation between chemokine receptor and T(h)1/T(h)2 cytokine expression by individual memory T cells. Int Immunol 2000;12:1659–67.
[102] Yong VW, Krekoski CA, Forsyth PA, et al. Matrix metalloproteinases and diseases of the CNS. Trends Neurosci 1998;21:75–80.
[103] Kieseier BC, Seifert T, Giovannoni G, et al. Matrix metalloproteinases in inflammatory demyelination: targets for treatment. Neurology 1999;53:20–5.
[104] Kieseier BC, Pischel H, Neuen-Jacob E, et al. ADAM-10 and ADAM-17 in the inflamed human CNS. Glia 2003;42:398–405.
[105] Rosenberg GA, Kornfeld M, Estrada E, et al. TIMP-2 reduces proteolytic opening of blood-brain barrier by type IV collagenase. Brain Res 1992;576:203–7.
[106] Leppert D, Waubant E, Galardy R, et al. T cell gelatinases mediate basement membrane transmigration in vitro. J Immunol 1995;154:4379–89.
[107] Cuzner ML, Gveric D, Strand C, et al. The expression of tissue-type plasminogen activator, matrix metalloproteases and endogenous inhibitors in the central nervous system in multiple sclerosis: comparison of stages in lesion evolution. J Neuropathol Exp Neurol 1996;55:1194–204.

[108] Maeda A, Sobel RA. Matrix metalloproteinases in the normal human central nervous system, microglial nodules, and multiple sclerosis lesions. J Neuropathol Exp Neurol 1996; 55:300–9.

[109] Hartung HP, Jung S, Stoll G, et al. Inflammatory mediators in demyelinating disorders of the CNS and PNS. J Neuroimmunol 1992;40:197–210.

[110] Black RA, Rauch CT, Kozlosky CJ, et al. A metalloproteinase disintegrin that releases tumour-necrosis factor-alpha from cells. Nature 1997;385:729–33.

[111] Proost P, Van Damme J, Opdenakker G. Leukocyte gelatinase B cleavage releases encephalitogens from human myelin basic protein. Biochem Biophys Res Commun 1993; 192:1175–81.

[112] Cuzner ML, Davison AN, Rudge P. Proteolytic enzyme activity of blood leukocytes and cerebrospinal fluid in multiple sclerosis. Ann Neurol 1978;4:337–44.

[113] Gijbels K, Masure S, Carton H, et al. Gelatinase in the cerebrospinal fluid of patients with multiple sclerosis and other inflammatory neurological disorders. J Neuroimmunol 1992; 41:29–34.

[114] Leppert D, Ford J, Stabler G, et al. Matrix metalloproteinase-9 (gelatinase B) is selectively elevated in CSF during relapses and stable phases of multiple sclerosis. Brain 1998; 121(Pt 12):2327–34.

[115] Lee MA, Palace J, Stabler G, et al. Serum gelatinase B, TIMP-1 and TIMP-2 levels in multiple sclerosis. A longitudinal clinical and MRI study. Brain 1999;122(Pt 2):191–7.

[116] Bar-Or A, Nuttall RK, Duddy M, et al. Analyses of all matrix metalloproteinase members in leukocytes emphasize monocytes as major inflammatory mediators in multiple sclerosis. Brain 2003;126(Pt 12):2738–49.

[117] Alter A, Duddy M, Hebert S, et al. Determinants of human B cell migration across brain endothelial cells. J Immunol 2003;170:4497–505.

[118] Genain CP, Cannella B, Hauser SL, et al. Identification of autoantibodies associated with myelin damage in multiple sclerosis. Nat Med 1999;5:170–5.

[119] Raine CS, Cannella B, Hauser SL, et al. Demyelination in primate autoimmune encephalomyelitis and acute multiple sclerosis lesions: a case for antigen-specific antibody mediation. Ann Neurol 1999;46:144–60.

[120] Piddlesden SJ, Lassmann H, Zimprich F, et al. The demyelinating potential of antibodies to myelin oligodendrocyte glycoprotein is related to their ability to fix complement. Am J Pathol 1993;143:555–64.

[121] Pender MP. The pathogenesis of primary progressive multiple sclerosis: antibody-mediated attack and no repair? J Clin Neurosci 2004;11:689–92.

[122] Berger T, Rubner P, Schautzer F, et al. Antimyelin antibodies as a predictor of clinically definite multiple sclerosis after a first demyelinating event. N Engl J Med 2003;349:139–45.

[123] Antel JP, Bar-Or A. Do myelin-directed antibodies predict multiple sclerosis? N Engl J Med 2003;349:107–9.

[124] O'Connor KC, Chitnis T, Griffin DE, et al. Myelın basic protein-reactive autoantibodies in the serum and cerebrospinal fluid of multiple sclerosis patients are characterized by low-affinity interactions. J Neuroimmunol 2003;136:140–8.

[125] Li W, Walus L, Rabacchi SA, et al. A neutralizing anti-Nogo66 receptor monoclonal antibody reverses inhibition of neurite outgrowth by central nervous system myelin. J Biol Chem 2004;279:43780–8.

[126] Miller DJ, Rodriguez M. A monoclonal autoantibody that promotes central nervous system remyelination in a model of multiple sclerosis is a natural autoantibody encoded by germline immunoglobulin genes. J Immunol 1995;154:2460–9.

[127] Miller DJ, Njenga MK, Murray PD, et al. A monoclonal natural autoantibody that promotes remyelination suppresses central nervous system inflammation and increases virus expression after Theiler's virus-induced demyelination. Int Immunol 1996;8: 131–41.

[128] Bar-Or A, Oliveira EM, Anderson DE, et al. Immunological memory: contribution of memory B cells expressing costimulatory molecules in the resting state. J Immunol 2001; 167:5669–77.
[129] Pender MP. Infection of autoreactive B lymphocytes with EBV, causing chronic autoimmune diseases. Trends Immunol 2003;24:584–8.
[130] Prineas JW. Multiple sclerosis: presence of lymphatic capillaries and lymphoid tissue in the brain and spinal cord. Science 1979;203:1123–5.
[131] Serafini B, Rosicarelli B, Magliozzi R, et al. Detection of ectopic B-cell follicles with germinal centers in the meninges of patients with secondary progressive multiple sclerosis. Brain Pathol 2004;14:164–74.
[132] Duddy ME, Alter A, Bar-Or A. Distinct profiles of human B cell effector cytokines: a role in immune regulation? J Immunol 2004;172:3422–7.
[133] Anderson AC, Reddy J, Nazareno R, et al. IL-10 plays an important role in the homeostatic regulation of the autoreactive repertoire in naive mice. J Immunol 2004;173:828–34.
[134] Fillatreau S, Sweenie CH, McGeachy MJ, et al. B cells regulate autoimmunity by provision of IL-10. Nat Immunol 2002;3:944–50.
[135] Aloisi F, Ria F, Penna G, et al. Microglia are more efficient than astrocytes in antigen processing and in Th1 but not Th2 cell activation. J Immunol 1998;160:4671–80.
[136] Williams K, Ulvestad E, Antel J. Immune regulatory and effector properties of human adult microglia studies in vitro and in situ. Adv Neuroimmunol 1994;4:273–81.
[137] Ulvestad E, Williams K, Bjerkvig R, et al. Human microglial cells have phenotypic and functional characteristics in common with both macrophages and dendritic antigen-presenting cells. J Leukoc Biol 1994;56:732–40.
[138] Kim HJ, Ifergan I, Antel JP, et al. Type 2 monocyte and microglia differentiation mediated by glatiramer acetate therapy in patients with multiple sclerosis. J Immunol 2004;172: 7144–53.
[139] Tuohy VK, Yu M, Yin L, et al. The epitope spreading cascade during progression of experimental autoimmune encephalomyelitis and multiple sclerosis. Immunol Rev 1998; 164:93–100.
[140] Giuliani F, Goodyer CG, Antel JP, et al. Vulnerability of human neurons to T cell-mediated cytotoxicity. J Immunol 2003;171:368–79.
[141] Neumann H, Medana IM, Bauer J, et al. Cytotoxic T lymphocytes in autoimmune and degenerative CNS diseases. Trends Neurosci 2002;25:313–9.
[142] Waxman SG. Nitric oxide and the axonal death cascade. Ann Neurol 2003;53:150–3.
[143] Waxman SG. Acquired channelopathies in nerve injury and MS. Neurology 2001;56: 1621–7.
[144] Chari DM, Blakemore WF. New insights into remyelination failure in multiple sclerosis: implications for glial cell transplantation. Mult Scler 2002;8:271–7.
[145] Reddy H, Narayanan S, Matthews PM, et al. Relating axonal injury to functional recovery in MS. Neurology 2000;54:236–9.
[146] Schwartz M. Protective autoimmunity as a T-cell response to central nervous system trauma: prospects for therapeutic vaccines. Prog Neurobiol 2001;65:489–96.
[147] Sakaguchi S, Sakaguchi N, Asano M, et al. Immunologic self-tolerance maintained by activated T cells expressing IL-2 receptor alpha-chains (CD25). Breakdown of a single mechanism of self-tolerance causes various autoimmune diseases. J Immunol 1995;155:1151–64.
[148] Anderton S, Burkhart C, Metzler B, et al. Mechanisms of central and peripheral T-cell tolerance: lessons from experimental models of multiple sclerosis. Immunol Rev 1999;169: 123–37.
[149] Kohm AP, Carpentier PA, Anger HA, et al. Cutting edge: CD4 + CD25 + regulatory T cells suppress antigen-specific autoreactive immune responses and central nervous system inflammation during active experimental autoimmune encephalomyelitis. J Immunol 2002; 169:4712–6.

[150] Viglietta V, Baecher-Allan C, Weiner HL, et al. Loss of functional suppression by CD4 + CD25 + regulatory T cells in patients with multiple sclerosis. J Exp Med 2004;199: 971–9.
[151] Baecher-Allan C, Viglietta V, Hafler DA. Human CD4 + CD25 + regulatory T cells. Semin Immunol 2004;16:89–98.
[152] Cottrez F, Groux H. Specialization in tolerance: innate CD(4 +) CD(25 +) versus acquired TR1 and TH3 regulatory T cells. Transplantation 2004;77(1 Suppl):S12–5.
[153] Hu D, Ikizawa K, Lu L, et al. Analysis of regulatory CD8 T cells in Qa-1-deficient mice. Nat Immunol 2004;5:516–23.
[154] Chess L, Jiang H. Resurrecting CD8 + suppressor T cells. Nat Immunol 2004;5:469–71.
[155] Kerschensteiner M, Gallmeier E, Behrens L, et al. Activated human T cells, B cells, and monocytes produce brain-derived neurotrophic factor in vitro and in inflammatory brain lesions: a neuroprotective role of inflammation? J Exp Med 1999;189:865–70.
[156] Stadelmann C, Kerschensteiner M, Misgeld T, et al. BDNF and gp145trkB in multiple sclerosis brain lesions: neuroprotective interactions between immune and neuronal cells? Brain 2002;125(Pt 1):75–85.
[157] Arnett HA, Mason J, Marino M, et al. TNF alpha promotes proliferation of oligodendrocyte progenitors and remyelination. Nat Neurosci 2001;4:1116–22.
[158] Miller DJ, Asakura K, Rodriguez M. Experimental strategies to promote central nervous system remyelination in multiple sclerosis: insights gained from the Theiler's virus model system. J Neurosci Res 1995;41:291–6.
[159] Reindl M, Khantane S, Ehling R, et al. Serum and cerebrospinal fluid antibodies to Nogo-A in patients with multiple sclerosis and acute neurological disorders. J Neuroimmunol 2003; 145:139–47.
[160] Schwab ME. Nogo and axon regeneration. Curr Opin Neurobiol 2004;14:118–24.
[161] Herx LM, Rivest S, Yong VW. Central nervous system-initiated inflammation and neurotrophism in trauma: IL-1 beta is required for the production of ciliary neurotrophic factor. J Immunol 2000;165:2232–9.
[162] Mason JL, Suzuki K, Chaplin DD, et al. Interleukin-1beta promotes repair of the CNS. J Neurosci 2001;21:7046–52.
[163] Wosik K, Antel J, Kuhlmann T, et al. Oligodendrocyte injury in multiple sclerosis: a role for p53. J Neurochem 2003;85:635–44.
[164] Niehaus A, Shi J, Grzenkowski M, et al. Patients with active relapsing-remitting multiple sclerosis synthesize antibodies recognizing oligodendrocyte progenitor cell surface protein: implications for remyelination. Ann Neurol 2000;48:362–71.
[165] Rudick RA, Ransohoff RM, Peppler R, et al. Interferon beta induces interleukin-10 expression: relevance to multiple sclerosis. Ann Neurol 1996;40:618–27.
[166] Kilinc M, Saatci-Cekirge I, Karabudak R. Serial analysis of soluble intercellular adhesion molecule-1 level in relapsing-remitting multiple sclerosis patients during IFN-beta1b treatment. J Interferon Cytokine Res 2003;23:127–33.
[167] Karabudak R, Kurne A, Guc D, et al. Effect of interferon beta-1a on serum matrix metalloproteinase-9 (MMP-9) and tissue inhibitor of matrix metalloproteinase (TIMP-1) in relapsing remitting multiple sclerosis patients. One year follow-up results. J Neurol 2004; 251:279–83.
[168] Galboiz Y, Shapiro S, Lahat N, et al. Matrix metalloproteinases and their tissue inhibitors as markers of disease subtype and response to interferon-beta therapy in relapsing and secondary-progressive multiple sclerosis patients. Ann Neurol 2001;50: 443–51.
[169] Yong VW. Differential mechanisms of action of interferon-beta and glatiramer aetate in MS. Neurology 2002;59:802–8.
[170] Teitelbaum D, Meshorer A, Hirshfeld T, et al. Suppression of experimental allergic encephalomyelitis by a synthetic polypeptide. Eur J Immunol 1971;1:242–8.

[171] Miller A, Shapiro S, Gershtein R, et al. Treatment of multiple sclerosis with copolymer-1 (Copaxone): implicating mechanisms of Th1 to Th2/Th3 immune-deviation. J Neuroimmunol 1998;92:113–21.

[172] Qin Y, Zhang DQ, Prat A, et al. Characterization of T cell lines derived from glatiramer-acetate-treated multiple sclerosis patients. J Neuroimmunol 2000;108:201–6.

[173] Neuhaus O, Farina C, Yassouridis A, et al. Multiple sclerosis: comparison of copolymer-1-reactive T cell lines from treated and untreated subjects reveals cytokine shift from T helper 1 to T helper 2 cells. Proc Natl Acad Sci USA 2000;97:7452–7.

[174] Farina C, Then Bergh F, Albrecht H, et al. Treatment of multiple sclerosis with Copaxone (COP): Elispot assay detects COP-induced interleukin-4 and interferon-gamma response in blood cells. Brain 2001;124(Pt 4):705–19.

[175] Karandikar NJ, Crawford MP, Yan X, et al. Glatiramer acetate (Copaxone) therapy induces CD8(+) T cell responses in patients with multiple sclerosis. J Clin Invest 2002;109: 641–9.

[176] Schmied M, Duda PW, Krieger JI, et al. In vitro evidence that subcutaneous administration of glatiramer acetate induces hyporesponsive T cells in patients with multiple sclerosis. Clin Immunol 2003;106:163–74.

[177] Hafler DA. Degeneracy, as opposed to specificity, in immunotherapy. J Clin Invest 2002; 109:581–4.

[178] Duda PW, Schmied MC, Cook SL, et al. Glatiramer acetate (Copaxone) induces degenerate, Th2-polarized immune responses in patients with multiple sclerosis. J Clin Invest 2000;105:967–76.

[179] Kim HJ, Biernacki K, Prat A, et al. Inflammatory potential and migratory capacities across human brain endothelial cells of distinct glatiramer acetate-reactive T cells generated in treated multiple sclerosis patients. Clin Immunol 2004;111:38–46.

[180] Ziemssen T, Kumpfel T, Klinkert WE, et al. Glatiramer acetate-specific T-helper 1- and 2-type cell lines produce BDNF: implications for multiple sclerosis therapy. Brain-derived neurotrophic factor. Brain 2002;125(Pt 11):2381–91.

[181] Chen M, Valenzuela RM, Dhib-Jalbut S. Glatiramer acetate-reactive T cells produce brain-derived neurotrophic factor. J Neurol Sci 2003;215:37–44.

ELSEVIER
SAUNDERS

Neurol Clin 23 (2005) 177–187

NEUROLOGIC
CLINICS

Managing Symptoms of Multiple Sclerosis

Randall T. Schapiro, MD[a,b,*]

[a] *University of Minnesota, Minneapolis, MN, USA*
[b] *The Schapiro Center for Multiple Sclerosis, The Minneapolis Clinic of Neurology, Minneapolis, MN, USA*

During the past 10 years, clinicians have emphasized the disease-altering approach to multiple sclerosis (MS). The birth of therapeutic immune-modulating treatments, which have the potential to alter the course of MS, changed the emphasis from supportive symptom management to disease management of patients. Until that time, supportive care was all that was available. Symptomatic management often took a back seat in the minds of physicians. It has not taken that seat in patient's thoughts, however. Even though people who have MS want to see their disease halted, quality of life means just as much to most patients, and that entails effective treatment of the primary symptoms of MS (resulting from actual demyelination and axonal loss), the secondary symptoms of MS (eg, contractures, bladder infections, osteoporosis, and decubiti resulting from failure to treat the primary problems), and the tertiary symptoms of MS (personal, vocational, relationship issues). This article is devoted to those issues that make the life of a person who has MS more comfortable.

Fatigue

The single most common and most disabling symptom of MS is fatigue. Fatigue roars its ugly head in almost all patients who have MS [1]. To manage fatigue effectively, it is essential to recognize that there are different types of fatigue that can occur independently or in combination. There are five forms of fatigue frequently seen in MS.

Fatigue 1 may be called normal fatigue. Having MS does not protect a person from becoming tired after a trying, hard day of work or play. Sometimes it is not recognized that having MS does not protect one from

* The Schapiro Center for Multiple Sclerosis, The Minneapolis Clinic of Neurology, 4225 Golden Valley Road, Minneapolis, MN 55422.

E-mail address: schap003@umn.edu

0733-8619/05/$ - see front matter
doi:10.1016/j.ncl.2004.09.001 ***neurologic.theclinics.com***

having this type of fatigue. We teach that it is a good fatigue and that people who have MS are not fragile and do not break because they have worked hard. Often the emphasis in MS is rest, rest, rest. Clearly, pushing the envelope to see how fatigued one can become before breaking is not appropriate, but the person who has MS certainly can become fatigued every now and again and can recover and do well after a rest.

Fatigue 2 may be called deconditioning fatigue. People who do not have MS become fatigued if they are out of shape and the same is true for those who have MS. Studies show that those who have MS can and should exercise (see later discussion on exercise). To gain endurance, aerobic exercise is essential. Without endurance, attempting to perform an out-of-the-ordinary activity results in fatigue.

Fatigue 3 may be called neuromuscular or short-circuiting fatigue. The demyelinated nerve fires again and again until it shorts when it is called upon to do a repetitive task. Thus, progressive resistive exercises (weight lifting) often result in a feeling of increased fatigue and weakness rather than a feeling of increased strength. Short breaks with energy conservation can make this fatigue less prominent.

Fatigue 4 may be called depression fatigue. People who are depressed, whether they have or do not have MS, often do not sleep properly, eat properly, or feel well. They may describe this as fatigue, but the treatment revolves around the treatment of depression [2].

Fatigue 5 is the most common fatigue seen in MS, occurring in 85% to 90% [3]. It often is called lassitude or MS-related fatigue. It presents as an overwhelming feeling of tiredness in those who have done little and are not depressed. Neurochemistry has contributed treatments that have been partially successful in its management (Table 1). Amantidine, pemoline, methylphenidate, fluoxetine, and now, most commonly, modafinil, have been of some value in modulating this common problem of MS [4–6].

When developing a strategy for fatigue, the clinician must look for mitigating circumstances that can be corrected to ease the fatigue. Occupational therapists can be helpful in finding these and teaching simple approaches to activities of daily living. After correcting those issues and treating concomitant medical problems that may be contributing (eg, heart disease, sleep disorders, or bladder infections), the fatigue may be addressed with a combination of physical and pharmacologic approaches. Amantidine at 100 mg twice a day helps approximately 30% of patients but often loses its effectiveness over time. Pemoline has black box warnings from the Food and Drug Administration because of the potential for liver disease and is not used often. The energizing antidepressants can be helpful but not significantly. Stimulants, such as amphetamines and methylphenidate, are habit forming and often require increasing doses to remain effective. Modafinil has become a popular alternative at a dose of 200 mg a day. It seems to have little habit forming potential and does not seem to lose its effectiveness over time.

Table 1
Select symptomatic medications

Generic name	Brand name	Usage in multiple sclerosis
Alprostadil	Caverject, Muse	Erectile dysfunction
Amantadine	Symmetrel	Fatigue
Amitriptyline	Elavil	Pain (dysesthesias)
Baclofen	Lioresal	Spasticity
Carbamazepine	Tegretol	Pain (trigeminal neuralgia)
Clonazepam	Klonopin	Tremor, pain, spasticity
Desmopressin	DDAVP	Decrease urine production
Diazepam	Valium	Spasticity (muscle spasms)
Fluoxetine	Prozac	Depression, fatigue
Gabapentin	Neurontin	Pain, dysesthesias, spasticity
Imipramine	Tofranil	Bladder dysfunction, pain
Modafinil	Provigil	Fatigue
Oxybutynin	Ditropan, Ditropan XL	Bladder dysfunction
Oxybutynin (transdermal patch)	Oxytrol	Bladder dysfunction
Pemoline	Cylert	Fatigue
Phenytoin	Dilantin	Pain (paresthesias)
Sertraline	Zoloft	Depression, anxiety
Sildenafil	Viagra	Erectile dysfunction
Tizanidine	Zanaflex	Spasticity
Tolterodine	Detrol (LA)	Bladder dysfunction
Topiramate	Topamax	Pain, tremor
Venlafaxine	Effexor	Depression

Spasticity

Spasticity, velocity-dependent stiffness about a joint, is another common problem in MS [7]. It can vary from nonexistent to severe, even in the same person, and from moment to moment, making its management challenging. It seems to be the result of disequilibrium in the ascending and descending excitatory and inhibitory pathways in the brain and spinal cord. Gamma-aminobutyric acid and other neurotransmitters are involved. When evaluating spasticity, the examiner must take into consideration how the stiff extremity is used. Often those who have significant spasticity use their spasticity to walk, transfer, and manage their daily living. Treatment becomes an issue only if the spasticity is causing discomfort, pain, or problems with daily living.

Pain, either from an injury or from a bladder infection, exacerbates spasticity. Thus, the management of spasticity begins with the removal of noxious stimuli. Then an exercise program emphasizing stretching, range of motion, and aerobic function is initiated. If the spasticity remains problematic, a pharmacologic approach is begun, usually with baclofen [8]. Increasing doses up to 160 mg or more a day in divided doses can decrease spasticity. At higher dosing, stiffness may be traded for weakness. Tizanidine often is more difficult to tolerate. It is as effective as baclofen but leads to more fatigue and dry mouth. Initiation with 2 mg and slowly increasing up to 36 mg can be helpful, especially if the spasticity is nocturnal and the medication is given at night [9]. The fatiguing side effect then becomes an advantage. Both of these treatments have short half-lives; thus, when used chronically, they need to be dosed frequently (every 4–6 hours).

Spasms may accompany the spasticity and usually are more severe and frequent at night. They often interrupt the sleep cycle even in those who do not recognize their awakenings. This may lead to severe fatigue the next day; thus, minimizing nocturnal spasms is important. Clonazapam (0.5–1.5 mg), given at bedtime, can aid in sleep initiation and decrease spasms with minimum side effects. Diazepam (5–7.5 mg) has a similar effect. Dose escalation should be avoided. Dopamine agonists and dopamine itself also decrease nocturnal spasms reasonably effectively at low dosages.

Spasms occurring during the day usually are handled best by the addition of the newer antiepileptic medications, including gabapentin and topiramate. The sedation afforded by the nocturnal treatments should be avoided as much as possible.

In some patients, spasticity can be intractable. The high doses of medications necessitated by this circumstance sedate and cause disability on their own. The judicious use of botulinum toxin may relieve focal muscle spasm. Unfortunately, the intractable spasticity usually seen in MS often involves an entire extremity rather than an isolated muscle. Thus, the amount of toxin becomes inappropriate to deliver safely [10]. Cannabinoids have been regarded as an additional spasticity treatment. Controversy has developed regarding that use. Although studies have been performed, no definitive answer has been forthcoming [11,12]. The replacement of oral spasticity medications with intrathecal baclofen (ITB) may be sensational if a careful selection process is undertaken [13]. Any spasticity the patient is using for activities of daily living may be altered. Thus, transferring techniques may require a different approach. The perception of strength that may be given by stiffness may disappear, giving the perception of weakness. This can be alarming to those who are not prepared. A test dose of 50 to 100 μg of ITB is delivered preimplantation via a spinal tap. If there is a change in the spasticity with the test dose, implantation may proceed. The Medtronic Syncromed© pump allows specific programming of dose and timing to maximize the therapeutic effects. Refilling the pump may take place in the office. Microgram dosing allows for significant effect without generalized side effects.

Paroxysmal symptoms

Unique symptoms in MS are called paroxysmal because they come in bouts. Sometimes they are sensory in nature and may be painful. Trigeminal neuralgia is a common example of this type of painful, paroxysmal symptom. This lancinating, electrical sensation along the distribution of a branch of the trigeminal nerve can be terribly disabling. It may be a standalone problem in some patients but also is a symptom associated with MS. Periodic electrical sensation down the spine with the bending of the neck is called Lhermitte's sign, another paroxysmal sensory symptom. These types of sensations occasionally may be felt in other parts of the body. Often the paroxysmal symptoms are motor in nature. They may be twitching of an eyelid or myokymia in the facial muscles. They may manifest as a true spasm of an arm in an extended or, occasionally, flexed position lasting for seconds. They can occur frequently, several times an hour. The spasm may occur with speech, a paroxysmal dysarthria or speech arrest. All of these can be disconcerting to the patient and the clinician. Surprisingly, they usually are easy to treat once recognized. Carbamazepine, topiramate, gabapentin, and other antiseizure treatments usually are effective at low dosages. Misoprostol also has been discussed as an alternative treatment [14]. After the spasms are settled, the drugs may be withdrawn and only started again if the symptoms recur.

Pain

Pain is surprisingly common in MS, occurring in 50% of patients [15]. The pain usually is a burning neuropathic type. It may be disturbing, and pain medicine offers little if any relief. The distribution of the pain may not follow any recognizable neurologic distribution. It can be paroxysmal in nature but often is fairly constant with nocturnal worsening when the body is at rest in bed.

The antiepileptic agents and antidepressant treatments often are effective in modulating the painful symptoms. Gabapentin, in doses of 1800 to 2400 mg, often is necessary for the desired effect. All of these treatments require adjustment from time to time to maintain some relief. Amitriptyline is helpful especially at night as it can sedate and provide pain relief.

Ataxia and tremor

Balance and coordination (ataxia) problems often accompany tremor and are among the most difficult symptoms to manage. Compensatory techniques taught via exercises can be helpful but rarely enough to satisfy. The use of a Swiss Ball or Balance Master technology allows for higher-level treatments. There are no medications that are useful for balance and coordination issues.

Many medications have been used for tremor with little success. None of these were developed for tremor and each was discovered empirically. β-Blockers can decrease tremor in some patients. Antianxiety agents (buspirone and clonazapam) can be helpful in other patients. There are assorted other treatments, including isoniazid, primidone, ondansetron, and glutethemide, that are reported as helpful in an occasional patient.

The use of weights strategically placed on the extremity and bracing the effected joints provide some relief without significant discomfort. Developing compensatory techniques for activities of daily living with tremor is important.

There are isolated reports on the use of thalamic stimulation for those who have severe tremors secondary to MS. The aggressiveness of this technique requires better and bigger studies before it can be considered a reasonable therapy, even for this severely disabling symptom.

The bladder

Bladder issues are prominent in those who have MS [16]. The bladder can present itself with frequency, urgency, hesitancy, and incontinence with differing mechanisms. Most frequent is the small, failure-to-store bladder. It often has uncontrollable contractions, including many of those symptoms listed. A large, failure-to-empty bladder overfills and presents with the same symptomatology despite looking different anatomically and physiologically. Frequently, there is a dysynergia between the bladder and the urinary sphincter, causing similar symptoms from yet another mechanism. Complicating these symptoms are frequent bladder infections, which exacerbate the problems significantly.

The small, failure-to-store bladder is characterized by a low postvoid residual. This can be measured by catheterization or ultrasound. This type of bladder often can be managed effectively with the use of anticholinergic medications (eg, tolteridine or oxybutynin). Dosing needs to be enough to decrease the spasms but not turn off other cholinergic functions, such as sweating or bowel function. The research use of botulinum toxin injected in the hyperactive bladder wall is being evaluated.

More problematic from a management point of view is the large, failure-to-empty bladder. There may be residuals from 200 to 900 mL. Impairing the contractility of the bladder wall with anticholinergic treatments is contraindicated in this situation unless there is the mechanical ability to empty the bladder. Self-catheterization or continuous catheterization becomes essential to prevent reflux toward the kidneys. Self-catheterization is preferable if upper extremity function is such that it can be done safely and cleanly (not sterilely). If coordination is not present, an indwelling catheter is preferable to diapers and ongoing wetness, which promotes skin breakdown. The same issue is present with the dysynergia bladder. Bladder pressures may be increased significantly as the sphincter closes against the contracting bladder. To relieve the pressure, mechanical emptying via catheter is necessary.

Sometimes the use of antidiuretic hormone (desmopressin, 0.2 mg hs) at night decreases urinary production and allow for a better night's sleep with improved urinary continence during the daytime [17].

The bowel

Bowel function is affected less than bladder function but can be problematic. Irritable bowel is a common associated problem and regulating the bowel often means changing treatments, depending on the circumstances. It is better to be slightly constipated than slightly loose. Bowel regulation often revolves around the judicious use of bulk formers (eg, psyllium). Adding more or less water to a regular amount of psyllium allows some control over the situation. If the bowel is loose, less water is added to the tablespoon of psyllium and, if constipated, a glass or two may be the accompanying drink. Stool softeners, glycerin suppositories, and an understanding of the gastrocolic reflex can allow for a scheduling a bowel movement. Knowing that the gastrocolic reflex is present approximately 30 minutes after a meal makes that the best time for that scheduled bowel movement.

Sexual expression

Sexual expression may require special attention in MS. Relationships remain of utmost importance and need to be stressed, without diminishing the importance of the actual sexual performance in the face of disability. In men, erectile dysfunction is frequent. The use of oral agents for erectile dysfunction has become popular and often is effective. Sildenafil citrate (Viagra), vardenafil HCl (Levitra), and tadalafil (Cialis) may be tried to improve erection. If they fail, the use of injectable prostaglandin, alprostadil (Caverject), under the auspices of a urologist, can allow for a good workable erection. The small needle is injected into the shaft of the penis before intercourse. This medication can be administered by urethral suppository (alprostadil [MUSE]) with somewhat less effectiveness but with ease.

Occasionally, penile prostheses may be placed. This is less common today because of alternative treatment options.

Female sexual expression may be diminished by vaginal dryness or decreased or altered sensation in the vaginal area. Vaginal lubricants that are water-soluble are readily available in drugstores and are helpful. Increased stimulation, using vibration, or gentle cooling by massaging with a cooled object (such as a frozen bag of peas) to the vaginal area may produce the desired effect of overcoming the decreased sensation. There is a device that combines the effect of a vibrator with gentle suction to pull blood into the clitoris [18]. This FDA approved tool is called the Eros device.

Antidepressant use may decrease libido and is a difficult clinical problem with no good solution. Sometimes a change in medication can be helpful but they all seem to have this potential.

Depression

Depression is a primary symptom of MS occurring because of actual changes in the brain and its chemistry [19]. There is no question that reactive (exogenous) depression occurs frequently in MS and is amenable to counseling and other nonpharmacologic techniques, but the brain disease seen in MS clearly leads to chemical (endogenous) depression in many. The suicide rate for MS seems greater than that for many other neurologic diseases, some of which have a worse perceived prognosis [20–22]. The aggressive use of appropriate antidepressant medication coupled with counseling can make a difference in the quality of life for those affected by this common symptom.

Exercise

The concept of exercise in neurologic disease seems intuitive. If exercise is applied in an inappropriate manner, however, it can lead to increasing fatigue and disability. For decades, exercise in MS was downplayed because of these issues. In the past 15 to 20 years, much knowledge of appropriate exercise techniques has been gained [23]. This knowledge can be applied to MS with some success.

When beginning an exercise program, it is important to understand what the goal of the exercise is. Different exercises are used for different goals, for instance, endurance training or strength building. If balance is a problem, the exercise is different from that if spasticity is a problem. An exercise prescription begins with the type of exercise, based on the goal. Then the duration, frequency, and intensity of training should be specified.

Exercise science and physiology have been applied to MS with new understanding that confirms the ability to build strength if there is nerve supply to sustain the muscle. If there is not, a compensatory strategy to maintain and allow as much function as possible is developed.

Cognition

For many decades, it was believed that there were no cognitive problems in MS, which is amazing, given that 50% of those who have MS have recognizable cognitive issues [24,25]. Ten percent have major problems that can impair normal living [26], involving memory, planning, foresight, and judgment. Because so much thinking involves the movement of information via myelinated tracts, it should be no surprise that the problem is prominent.

Neuropsychologic testing can detect and show areas of impairment. Speech pathologists and occupational therapists also can aid in codifying specific problems and developing strategies to compensate. These may be as simple as socialization exercises or may include repetitive tasking to attempt to work around the structural issues in the brain. Occasionally, treatments used in patients who have Alzheimer's disease can provide help, but they have not been dramatic in the MS subcortical type dementia.

Medication use for other symptoms may contribute to the cognitive problems with sedation and confusion; thus, these must be reviewed regularly in those who have dulled cognition. Depression may be an additive culprit and is treatable if recognized.

Weakness

Weakness in MS usually is a result of decreased neuromuscular impulses secondary to demyelination and axonal loss. As discussed previously, progressive resistive exercises may contribute to fatigue and give the appearance of increasing weakness. If there is enough innervation centrally, the muscle can be strengthened with appropriate exercise. If this is lacking, atrophy is likely to occur. Keeping the range of motion adequate may slow the process and allow for compensatory movements to improve function.

4-Aminopyridine, a potassium channel blocker, has been shown to have an effect on nerve transmission, allowing for modest improvement in strength and function [27]. This chemical is available in a raw form but has not been approved for this use by the Food and Drug Administration.

Heat, either from increased ambient temperature or fever, often increases weakness. This may be the result of a conduction block. Cooling often allows more efficient conduction and improved strength if there is appropriate innervation [28].

Side effects of injectables

The aggressive use of immune-modulating agents to slow down the actual disease process has contributed to the development of a whole new set of symptoms that the clinician must recognize and manage.

Interferon initiation often brings about a fever reaction, which may be disabling to the person who has MS. It often is recommended that interferon be administered in the evening before going to bed. This allows for the impact of the fever during the night, when it may be less disabling to activities of living. Antipyretic medications (ibuprofen or acetaminophen) may be administered 4 hours before the infection, at the time of injection, and then, if necessary, 4 hours after the injection.

Subcutaneous injections can lead to immune reactions within the skin with inflammation, redness, and significant irritation. Good injection technique is essential. This may involve icing the area before injecting. A common error is injecting too shallowly. Injection devices use improved techniques and have decreased many of these side effects but may contribute to the problem if they are set to deliver the medication too shallowly within the skin rather than beneath it. It is important to allow the air bubble in the syringe to remain to push the medication through the skin and it is recommended that the needle be free of lingering medication as it pierces the skin.

Rotation of the injections is an absolute necessity to preserve as much skin area as possible and allow healing between injections. For some patients, the addition of a cortisone cream or a local anesthetic cream may be helpful [15,29].

With some treatments, pain can linger after the injection. Applying cooling can offer symptomatic relief. Understanding the issues often is helpful in the development of compensation strategies.

Glatiramer acetate occasionally induces a systemic reaction. This rare, but real, symptom complex presents with a feeling of panic, chest discomfort, shortness of breath and a feeling of doom and gloom. It usually lasts for 20 minutes and then clears rapidly, but if panic sets in and an emergency is called, the issue may be magnified and complicated. The treatment is to realize that the problem is associated with the medication and requires resting for the duration of the symptoms to allow them to abate on their own. This usually is not a recurrent problem but occasionally can repeat.

Swallowing

Dysphagia needs evaluation if signs of gurgling, coughing, weight loss, pneumonia, choking, or a weak voice become present. The speech pathologist and the radiologist team perform a videofluoroscopy, which can demonstrate the exact location and the type of food that contributes to the swallowing defect. Once identified, a management plan can be constructed. This may involve modifying the texture, moistening, cooling, and so forth. Together with these changes, techniques of swallowing can be taught that may involve positioning of the head.

References

[1] Fisk JD, Pontefract A, Ritvo PG, et al. The impact of fatigue on patients with MS. Can J Neurol Sci 1994;21:9–14.

[2] Attarian HP, Brown KM, Duntley SP, et al. The relationship of sleep disturbances and fatigue in multiple sclerosis. Arch Neurol 2004;61:525–8.

[3] Krupp LB, Alvarez LA, LaRocca NB, et al. Fatigue in multiple sclerosis. Arch Neurol 1988; 45:435–51.

[4] Murray TJ. Amantidine therapy for fatigue in multiple sclerosis. Can J Neurol Sci 1985;12: 251–4.

[5] Bass B, Weinshenker BG, Penman M, et al. A double-blind, placebo-controlled trial to compare the efficacy of cylert (pemoline) and placebo in the control of fatigue in multiple sclerosis. Neurology 1990;40(Suppl 1):261.

[6] Rammohan KW, Rosenberg JH, Lynn DJ, et al. Efficacy and safety of modafinil (Provigil) for the treatment of fatigue in multiple sclerosis: a two center phase 2 study. J Neurol Neurosurg Psychiatry 2002;72:179–83.

[7] Schapiro RT. The management of MS symptoms. New York: Demos Medical Publishing; 2003.

[8] Young RR. Treatment of spastic paresis. N Engl J Med 1985;320:1953–5.

[9] Hokystrater MC, van der Ploeg RJD, van der Burg W, et al. Treatment of spasticity in multiple sclerosis patients. Acta Neurol Scand 1988;77:224–30.

[10] Borg-Stein J, Fine Z, Mille RJ, et al. Botulinum toxin for the treatment of spasticity in multiple sclerosis. Am J Phys Med Rehabil 1993;72:364–8.

[11] Killestein J, Uitdehaag BM, Polman CH. Cannabinoids in multiple sclerosis: do they have a therapeutic role? Drugs 2004;64:1–11.

[12] Beard S, Hunn A, Wight J. Treatments for spasticity and pain in multiple sclerosis: a systematic review. Health Technol Assess 2003;7:iii, ix–x, 1–111.
[13] Penn RD, Savoy SM, Corcos D, et al. Intrathecal baclofen for severe spinal spasticity. N Engl J Med 1989;320:1517–21.
[14] DMKG Study Group. Misoprostol in the treatment of trigeminal neuralgia associated with multiple sclerosis. J Neurol 2003;250:542–5.
[15] Warnell P. The pain experience of a multiple sclerosis population: a descriptive study. Axone 1991;13:26–8.
[16] Giannantoni A, Scivoletto G, DiStasi SM, et al. Lower urinary tract dysfunction and disability status in multiple sclerosis. Arch Phys Med Rehabil 1999;80:437–41.
[17] Valiquette G, Herbert J, Maede-D'Alisera P. Desmopressin in the management of nocturia in patients with multiple sclerosis, a double blind crossover trial. Arch Neurol 1996;53: 1270–5.
[18] Billups K, Berman L, Berman J, et al. A new non-pharmacological vacuum therapy for female sexual dysfunction. J Sex Marital Ther 2001;27.
[19] Ron MA, Logsdail SJ. Psychiatric morbidity in multiple sclerosis: a clinical and MRI study. Psychol Med 1989;19:887–95.
[20] Patten SB, Beck CA, Williams JV, et al. Major depression in multiple sclerosis: a population-based perspective. Neurology 2003;61:1524–7.
[21] Sadovnik AD, Remick RA, Allen J, et al. Depression and multiple sclerosis. Neurology 1996; 46:628–32.
[22] Schiffer RB, Babigian HM. Behavioral disorders in multiple sclerosis, temporal lobe epilepsy, and amyotrophic lateral sclerosis, an epidemiologic study. Arch Neurol 1984;41: 1067–9.
[23] Petajan JH, White AT. Recommendations for physical activity in multiple sclerosis. Sports Med 1999;27:179–91.
[24] Rao S, Leo GT, Bernardin L, et al. Cognitive dysfunction in multiple sclerosis I. Frequency, pattern and predictors. Neurology 1991;41:685–91.
[25] Bagert B, Camplair P, Bourdette D. Cognitive dysfunction in multiple sclerosis: natural history, pathophysiology and management. CNS Drugs 2002;16:445–55.
[26] Peyser JM, Edmals KR, Poser CM, et al. Cognitive function in patients with multiple sclerosis. Arch Neurol 1980;47:94–7.
[27] Polman CH, Bertelsmann FW, van Loenen AC, et al. 4-Aminopyridine in the treatment of patients with multiple sclerosis. Long-term efficacy and safety. Arch Neurol 1994;51:292–6.
[28] Syndulko K, Woldanski A, Baumhefner RW, et al. Preliminary evaluation of lowering tympanic temperature for the symptomatic treatment of multiple sclerosis. J Neurol Rehab 1995;9:205–14.
[29] Svendsen KB, Jensen TS, Overvad K, et al. Pain in patients with multiple sclerosis: a population-based study. Arch Neurol 2003;60:1089–94.

ELSEVIER
SAUNDERS

NEUROLOGIC CLINICS

Neurol Clin 23 (2005) 189–214

Interferons in Multiple Sclerosis

Ludwig Kappos, MD

Department of Neurology, University Hospitals, Kantonsspital, CH-4031 Basel, Switzerland

Since 1993, when the first interferon, interferon-β1b (IFN-β1b), was approved for treatment of multiple sclerosis (MS) [1,2], interferons have gained a central position in the therapeutic armamentarium. In nearly all countries, three different IFN-β products have been introduced into the market for treatment of relapsing-remitting MS (RRMS) and, to some extent, of secondary progressive MS (SPMS). IFN-β now has a key role in the management of patients who have MS. In this article, the available evidence of the mode of action of IFNs in MS, their efficacy on clinical and laboratory measures, and current knowledge about their emerging differential indication are reviewed.

Mode of action in multiple sclerosis

IFNs are pleiotropic molecules with a wide range of pro- and antiproliferative, pro- and antiapoptotic, antiviral, and complex immunoregulatory activities. Although first attempts to use IFNs as therapeutic agents in MS were based on their antiviral effect [3–6], more recent attention has focused on their direct effect on the blood-brain barrier and their immunomodulatory and antiproliferative effects [7–10]. After a first trial with IFN-γ showed a sharp increase of exacerbations [11], most likely related to upregulation of major histocompatibility complex (MHC) molecule expression, which facilitates antigen presentation and thereby augments and accelerates immune responses, type II IFNs were abandoned as MS therapeutics. Type I IFNs (IFN-α and IFN-β) share components of the same receptor. They are produced by almost all mammalian cells upon stimulation. They trigger the synthesis of many host cell proteins that contribute to the inhibition of viral replication and are believed to mediate most of the biologic effects of IFNs. Like IFN-γ, type I IFNs increase

E-mail address: lkappos@uhbs.ch

doi:10.1016/j.ncl.2004.10.004 *neurologic.theclinics.com*

expression of MHC class I, thereby enhancing the ability of virus-infected cells to present viral peptides to CD8+ T cells. In contrast to IFN-γ, type I IFNs do not induce, rather they suppress, the synthesis of MHC class II proteins. Apart from the inhibition of MHC class II expression, IFN-β has been shown to upregulate interleukin (IL)-10 expression. This also has been shown in MBP-specific CD4+ T-cell lines, where, in addition, proliferation and production of lymphotoxin is suppressed. Another important aspect of interferon activity is inhibition of T-cell migration across basement membranes in vitro, as a result of the decrease of secretion of matrix-degrading enzymes (metalloproteases) [12]. This is believed pertinent to the fast suppression of inflammation as depicted by reduced numbers of enhancing MRI lesions after interferon treatment. Additional mechanisms include increase in soluble vascular cell adhesion molecule and down-regulation of its corresponding partner adhesion molecule, very late activation antigen [13]. Many other effects, especially of IFN-β, are described (Table 1): inhibition of T-cell proliferation, different immunomodulatory effects on microglia, reduction of circulating CD8+ T cells and B cells, stimulation of nerve growth factor production by astrocytes, inhibition of human glial–inducible nitric oxide synthase, inhibition of mitogen-induced astrocyte proliferation, and many more. Because IFN-α and IFN-β bind to the same receptor, similar effects would be expected in MS. But they bind at different sites of the receptor, and induction of signaling by IFN-α requires the simultaneous binding to the IFN receptor α and β chains. These differences could translate into different clinical effects and side effects. Small studies suggest similar effects of IFN-α and IFN-β on relapse rates [35–37]. Experience in other diseases, such as hepatitis, and in oncology suggests a higher incidence of encephalopathic side effects amd moderate to severe reversible hair loss with IFN-α.

In summary, the beneficial effects of IFN-β in MS are believed mainly related to its anti-inflammatory effect, based on reduced MHC class II expression, shift of cytokine production from Th1 to Th2, and direct effects preserving the integrity of the blood-brain barrier.

Clinical evidence of efficacy

The rationale, design, and key results of phase I, phase II, and the pivotal phase III studies of IFN-β in RRMS have been reviewed comprehensively [38]. Fig. 1 and Tables 2 and 3 provide a summary of the pivotal trials of IFN-β in RRMS. Additional evidence has accumulated concerning the efficacy of IFN-β in SPMS, longer-term observations of patients included in the pivotal trials, and studies comparing different doses and products directly in prospective controlled or observational studies. Some evidence from first phase II studies in primary progressive MS has been presented but was either inconclusive or awaits peer reviewed publication [39,40]. In addition, two placebo-controlled studies address the efficacy of IFN-β1a

Table 1
Effects of interferon-β on the immune system

Parameter	Reported effects
MHC class I expression	Increased
MHC class II expression	Increased/decreased/no change
B7-1 expression (B cells)	Decreased [14]
B7-2 expression (macrophages)	Increased [14]
CD40 expression (T cells, B cells; monocytes)	Decreased; increased [14]
CD40 ligand expression (T cells)	Decreased [15]
FcR expression, phagocytosis, antibody-dependent cellular cytotoxicity (macrophages)	Increased
Antigen presentation (macrophages/microglia)	Increased/decreased
Proliferation (T cells)	Decreased/increased
Apoptosis (T cells)	Decreased/increased [16–21]
Fas expression (T cells)	Increased [22]
Cytotoxic T-lymphocyte function	Increased
Production of complement-fixing antibody isotypes (B cells)	Increased
Dendritic cell maturation	Increased
Natural killer cell numbers	Decreased [23]
Complement activation	Increased initially
Adhesion molecule expression (T cells, endothelia)	Decreased [24]
Matrix metalloproteinase-9 activity (T cells)	Decreased [12]
Tissue inhibitor of matrix metalloproteinase expression (T cells)	Increased [25]
IL-2 production (T cells)	Increased
IL-2 receptor expression (T cells)	Decreased
IFN-γ production (T cells, natural killer cells)	Increased/decreased [26]
IL-4 production (PBMCs, T cells)	Increased [27]
Lymphotoxin production (T cells)	Decreased
Interleukin-1 production (macrophages)	Increased
Interleukin-1 receptor antagonist production (macrophages)	Increased [28]
Transforming growth factor β production (PBMCs)	Increased
Tumor necrosis factor α production (macrophages/microglia)	Increased/decreased
RANTES, macrophage inflammatory protein-1α expression (T cells)	Decreased [29,30]
CCR5 expression (T cells)	Decreased [29]
Prostaglandin E_2 production (macrophages)	Decreased
Nitric oxide secretion (macrophages, microglia)	Increased/decreased [31]
IL-10 production (T cells)	Increased [32–34]
IL-12 production (monocyte/macrophages, DCs)	Decreased [34]

Abbreviations: PBMC, peripheral blood mononuclear cell; RANTES, regulated upon activity, normal T-cell expressed and secreted (chemokine).

Adapted from Karp CL, van Boxel-Dezaire AH, Byrnes AA, et al. Interferons beta in multiple sclerosis: altering the balance of interleukin-12 and interleukin-10? Curr Opin Neurol 2001;14:361–8.

once weekly after the first clinical event suggestive of MS. With the extended observations in controlled trials and with widespread open-label use of IFN-β, more evidence has accumulated about the side-effect profile and, especially, the frequency and possible impact of neutralizing antibodies (NAB) to interferon.

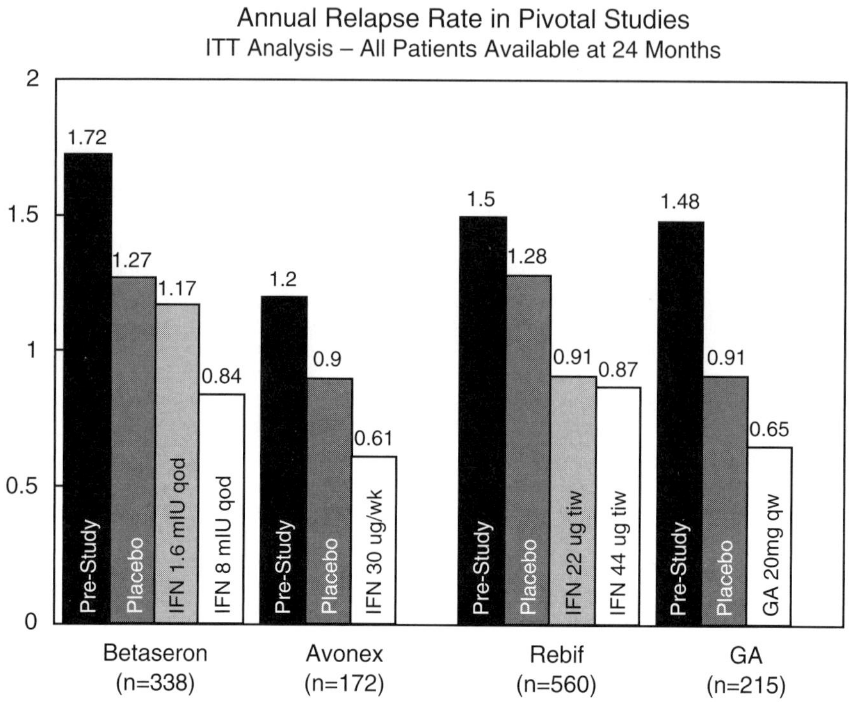

Fig. 1. Pivotal trials summary.

Impact of dosing, frequency, and route of administration

The pivotal trials with IFN-β1b (Betaseron (Berlex Laboratories, Inc., Montville, New Jersey, USA)/Betaferon, Schering AG, Berlin, Germany), IFN-β1a (Avonex, Biogen IDEC, Inc., Cambridge, Massachusetts, USA), and IFN-β1a (Rebif, Serono, Geneva, Switzerland) all recruited patients who had established RRMS after a mean disease duration of between 4 and 8 years, no or mild disability at entry, and relatively high relapse rates

Table 2
Evidence from pivotal trials of interferon-β in relapsing-remitting multiple sclerosis

	Populations studied						
			IFN-β1a				
	IFN-β1b		Rebif			IFN-β1a	
	Betaseron 8 mIU qod	PBO	22 μg tiw	44 μg tiw	PBO	Avonex 30 μg qw	PBO
Duration of disease (mean)	4.7	3.9	7.7	7.8	6.1	6.6	6.4
Prior 2-year relapse rate	1.7	1.8	1.5	1.5	1.5	1.2	1.2
EDSS at entry	3.0	2.8	2.5	2.5	2.4	2.4	2.3
EDSS range	0–5.5			0–5.0		1–3.5	

Table 3
Evidence from pivotal trials of interferon-β in relapsing-remitting multiple sclerosis

Duration of follow-up: number of patients (%) continuing in active treatment arm				
		IFN-β1a		
	IFN-β1b	Rebif		IFN-β1a
	Betaseron, 8 mIU qod	22 μg tiw	44 μg tiw	Avonex 30 μg qw
No. of patients	124	198	184	158
24 months	95 (77%)	177 (94%)	179 (97%)	85 (50)
36 months	89 (72%)			15 (10%)
48 months	58 (47%)	154 (78%)	148 (80%)	

(Tables 2 and 3). In these patients, the effect on the relapse rate was consistent with an approximately 30% reduction across all studies. There is some controversy about the real rate of relapse reduction in the pivotal Avonex trial, related to whether or not calculations were based on all patients recruited (−18%) or on all patients on treatment for 2 years until the trial's early termination (−32%) [38].

The PRISMS trial [30,41–43] compared IFN-β1a (Rebif) 22 μg or 44 μg three times weekly with placebo (PBO) over 2 years. Although both doses of IFN-β1a demonstrated clear-cut effects compared with PBO, they failed to show a significant dose response on relapse rate or progression in disability, whereas significant dose-related differences were shown for MRI-defined activity and disease burden. Together with a tendency for better efficacy of the higher dose in most clinical parameters, this raises the possibility that important clinical differences could have been delayed beyond the 2-year follow-up. The PRISMS-4 study [44] addresses this question. Patients completing the 2-year PBO-controlled trial were offered to continue for another 2 years in the study. Patients taking PBO were randomized to either 22 μg or 44μg, whereas IFN-β1a–treated patients were reassigned the same dose taken in the first 2 years. Of the patients originally randomized in PRISMS, 90% entered PRISMS-4 and approximately 80% completed the 4-year follow-up. Patients who switched from PBO to active treatment had a significant reduction in relapse count, MRI activity, and lesion burden accumulation compared with their PBO period. In the high- and low-dose groups, the dose effect regarding relapse rates for 4 years approached significance (P = 0.069; risk ratio, 0.88), favoring the higher dose. Time to sustained disability progression was prolonged significantly over 4 years for the 44-μg group compared with the crossover group (P = 0.047). In an Intention to Treat (ITT) analysis, time to first confirmed Expanded Disability Status Scale (EDSS) progression was prolonged significantly (42.1 months) in the 44-μg group, compared with 24.2 months in the crossover group (40th percentile; P = 0.047). Time to first confirmed progression did not differ significantly between the 22-μg group (35.9 months) and the crossover group (P = 0.289), or between the 44-μg and 22-μg groups ($P = 0.33$). A dose response between 44 μg and 22 μg was observed for time to first progression only in years 3 and 4 (with month 24 reset as baseline).

In summary, the 4-year PRISMS study results support superiority of early treatment with IFN-β versus delayed treatment and also superiority of higher dose, although the differences for the primary endpoint, relapse rate over 4 years, and time to progression in disability over 4 years did not reach significance. The differences observed in several secondary clinical and MRI-based measures, all favoring the higher dose, have led to the recommendation of 44 μg as standard dose for patients treated with IFN-β1a (Rebif). In spite of the higher pricing (approximately 30% more than Rebif 22 μg or the other competitors), this standard dose recommendation has been endorsed by most funding agencies.

The European IFN beta-1a (Avonex) Dose-Comparison Study [45,46] was planned and conducted to determine if 60 μg could improve on the efficacy of 30-μg IFN-β1a (Avonex) given by intramuscular weekly injection in reducing the rate of sustained disability progression in patients who have RRMS. Compared with the pivotal trials of interferon, patients included in this study had a higher EDSS at entry (mean 3.6), 40% were in the EDSS range of 4.0 to 5.5, and 15% in each group were within 6 months of switching into SPMS. After 3 years, 81% of the 402 patients randomized to 30 μg and 82% of those randomized to 60 μg still were on study. No significant dose response was detected for the primary endpoint (time to disability progression, confirmed after 6 months). In both groups, the proportion of subjects with progression of disability by 36 months, estimated from Kaplan-Meier curves, was 37%. No dose effects were observed on any of the secondary clinical endpoints, including relapses, number of steroid treatments, change in 9-hole peg test, and others. Only one MRI at one time point, which measured the number of new or enlarging T2 lesions at month 36 compared with month 24, showed a difference favoring the 60-μg dose. Both doses were tolerated well; however, a slightly higher incidence of flu-like symptoms and muscle weakness was observed in the 60-μg group. The incidence of NAB was 2.3% in the 30-μg group and 5.8% in the 60-μg group. A 4-year follow-up is available for more than 60% of the patients recruited initially (not all centers participated during the 4th year) that supports the findings at 3 years [47].

A comparative trial of 44-μg IFN-β1a thrice weekly and 30-μg IFN-β1a weekly was designed to show superiority of the higher and more frequent dose for a period of 24 weeks with an extension for a total of 48 weeks [48,49]. In this EVIDENCE trial, 339 patients who had RRMS were randomized to Rebif and 338 to Avonex treatment. Because of the different routes and frequency of administration, treatment was not blinded for patients and their treating physicians. A second physician, not involved in the care of the patients, was responsible for assessment of relapses and neurologic impairment or disability. After 24 weeks, a significant difference favoring Rebif was observed in the frequency of relapses. This difference was sustained for 48 weeks, although relapse counts in the second 24 weeks were nearly identical for both treatments. A clear advantage of the high dose also was seen on MRI measures of enhancing lesions and T2 lesion numbers and volumes. Although criticized because of possible bias as a result of unblinding of patients and treating physicians, this study convincingly shows that the clinical and MRI-measured effects of IFN-β1a occur earlier with more frequent and higher dosing. The similar behavior of both treatment groups' relapse activity in the second half year [49] may indicate that this advantage diminishes over time. MRI-measured differences, however, although less pronounced, still favor the higher dose in the second 24 weeks. As intended by the sponsor, this study led to approval of Rebif in the United States, overruling the orphan drug status of Avonex.

An investigator initiated study supported by the Italian Multiple Sclerosis Society compared alternate-day 8-mIU IFN-β1b (Betaseron) and weekly 30-μg IFN-β1a (Avonex) over 2 years [50]. In this INCOMIN trial, patients who had RRMS were randomized to either treatment and followed prospectively by clinical evaluations every 3 months and by MRI assessment every year. No effort was made to blind patients or treating and evaluating physicians, but MRIs were analyzed in the study's lead and coordinating center without knowledge of treatment assignment. Fully 94 of 96 subjects assigned to IFN-β1b and 88 of 92 of those assigned to IFN-β1a completed clinical follow-up. The annualized relapse rate in the IFN-β1b group was 0.5 (a 76% reduction from baseline), whereas it was 0.7 in the IFN-β1a group, representing a 37% reduction from baseline. Forty nine percent of patients in the IFN-β1b group and 64% in the IFN-β1a group had at least one relapse; 14% and 30%, respectively, had progression by one or more steps in the EDSS for more than 3 months and progression was confirmed at 24 months. Forty nine percent of patients taking IFN-β1b and 75% of those taking IFN-β1a had active scans (scans with new or enlarging T2 or Gd-enhancing lesions). In this study, the difference favoring IFN-β1b increased with the duration of the trial for relapse rate and disability progression, in contrast to the findings of the EVIDENCE trial. As the study was not blinded, part of this effect might be because of increasing subject and investigator bias, as the results of the first year analysis were presented while the study was ongoing [51].

A population-based study recently was presented by Koch-Henriksen et al [53]. All Danish patients who had RRMS and applied for IFN-β treatment between June 1996 and November 1997 were asked to participate in a randomized open-label observational study. If they agreed, they were assigned randomly either to weekly 22-μg IFN-β1a (Rebif; n = 143) or alternate-day 8-mIU IFN-β1b (Betaseron; n = 160). Those who were unwilling to be randomized were treated with Betaseron (n = 125). Only 76%, 72%, and 63% of the patients in these three respective treatment groups completed 24 months of planned follow-up. The annualized relapse rates were 0.70, 0.71, and 0.84, respectively, representing a 55%, 53%, and 39%

reduction from baseline. Reasons for dropout included more frequent side effects in the Betaseron groups and perceived lack of efficacy in the low 22-μg weekly Rebif group. Annual MRI scans were performed, but results and publication of the study are not yet available. The open-label design and lack of methodologic study details limit interpretation of these preliminary results.

Several observational studies were reported at scientific meetings; most have not been published fully. Khan et al [52], in an observational open-label study, compared patients who had RRMS and selected alternate-day IFN-β1b (Betaseron), 30-μg weekly IFN-β1a (Avonex), 20-mg daily glatiramer acetate (glatiramer acetate), or no treatment. No blinding was attempted, and the criteria for treatment allocation to different groups were not clearly defined. Eighteen months' follow-up was available for nearly 80% of the patients in each group. Significant reductions of annualized relapse rates from baseline were reported for the Betaseron (−54%) and glatiramer acetate (−60%) groups, whereas the reduction by 29% in the Avonex group did not reach significance, and patients who did not have treatment had no change in their relapse rates. Trojano and coworkers in Southern Italy [54] followed patients treated with Betaseron or Avonex in approved dosages at their centers for up to 2 years. Two hundred nine of 234 patients in the Betaseron group and 169 of 217 in the Avonex group were available for 2-year follow-up. Fifty-one percent of patients taking Betaseron and 67% of patients taking Avonex had one or more relapses on treatment; the respective reduction of the annualized relapse rate was 52% and 39% in the first year and 54% and 46% over 2 years. Because of the nonrandomized open-label design, the results of all these studies, although reflecting "real life" in their respective centers and countries, are difficult to interprete.

In summary and conclusion, available data on direct head-to-head comparisons of the three IFN-β products show that doubling the dose of once-weekly IFN-β1a does not add to the drug's efficacy. During observation periods of up to 4 years, higher doses of more frequently administered IFN-β1a show advantages of earlier and more pronounced suppression of disease activity. The results also indicate a ceiling effect of dose response, however. One large, double-blind, randomized study (BEYOND trial) compares alternate-day 500-μg IFN-β1b with currently approved 250-μg IFN-β1b to assess if efficacy can be improved in RRMS while maintaining safety and tolerability [55]. By including a third arm, the difference between conventional-dose IFN-β1b and glatiramer acetate also will be addressed in a single-blinded design over 2 years. It remains to be shown in this and other large-scale comparative studies if the shape of the dose response curve is different in different individuals who have RRMS or in different phases or types of disease evolution. Regarding the direct comparison of frequent and once-weekly IFN-β dosing, available data from the reanalysis of the pivotal trials and the head-to-head studies support an earlier and probably more pronounced effect of more frequent than once-weekly dosing. This possible advantage is not consistent across studies; its real magnitude and clinical importance still is a matter of debate.

Studies of secondary progressive multiple sclerosis

Four large controlled trials address whether or not IFN-β1b also is effective in more disabled patients, especially in the secondary progressive phase of the disease, when disability continuously increases with or without superimposed relapses. Key data referring to baseline variables, study conduct, and the main results of these studies are summarized in Tables 4, 5, and 6.

The European SPMS trial, which compares alternate-day 8-mIU IFN-β1b with PBO, reports a highly significant effect on the primary endpoint, the time to disability progression by one or more steps in the EDSS confirmed after 3 months [64,67]. In the active treatment group, progression was delayed by 9 to 12 months in this study, which was stopped early for efficacy. The effect was apparent equally across disability grades (EDSS 2.5–6.5) and in patients who had superimposed relapses and in those who had only progressive deterioration and who did not have relapses. Results favoring treatment also were obtained for time to becoming wheelchair bound, relapse rate and severity, number of steroid treatments, hospital admissions, and some measures of quality of life and neuropsychologic deficits. The highly significant but modest clinical effect on the primary outcome was accompanied by more pronounced effects on MRI measures of inflammation [67]. Markers of tissue destruction (atrophy of brain and spinal cord [68] and magnetization transfer histograms) studied in smaller subgroups, however, did not show treatment effects. The only exception was T1-weighted hypointense lesions that reflected inflammatory and tissue matrix changes, where a significant treatment effect was shown [69]. Recently published data of the final analysis of this study confirm the original results [70].

Other trials of IFN-β in SPMS include one with IFN-β1b conducted in North America (NASPMS) that had a third arm with body surface–adapted doses (5 mIU/m^2 on alternate days) [43], one comparing IFN-β1a (Rebif) 22 μg and 44 μg thrice weekly with placebo (SPECTRIMS) [46,65], and one comparing IFN-β1a 60 μg weekly (Avonex) with PBO (IMPACT) [66]. All failed to demonstrate an effect on disability progression as reflected by the EDSS. In the IMPACT study, EDSS was not the primary endpoint, but the Multiple Sclerosis Functional Composite (MSFC) was. In IMPACT, active treatment resulted in a significantly lower change in this composite measure (PBO $= -0.495 \pm 1.58$ versus IFN-β1a $= 0.362 \pm 1.41$; $P = 0.033$). This measure is less familiar to most neurologists and the clinical implications of such differences are less well understood. Looking at the results for the three components of the MSFC, no significant effect was found for the timed 25-feet walk, and there was only a trend in favor of active treatment for the PASAT, a measure of some neuropsychologic functions. The treatment

Table 4
Major randomized controlled studies of interferon-β in multiple sclerosis—effect on exacerbation and MRI lesion rates

Relapsing-remitting multiple sclerosis or early multiple sclerosis		Exacerbations				MRI active lesion rate*			
Drug/study	Doses studied	PBO	IFN-1	IFN-2	Notes	PBO	IFN-1	IFN-2	Notes
IFN-β1b/Betaseron [5,6,56]	PBO, 1.6 mIU, 8 mIU qod	1.31	1.14	0.9	Annualized exacerbation rate over 2 years	4.9	1.8	2	Active lesions per year in small subset
IFN-β1a/Avonex Pivotal trial [57–59]	PBO, 30 μg qw	0.82	0.67		Over 2 years annualized rate	4.8	3.2		Only 2 years subset
Avonex/CHAMPS [60]	PBO, 30 μg qw	50%	35%		Proportion with at least 1 exacerbation	2.8	1.5		No. of active lesions in first 6 months
IFN-β1a/PRISMS [41,42]	PBO, 22 μg, 44 μg tiw	1.28 (NA)	0.91 (0.80)	0.87 (0.72)	Annualized relapse rate over 2 [4] years	0.88	0.17	0.11	CU lesions freq MRI subset
IFN-β1a/ETOMS [61,62]	PBO, 22 μg qw	0.43	0.33		Annualized relapse rate over 2 years	3	2		Median T2 active lesions
IFN-β1a/OWIMS [63]	PBO, 22 μg, 44 μg qw	1.08	1.08	0.87	Relapse rate over 1 year	1.7	1.3	0.8	6-month MRI CU lesions
Secondary progressive multiple sclerosis									
IFN-β1b/EUSPMS [45,64]	PBO, 8 mIU qod	0.57	0.42		Annualized relapse rate across 3 years	8.82	3.77		No. new or enlarging T2 lesions during first 6 months, monthly MRI subset
IFN-β1b/NASPMS [43]	PBO, 8 mIU, 5 mIU/m^2 qod	0.28	0.2	0.16	Annualized relapse rate across 3 years	17	4	6	Annualized rate of new enhancing lesions during 3 years
IFN-β1/SPECTRIMS [46,65]	PBO, 22 μg, 44 μg tiw	0.71	0.5	0.5	Annualized relapse rate across 3 years	1	0.22	0.11	Combined unique (CU) lesions in MRI subset
IFN-β1a/IMPACT [66]	Pbo, 60 μg qw	0.30	0.20		Annualized relapse rate across 2 years	2.74	1.49		No. new or enlarging T2 lesions during 2 years

Abbreviation: NA, not available.

* MRI results based on differing methods between studies, and differing parameters reported in publications (eg, mean versus median).

Modified from Rask C, Unger E, Walton M. Comparative study of Rebif to Avonex and orphan exclusivety: comparative memorandum. FDA, Division of Clinical Trial Design and Analysis; 2002. Available at: www.fda.gov/cder/biologics/review/ifnbser030702r14.pdf.

Table 5
Major randomized controlled studies of interferon-β in multiple sclerosis—treatment effect expressed as relative rates versus placebo

Relapsing-remitting multiple sclerosis or early multiple sclerosis		Exacerbations			MRI active lesion rate*		
Drug/study	Doses studied	IFN-1/PBO	IFN-2/PBO	IFN-2/IFN-1	IFN-1/PBO	IFN-2/PBO	IFN-2/IFN-1
IFN-β1b/Betaseron [5,6,56]	PBO, 1.6 mIU, 8 mIU qod	0.87	0.69	0.79	0.37	0.41	1.11
IFN-β1a/Avonex Pivotal trial [56–58]	PBO, 30 μg qw	0.82			0.67		
Avonex/CHAMPS [60]	PBO, 30 μg qw	0.70			0.54		
IFN-β1a/PRISMS [41,42]	PBO, 22 μg, 44 μg tiw	0.71	0.68	0.95	0.19	0.13	0.65
IFN-β1a/ETOMS [61,62]	PBO, 22 μg, qw	0.77			0.67		
IFN-β1a/OWIMS [63]	PBO, 22 μg, 44 μg tiw	1.00	0.81	0.81	0.76	0.47	0.62
Secondary progressive multiple sclerosis							
IFN-β1b/EUSPMS [45,64]	PBO, 8 mIU qod	0.74			0.43		
IFN-β1b/NASPMS [43]	PBO, 8 mIU, 5 mIU/m^2 qod	0.71	0.57	0.80	0.24	0.35	1.50
IFN-β1/SPECTRIMS [46,65]	PBO, 22 μg, 44 μg tiw	0.70	0.70	1.00	0.22	0.11	0.50
IFN-β1a/IMPACT [66]	PBO, 60 μg, qw	0.67			0.54		

* MRI results based on differing methods between studies and differing parameters reported in publications (eg, mean versus median). Relative rates calculated from parameters.

Modified from Rask C, Unger E, Walton M. Comparative study of Rebif to Avonex and orphan exclusivety: comparative memorandum. FDA, Division of Clinical Trial Design and Analysis; 2002. Available at: www.fda.gov/cder/biologics/review/ifnbser030702r14.pdf.

Table 6
Studies comparing different products, doses, frequencies, and routes of administration of interferon-β

Study	Drug dose schedule compared	No. included/ followed-up	Design, duration	Annualized relapse rate (% reduction versus baseline)	% with relapse	% Confirmed progression	% with active scans
European Dose Comparison [45,64]	Avonex 30 µg qw versus 60 µg qw	402/318 400/316	Double-blind, 36 months	0.77 (−41.0%) 0.81 (−37.7%)	77 77	2nd y 29/3rd y 37 2nd y 28/3rd y 37	2nd y 73/3rd y 77 2nd y 66/3rd y 61
EVIDENCE [48]	Rebif 3 × 44 µg qw versus Avonex 30 µg qw	339/331 338/328	(Double)-blind, 24/48 weeks	0.63/0.58 (−55%) 0.85/0.68 (−48%)	25/38 37/48	NA NA	Mo 0–6 31, 7–12 25 Mo 0–6 51, 7–12 37
INCOMIN [50]	Betaseron 8 mIU eod versus Avonex 30 µg qw	96/94 92/88	Randomized, open-label, 24 months	0.5 (−76%) 0.7 (−37%)	49 64	14 30	49 75
Danish IFN-β [53]	Randomized Betaseron 8 mIU eod versus nonrandomized. Betaseron 8 mIU eod versus randomized Rebif 22 µg qw	160/116 125/79 143/109	Randomized (2 arms), population-based, Open-label, 24 months	0.71 (−53%) 0.84 (−39%) 0.70 (−55%)	NA NA NA	NA NA NA	NA NA NA

Abbreviation: NA, not available.

difference appeared mainly because of the results of the 9-hole peg test, a measure of dexterity and upper extremity motor dysfunction.

Across all four SPMS studies, significant beneficial effects were observed for relapses and markers of MRI-based inflammatory activity. Although the studies have similar inclusion criteria and definitions of progression, comparison of baseline variables across studies (Table 7) shows that the European SPMS study recruited younger patients and more patients who had relapses superimposed on their progressive course. Only approximately 30% of the European SPMS patients were exacerbation free during the 2 years preceding inclusion, whereas higher percentages were reported for SPECTRIMS (50%), NASPMS (55%), and IMPACT (approximately 50%). Part of this baseline difference could be biased, because with similar relapse definitions, relapse frequencies on study in the PBO groups of the European SPMS trial and SPECTRIMS were nearly identical, whereas the difference increased with even lower relapse rates during the trial in the PBO groups of IMPACT and NASPMS (Tables 7, 8, and 9).

In summary, these studies of SPMS show that any therapeutic benefit of IFN-β in advanced MS seems limited to patients who have particular disease characteristics. Subgroup analyses in individual studies yield somewhat conflicting results, as in the initial analysis of the European SPMS study the treatment effect was found equally in patients who had and did not have relapses, whereas the SPECTRIMS study indicated a better effect of treatment in patients who had superimposed relapses. A combined analysis of the European SPMS and NASPMS IFN-β1b studies shows that the most robust predictor of a favorable response is relapse activity. A greater than average EDSS progression in the 2 years preceding inclusion (>1 step in the EDSS) also is predictive of response. Other disease-related baseline characteristics, including age, duration of MS, EDSS, T2 lesion load, and enhanced lesion numbers, are less consistently associated with therapeutic effect in SPMS [45].

The reason for this reduced or possible lack of efficacy in SPMS is not completely clear. Accumulating evidence shows that inflammation is less important as a pathogenic component in the later phases of the disease. In addition, destructive and degenerative processes, induced by (autoimmune) inflammation, can continue at least for several months or years, even if inflammation is attenuated. A putative stabilizing effect, therefore, might be detected only with prolonged follow-up. Well-controlled, long-term follow-up studies have been deemed not feasible and observational studies without true control groups may yield uninterpretable results. The problem remains for clinicians as to how to reliably identify possible treatment responders. Despite the known limitations of retrospective analyses, the data from the meta-analyses of the European SPMS and NASPMS studies suggest that pronounced disability progression or continuing superimposed relapses in SPMS may help identify patients who may benefit from treatment. By analogy, but less clearly supported by the data because of more divergent results in the two studies, the opposite features of no superimposed relapses

Table 7
Four studies of interferon-β in secondary progressive multiple sclerosis: EUSPMS, SPECTRIMS, NASPMS, and IMPACT—baseline variables

	EUSPMS [45,63]	SPECTRIMS [46,64]	NASPMS [43]	IMPACT [65]	EUSPMS	SPECTRIMS		NASPMS		IMPACT
	PBO	PBO	PBO	PBO	8 mIU qod	22 μg tiw	44 μg tiw	8 mIU qod	5 mIU/m^2 qod	60 μg qw
n	358	204	308	218	360	209	205	317	314	217
% Female	64	60	60	64	58	62	67	66	61	64
Age	40.9	42.7	47.6	47.9	41.1	43.1	42.6	46.1	46.8	47.2
Mean EDSS	5.2	5.4	5.1	5.2	5.1	5.5	5.4	5.2	5.1	5.2
Disease duration (from diagnosis)	13.4	13.7	14.9	10.5	12.8	13.3	12.9	14.6	14.5	10.2
Secondary progressive phase duration	3.8	4.1	4.1	NA	3.8	4.2	3.7	4.0	4.0	NA
% Exacerbation free	28.2	52	56	44/62[a]	31.9	54	51	54	55	37/59[a]

Abbreviation: NA, not available.
[a] Values for prior 3/1 years.

Table 8
Four studies of interferon-β in secondary progressive multiple sclerosis EUSPMS, SPECTRIMS, NASPMS, and IMPACT—study conduct

	EUSPMS [45,63]	SPECTRIMS [46,64]	NASPMS [43]	IMPACT [65]	EUSPMS	SPECTRIMS		NASPMS		IMPACT
	PBO	PBO	PBO	PBO	8 mIU qod	22 μg tiw	44 μg tiw	8 mIU qod	5 mIU/m^2 qod	60 μg qw
% Lost to follow-up	8.7	9.3	10.4	10.5	7.2	7.7	6.9	13.9	8.9	13.3
% Discontinued treatment	27.1	15.6	24.4	24.7	25.0	17.7	21.1	24.9	23.9	28.1
Blinding (patients)[a]	54%	52%	38%	NA	66%	59%	59%	51%	56%	NA
Blinding (EDSS-Physician)[a]	19%	26%	9%	NA	21%	29%	29%	7%	6%	NA

Abbreviation: NA, not available.
[a] Percent correct guesses about assigned treatment.

Table 9
Four studies of interferon-β in secondary progressive multiple sclerosis: EUSPMS, SPECTRIMS, NASPMS, and IMPACT—results

	EUSPMS [45,63] PBO	SPECTRIMS [46,64] PBO	NASPMS [43] PBO	IMPACT [65] PBO	EUSPMS	SPECTRIMS		NASPMS		IMPACT
					8 mIU qod	22 μg tiw	44 μg tiw	8 mIU qod	5 mIU/m^2 qod	60 μg qw
% Confirmed progression	54	65	37	27	45*	60	59	37	44	26
% Exacerbation free	36	37	62	63	43*	42*	44*	71*	67*	74*
Median time to first relapse	385	281	NR	NR	644	476	494	NR	NR	NR
% No MRI activity (new and enlarging T2 lesions)	16	24	31	42	36*	36*	41*	30*	44*	63*
Median % change in T2 volume	9.7	10.0	10.9	NA	−5.3	−0.5	−1.3	0.4	NA	NA

Abbreviations: NA, not available; NR, not reached.
* $P < 0.05$–0.001.

and a slow pace of disability progression may help characterize patients less likely to respond to IFN-β treatment.

Treatment of clinically isolated syndromes

Two studies address the effects of IFN-β1a initiated at the time of a first clinical demyelinating event (Tables 4, 5, and 10) [60–62,71]. In the CHAMPS study by Jacobs et al, 383 patients who had a first acute clinical demyelinating event were randomized to IFN-β1a (Avonex) 30 μg weekly or PBO after initial treatment with high-dose corticosteroids [60]. During up to 2 years of follow-up, the cumulative probability of the development of another clinical relapse that defined clinically definite MS (CDMS) was significantly lower in the IFN-β1a group (rate ratio = 0.56; 95% confidence interval, 0.38–0.81; $P = 0.002$). When compared with the PBO group, patients taking IFN-β1b had a relative reduction in the volume of brain lesions, fewer new or enlarging T2 lesions, and fewer enhanced lesions at 18 months (Table 10). In the ETOMS study reported by Comi et al, patients who had a first episode of neurologic dysfunction suggesting MS within the previous 3 months and brain MRI lesions compatible with MS were randomized to weekly subcutaneous 22-μg IFN-β1a (Rebif) or PBO. Of 308 randomized patients, 78% received study treatment for 2 years and 90% were evaluable at study termination [61,62]. Fewer patients developed CDMS in the IFN-β1a group (IFN-β1a = 34%, PBO = 45%; $P = 0.047$). The time at which 30% of patients converted to CDMS was 569 days with IFN-β1a and 252 days with PBO ($P = 0.034$).

Both studies show that IFN-β1a treatment at an early stage of MS has significant positive effects on clinical and MRI outcomes. Although reassuring, the results of these two studies leave open whether or not the

Table 10
Comparison of two studies of patients who had first episode suggestive of multiple sclerosis

	ETOMS [60,61]	CHAMPS [59]
N	309	383
Mean age	28	33
% Female	64	75
Time from first symptoms to IFN treatment (mean)	79 days	20 days
Polysymptomatic onset	27%	0%
Optic neuritis	32%	50%
Brain stem/cerebellum	29%	28.5%
Spinal cord	27%	21.5%
T1-Gd + at onset	59%	29%*
% Treated with steroids for first episode	70%	All
IFN (brand/dosage/route)	IFN-β1b (Rebif/22 μg/1 qw sc)	IFN-β1a (Avonex/30 μg/1 qw im)

* All patients treated with high-dose steroids.

delay of the second demyelinating event has an impact on long-term disability progression and how to best define those patients at the highest risk for progression to CDMS or development of disease-related disability. Subgroup analyses identify the number of T2 lesions on the initial scan ($\geq$9 in CHAMPS; $\geq$8 in ETOMS) and identification of at least one Gd-enhancing lesion at baseline as the most robust prognostic criteria for a rapid progression to CDMS [61,71]. In ETOMS, patients who had polysymptomatic first episodes were at higher risk for CDMS; such patients were excluded from CHAMPS. In ETOMS, severity of the first relapse also emerged as a negative prognostic factor. Long-term observation of patients included in these two studies and the results of an ongoing study (BENEFIT) of early intervention with 8-mIU alternate-day IFN-β1b compared with PBO, which is planned to provide individual subject follow-up to 5 years, hopefully will provide some answers to these open issues [72].

Adverse event profile

Approximately 70% to 80% of patients experience flu-like symptoms of fever, myalgia, headache, fatigue, and chills when starting IFN-β treatment [73,74]. These side effects begin 3 to 4 hours after injection and improve spontaneously within 24 hours; they seem related to upregulation of inflammatory cytokines, such as IL-6, tumor necrosis factor α, and even IFN-γ. For 80% or more of patients, these flu-like symptoms resolve during the first 2 to 3 months of therapy. Slow stepwise increase of dosage and preventive administration of nonsteroidal anti-inflammatory drugs or low-dose steroids in most cases attenuate these side effects until they resolve spontaneously within 2 to 3 months [74]. Less than 20% of patients treated with IFN-β needs continuous or intermittent treatment with nonsteroidal anti-inflammatory drugs. Skin reactions occur in more than 50% of the patients after subcutaneous IFN-β administration. Meticulous instruction in injection technique, frequent change of the injection site, local cooling, and avoiding excessive exposure to sunlight may reduce these side effects and prevent skin necrosis. Skin necrosis at subcutaneous injection sites occurs in up to 5% of treated patients in the pivotal clinical trials.

Neutralizing antibodies

NAB are observed in some patients who have MS and are treated with IFN-β [41,44,75,76]. Several reports address the impact of NAB on a variety of outcome measures; most suggest some attenuation of treatment effects. It is difficult to draw clear conclusions, however, from the incidence and clinical significance of NAB positivity based on the available data, especially in light of differences in assay methods, definitions of positivity to NAB, sampling rates, and patient populations [76–78]. The reported frequencies of NAB in controlled studies are given in Table 11. The lower incidence of

Table 11
Rate of neutralizing antibodies (%)

	1 year [61]	2–3 years	4 years
Avonex 30/qw [76]	14.0	22.0	
Avonex 30/qw [45]		2.2	
Avonex 60/qw [45]		5.8	
Avonex 60/qw [45]		3.3	
Rebif 3 × 22/qw [63]	5.3		
Rebif 3 × 44/qw [63]	16.3		
Rebif 3 × 22/qw [41,42]	15.8	23.8	23.7
Rebif 3 × 44/qw [41,42]	13.6	12.5	14.3
Rebif 3 × 22/qw [65]		20.6	
Rebif 3 × 44/qw [65]		14.7	
IFN-β1b 8 mIU/eod [75]	31	38	
IFN-β1b 8 mIU/eod [45,79]	18.3	27.8	

NAB with IFN-β1a (Avonex) in all but the pivotal trial has been explained by a different manufacturing procedure, which allowed for less aggregate formation. Possibly, antibody formation also is dependent on the route (intramuscular or subcutaneous), formulation, dosage, or frequency of dosing [78,80,81]. Guidelines for physicians who have patients taking IFN-β state that treatment decisions should be based mainly on clinical grounds [82].

In the IFN-β1b pivotal study of RRMS, NAB status was determined in sera drawn every 3 months [75]. In patients who were NAB positive, an attenuation of treatment effects was reported with respect to relapse rates and the T2 lesion load found on serial MRIs from month 18 on study and beyond, but mean scores on the EDSS showed a trend to worsening only among those patients who did not have NAB. Data then were analyzed with a more reliable assay based on the induction of the MXA protein. Sophisticated statistical methods addressed the question of whether or not change in NAB positivity and NAB negativity during treatment was associated with diminished efficacy [83,84]. In this approach, NAB-negative and NAB-positive periods were compared for individual patients. This analysis does not show a NAB-associated attenuation of efficacy for the registered dose of 8-mIU IFN-β1b on relapse rates, EDSS, or MRI measures. Only in the cross-sectional analysis was the rate of relapses attenuated by NAB [85]. The two studies of IFN-β1a also demonstrate trends toward reduced treatment effect on relapses and on MRI activity in patients who were NAB positive [41,76]. Although only a weak trend was described in the IFN-β1a (Avonex) trial, in the PRISMS 4-year analysis, an effect of NAB positivity on relapse rates and MRI parameters was shown from the third year on [44]. No study has demonstrated an effect of NAB positivity on disability progression. Recent data on the relation of NAB status to clinical efficacy from the European SPMS trial show varying effects of NAB on relapse rates, depending on the statistical approach and definition of positivity, but no effect on disability progression [79]. A substantial proportion of patients who were NAB positive seems to become NAB negative. In a subgroup of participants in the IFN-β1b pivotal trial, NAB antibodies disappeared at year 10 of treatment [86].

In conclusion, there is an important body of evidence suggesting that high-titer NAB activity has a negative impact on treatment efficacy with respect to relapses and MRI measures of inflammatory activity. Nevertheless, it is generally recommended to base treatment decisions primarily on clinical grounds.

Use of interferon-β in daily practice—is there a consensus?

The Therapeutics and Technology Assessment Subcommittee of the American Academy of Neurology and the MS Council for Clinical Practice Guidelines [87] summarized available evidence on IFN-β in MS (Table 12).

Table 12
Available evidence on IFN-β in MS

1. On the basis of several consistent Class I studies, IFN-β has been demonstrated to reduce the attack rate (measured either clinically or by MRI) in patients who have MS or who have CIS and who are at high risk for developing MS (Type A recommendation). Treatment of MS with IFN-β produces a beneficial effect on MRI measures of disease severity, such as T2 disease burden and probably also slows sustained disability progression (Type B recommendation).
2. As a result, it is appropriate to consider IFN-β for treatment in any patient who is at high risk for developing CDMS or who already has either RRMS or SPMS and still is experiencing relapses (Type A recommendation). The effectiveness of IFN-β in patients who have SPMS but do not have relapses is uncertain (Type U recommendation).
3. It is possible that certain populations of patients who have MS (eg, those who have more attacks or at earlier disease stages) may be better candidates for therapy than others, although, at the moment, there is insufficient evidence regarding these issues (Type U recommendation).
4. On the basis of Class I and II studies and several pieces of consistent Class III evidence, it is considered probable that there is a dose-response curve associated with the use of IFN-β for the treatment of MS (Type B recommendation). It is possible, however, that a portion of this apparent dose-effect instead may be the result of differences in the frequency of IFN-β administration (rather than dose) between studies.
5. On the basis of several Class II studies, the route of administration of IFN-β probably is not of clinical importance, at least regarding efficacy (Type B recommendation). The side-effect profile, however, does differ between routes of administration. There is no known clinical difference between the different types of IFN-β, although this has not been studied thoroughly (Type U recommendation).
6. On the basis of several Class I studies, treatment of patients who have MS with IFN-β is associated with the production of NAB (Type A recommendation). The rate of NAB production, however, probably is less with IFN-β1a treatment than with IFN-β1b treatment (Type B recommendation). The biologic effect of NAB is uncertain, although their presence may be associated with a reduction in clinical effectiveness of IFN-β treatment (Type C recommendation). Whether or not there is a difference in immunogenicity between subcutaneous and intramuscular routes of administration is unknown (Type U recommendation). The clinical usefulness of measuring NAB in an individual on IFN-β therapy is uncertain (Type U recommendation).

There is little to add to this consensus statement. All three IFN-β preparations are effective in reducing relapse rate and severity in patients who have RRMS. In patients who have average relapse rates of approximately one per year or two every 3 years, most neurologists indicate treatment. In patients who have less frequent relapses and minor or no evidence of disease progression in paraclinical investigations, the issue is more controversial, with a clear tendency in the past few years to extend the indication for treatment. The same is the case for clinically isolated syndromes (CIS), where evidence from CHAMPS and ETOMS trials supports the efficacy of weekly IFN-β1a. Because of the lack of data on the long-term impact of such treatment, few countries reimburse IFN-β therapy for CIS. Recently, the European Commission recommended reimbursement for patients who have CIS and who have more than 9 T2 lesions, one of them Gd-enhancing, because of their higher probability of conversion into CDMS.

In very active relapsing MS and when an early effect is mandatory, frequent and higher IFN-β1 dosing may be preferable. In treatment failures, defined by unchanged relapse rate or accumulating disability, switching from lower-dose to higher-dose IFN-β is an option, if systemic side effects of the IFN-β are not already an issue. In such cases, NAB against IFN-β might be sought. If positive, switching to another disease-modifying compound (glatiramer acetate or an immunosuppressant) might be appropriate, because IFN-β NAB are cross-reactive. In view of the lower immunogenicity of IFN-β1a (Avonex), some advocate switching to this treatment after a wash-out of 2 to 3 months [81]. In SPMS, treatment with IFN-β seems justified in patients who have additional relapses or evidence of rapid disability progression, if side effects of treatment have minor or no impact on patients' everyday life. IFN-β1b has been approved for this indication in several countries, including those in the European Community; some countries also allow IFN-β1a (Rebif) for patients who have SPMS and superimposed relapses. No indication exists for IFN-β treatment of primary progressive MS.

Ongoing research, including long-term follow-up of patients participating in controlled trials and long-term observational studies, if supplemented by sophisticated MRI and pharmacogenetic studies using advanced technologies, such as cDNA microarray and quantitative PCR, hopefully will enlighten future treatment decisions by helping to identify responders and nonresponders to IFN-β and expanding knowledge of the effects of interferon treatment [88].

References

[1] The IFNB Multiple Sclerosis Study Group. Interferon beta-1b is effective in relapsing-remitting multiple sclerosis. I. Clinical results of a multicenter, randomized, double-blind, placebo-controlled trial. Neurology 1993;43:655–61.

[2] Paty DW, Li DKB, UBC MS/MRI Study Group, IFNB Multiple Sclerosis Study Group. Interferon beta-1b is effective in relapsing-remitting multiple sclerosis. II. MRI analysis

results of a multicenter, randomized double-blind, placebo-controlled trial. Neurology 1993; 43:662–7.

[3] Isaacs A, Lindenmann J. Virus interference. I. The interferon. Proc R Soc Lond 1957;147: 258–67.

[4] Jacobs L, Johnson KP. A brief history of the use of interferons as treatment of multiple sclerosis. Arch Neurol 1994;51:1245–52.

[5] Jacobs L, O'Malley JA, Freeman A, et al. Intrathecal interferon reduces exacerbations of multiple sclerosis. Science 1982;214:1026–8.

[6] Jacobs L, O'Malley JA, Freeman A, et al. Intrathecal interferon in multiple sclerosis. Arch Neurol 1982;39:609–15.

[7] Arnason BGW. Interferon beta in multiple sclerosis. Clin Immunol Immunopathol 1996;81: 1–11.

[8] Weinstock-Guttman B, Ransohoff RM, Kinkel RP, et al. The interferons: biological effects, mechanisms of action, and use in multiple sclerosis. Ann Neurol 1995;37:7–15.

[9] Karp CL, van Boxel-Dezaire AH, Byrnes AA, et al. Interferon beta in multiple sclerosis: altering the balance of interleukin-12 and interleukin-10? Curr Opin Neurol 2001;14:361–8.

[10] Hohlfeld R. Biotechnological agents for the immunotherapy of multiple sclerosis. Brain 1997;120:865–916.

[11] Panitch HS, Hirsch RL, Haley AS, et al. Exacerbations of multiple sclerosis in patienzs treated with gamma interferon. Lancet 1987;I:893–5.

[12] Leppert D, Waubant E, Bürk MR, et al. Interferon beta-1b inhibits gelatinase secretion and in vitro migration of human T cells: a possible mechanism for treatment efficacy in multiple sclerosis. Ann Neurol 1996;40:846–52.

[13] Calabresi PA, Tranquill LR, Dambrosia JM, et al. Increases in soluble VCAM-1 correlate with a decrease in MRI lesions in multiple sclerosis treated with interferon beta-1b. Ann Neurol 1997;41:669–74.

[14] Liu Z, Pelfrey CM, Cotleur A, et al. Immunomodulatory effects of Interferon beta-1a in multiple sclerosis. J Neuroimmunol 2001;112:153–62.

[15] Teleshova N, Kivisakk P, Ozenci V, et al. Elevated CD40 ligand expressing blood T-cell levels in multiple sclerosis are reversed by interferon-beta treatment. Scand J Immunol 2000; 51:312–20.

[16] Marrack P, Kappler J, Mitchell T. Type I Interferons keep activated T-cells alive. J Exp Med 1999;189:521–30.

[17] Pilling D, Akbar AN, Girdlestone J, et al. Interferon beta mediates stromal cell rescue of T-cells from apoptosis. Eur J Immunol 1999;29:1041–50.

[18] Borthwick NJ, Lowdell M, Salmon M, et al. Loss of CD28 expression on CD8(+) T-cells is induced by IL-2 receptor gamma chain signalling cytokines and type I IFN, and increases susceptibility to activation-induced apoptosis. Int Immunol 2000;12:1005–13.

[19] Kaser A, Nagata S, Tilg H. Interferon alpha augments activation-induced T-cell death by upregulation of Fas (CD95/APO-1) and Fas ligand expression. Cytokine 1999;11: 736–43.

[20] Zipp F, Beyer M, Gelderblom H, et al. No induction of apoptosis by IFN-beta in human antigen-specific T-cells. Neurology 2000;54:485–7.

[21] Lombardi G, Dunne PJ, Scheel-Toellner D, et al. Type I IFN maintains the survival of anergic $CD4^{+}$ T-cells. J Immunol 2000;165:3782–9.

[22] Rep MHT, Schrijver HM, van Lopik T, et al. Interferon (IFN)-beta treatment enhances CD95 and interleukin 10 expression but reduces interferon-gamma producing T-cells in MS patients. J Neuroimmunol 1999;96:92–100.

[23] Perini P, Wadhwa M, Buttarello M, et al. Effect of IFN beta and anti-IFN beta antibodies on NK cells in multiple sclerosis patients. J Neuroimmunol 2000;105:91–5.

[24] Muraro PA, Leist TP, Bielekova B, et al. VLA4/CD49d downregulated on primed T lymphocytes during Interferon beta therapy in multiple sclerosis. J Neuroimmunol 2000;111: 186–94.

[25] Ozenci V, Kouwenhoven M, Teleshova N, et al. Multiple Sclerosis: pro- and anti-inflammatory cytokines and metalloproteinases are affected differentially by treatment of multiple sclerosis. J Neuroimmunol 2000;108:236–43.

[26] Furlan R, Bergami A, Lang R, et al. Interferon beta treatment in multiple sclerosis patients decreases the number of circulating T cells producing interferon-gamma and Interleukin-4. J Neuroimmunol 2000;111:86–92.

[27] Becher B, Giacomini PS, Pelletier D, et al. Interferon-gamma secretion by peripheral blood T-cell subsets in multiple sclerosis: correlation with disease phase and Interferon-beta therapy. Ann Neurol 1999;45:247–50.

[28] Sciacca FL, Canal N, Edoardo Grimaldi LM. Induction of IL-1 receptor antagonist by Interferon beta: implication for the treatment of multiple sclerosis. J Neurovirol 2000;6: 33–7.

[29] Zang YCQ, Halder JB, Samanta AK, et al. Regulation of chemokine receptor CCR5 and production of RANTES and MIP-1alpha by Interferon beta. J Neuroimmunol 2001;112: 100–7.

[30] Iaorlori C, Reale M, Lugaresi A, et al. RANTES production and expression is reduced in relapsing-remitting Multiple Sclerosis patients treated with Interferon beta-1b. J Neuroimmunol 2000;107:100–7.

[31] Hua LL, Liu JSH, Brosnan CF, Lee SC. Selective inhibition of human glial inducible nitric oxide synthase by Interferon beta: implications for multiple sclerosis. Ann Neurol 1998;43: 384–7.

[32] Rudick RA, Ransohoff RM, Peppler R, et al. Interferon beta induces interleukin-10 expression: relevance to multiple sclerosis. Ann Neurol 1996;40:618–27.

[33] Rudick RA, Ransohoff RM, Lee J-C, et al. In vivo effects of interferon beta-1a on immunosuppressive cytokines in multiple sclerosis. Neurology 1998;50:1294–300.

[34] Byrnes AA, McArthur JC, Karp CL. Interferon-beta therapy for Multiple Sclerosis induces reciprocal changes in Interleukin-12 and Interleukin-10 production. Ann Neurol 2002;51: 165–74.

[35] Hughes R. Wait for further evidence confirming effect of interferon beta in multiple sclerosis. BMJ 1997;314:1763.

[36] Durelli L, Bongioanni MR, Ferrero B, et al. Interferon alpha-2a treatment of relapsing-remitting multiple sclerosis: disease activity resumes after stopping treatment. Neurology 1996;47:123–9.

[37] Myhr KM, Riise T, Green Lilleas FE, et al. Interferon-alpha2a reduces MRI disease activity in relapsing-remitting multiple sclerosis. Neurology 1999;52:1049–56.

[38] Polman CH, Herndon R, Pozzilli C Interferons. In: Rudick RA, Goodkin DE, editors. Multiple sclerosis therapeutics. London: Martin Dunitz; 1999. p. 243–76.

[39] Leary SM, Miller DH, Stevenson VL, et al. Interferon beta-1a in primary progressive MS: an exploratory, randomized, controlled trial. Neurology 2003;60(1):44–51.

[40] Montalban X. Overview of European pilot study of interferon beta-1b in primary progressive multiple sclerosis. Multiple sclerosis 2004;10(S1):62–4.

[41] The PRISMS Study. Randomized double-blind placebo-controlled study of interferon β-1b in relapsing/remitting multiple sclerosis. Lancet 1998;352:1498–504.

[42] Li DKB, Paty DW, UBC MS/MRI Analysis Research Group, PRISMS Study Group. Magnetic resonance imaging results of the PRISMS Trial: a randomized, double-blind, placebo-controlled study of interferon-β1a in relapsing-remitting multiple sclerosis. Ann Neurol 1999;46:197–206.

[43] The North American Study Group on Interferon beta-1b in Secondary Progressive MS. Interferon beta-1b in secondary progressive ms: results from a 3-year controlled study. Neurology 2004;63:1788–95.

[44] The PRISMS Study Group, University of British Columbia MS/MRI Analysis Group. PRISMS-4: long-term efficacy of interferon-beta-1a in relapsing MS. Neurology 2001;56: 1628–36.

[45] Clanet M, Raduc EW, Kappos L, et al. A randomized, double-blind, dose-comparison study of weekly interferon beta-1a (Avonex) in relapsing-remitting MS. Neurology 2002;59: 1507–17.

[46] Li DKB, Zhao GJ, Paty D, University of British Columbia MS/MRI Analysis Research Group, SPECTRIMS Study Group. Randomized controlled trial of interferon beta-1a in secondary progressive MS—MRI results. Neurology 2001;56:1505–13.

[47] Kappos L, Clanet M. European IFN beta-1a (Avonex) Dose-Comparison Study. Sustained efficacy of Interferon beta-1a in relapsing multiple sclerosis: 4-year results from the European dose-comparison study. Neurology 2002;58:P03.069.

[48] Panitch H, Goodin DS, Francis G, et al. Randomized comparative study of interferon beta-1a treatment regimens in MS: The EVIDENCE trial. Neurology 2002;59:1496–506.

[49] Rask C, Unger E, Walton M. Comparative study of Rebif to Avonex and orphan exclusivety: comparative memorandum. FDA, Division of Clinical Trial Design and Analysis; 2002. Available at: www.fda.gov/cder/biologics/review/ifnbser030702r14.pdf.

[50] Durelli L, Verdun E, Barbero P, et al. Every-other-day interferon beta-1b versus once-weekly interferon beta-1a for multiple sclerosis: results of a 2-year prospective randomised multicentre study (INCOMIN). Lancet 2002;359:1453–60.

[51] Durelli L, Ferrero B, Oggero A, et al. A multicenter trial comparing clinical and MRI efficacy of interferon beta-1a and beta-1b in multiple sclerosis. J Neurol 2001;248(Suppl 2):II/62.

[52] Khan OA, Tselis AC, Kamholz JA, et al. A prospective, open-label treatment trial to compare the effect of IFN beta-1a (Avonex), IFN beta-1b (Betaseron), and glatiramer acetate (Copaxone) on the relapse rate in relapsing-remitting multiple sclerosis: results after 18 months of therapy. Mult Scler 2001;7:349–53.

[53] Koch-Henriksen N, Sorensen P, Christensen T. Comparison of interferon-beta-1a 22 mcg once a week and interferon-beta-1b 250 mcg every other day in a randomised head-to-head study. Mult Scler 2004;10(S2):S240–1.

[54] Trojano M, Liguori M, Paolicell D, et al. Interferon beta in relapsing-remitting multiple sclerosis: an independent post marketing study in southern Italy. Mult Scler 2003;9:451–7.

[55] Kappos L, Arnason B, Comi G, et al. The BEYOND (Betaferon/Betaseron Efficacy Yielding Outcomes of a New Dose) programme: investigating further benefits with high-dose high-frequency interferon-beta treatment. Multiple Sclerosis 2004;10:S247–8 (Abstract).

[56] The IFNB Multiple Sclerosis Study Group, The University of British Columbia MS/MRI Analysis Group. Interferon beta-1b in the treatment of multiple sclerosis. Neurology 1995; 45:1277–85.

[57] Jacobs LD, Cookfair DL, Rudick RA, et al. A phase III trial of intramuscular recombinant interferon beta as treatment for exacerbating-remitting multiple sclerosis: design and conduct of study and baseline characteristics of patients. Mult Scler 1995;1:118–35.

[58] Jacobs LD, Cookfair DL, Rudick RA, et al. Intramuscular interferon beta-1a for disease progression in relapsing multiple sclerosis. Ann Neurol 1996;39:285–94.

[59] Simon JH, Jacobs LD, Campion MK, et al. Magnetic resonance studies of intramuscular interferon beta-1a for relapsing multiple sclerosis. Ann Neurol 1998;43:79–87.

[60] Jacobs LD, Beck RW, Simon JH, et al. The effect of intramuscular interferon beta-1a treatment initiated at the time of a first acute clinical demyelinating event on the rate of development of clinically definite multiple sclerosis. N Engl J Med 2000;343:898–904.

[61] Comi G, Filippi M, Barkhof F, et al. Effect of early interferon treatment on conversion to definite multiple sclerosis: a randomised study. Lancet 2001;357:1576–82.

[62] Comi G, Barkhof F, Durelli L, et al. Early treatment of multiple sclerosis with Rebif (recombinant human interferon beta): design of the study. Mult Scler 1995;1(Suppl 1):S24–7.

[63] Freedman M, OWIMS Study Group. Evidence of Interferon beta-1a dose response in relapsing-remitting MS: the OWIMS Study. Neurology 1999;53:679–86.

[64] The European Study Group on IFN beta-1b in Secondary Progressive MS. Placebo-controlled multicentre randomised trial of interferon β-1b in treatment of secondary progressive multiple sclerosis. Lancet 1998;352:1491–7.

[65] Secondary Progressive Efficacy Clinical Trial of Recombinant Interferon-beta-1a in MS (SPECTRIMS) Study Group. Randomized controlled trial of interferon beta-1a in secondary progressive MS—clinical results. Neurology 2001;56:1496–504.
[66] Cohen JA, Cutter G, Fischer J, et al. Benefit of interferon beta-1a on MSFC progression in secondary progressive MS. Neurology 2002;59:679–87.
[67] Miller DH, Molyneux PD, Barker GJ, et al. Effect of interferon β-1b on magnetic resonance imaging outcomes in secondary progressive multiple sclerosis: results of a European multicentre, randomised, double-blind, placebo-controlled trial. Ann Neurol 1999;46:850–9.
[68] Molyneux PD, Kappos L, Polman CH, et al. The effect of interferon beta-1b treatment on MRI measures of cerebral atrophy in secondary progressive multiple sclerosis. Brain 2000; 123:2256–63.
[69] Barkhof F, van Waesberghe JH, Filippi M, et al. T1 hypointense lesions in secondary progressive multiple sclerosis: effect of interferon beta-1b treatment. Brain 2001;124: 1396–402.
[70] Kappos L, Polman CH, Pozzilli C, et al. Final analysis of the European multicenter trial on IFN beta-1b in secondary progressive MS. Neurology 2001;57:1969–75.
[71] Beck RW, Chandler DL, Cole SR, et al. Interferon beta-1a for early multiple sclerosis: CHAMPS trial subgroup analyses. Ann Neurol 2002;51:481–90.
[72] Freedman M, Edan G, Hartung HP, et al. Betaferon/Betaseron (Interferon beta-1b) in early treatment of multiple sclerosis: the BENEFIT study. Neurology 2003;60(suppl 1):A483 (abstract).
[73] Walther EU, Hohlfeld R. MS: side effects of IFN beta-therapy. Neurology 1999;53:1623–7.
[74] Lublin FD, Whitaker JN, Eidelman BH, et al. Management of patients receiving interferon beta-1b for multiple sclerosis: report of a consensus conference. Neurology 1996;46:12–8.
[75] The IFNB Multiple Sclerosis Study Group, The University of British Columbia MS/MRI Analysis Group. Neutralizing antibodies during treatment of multiple sclerosis with interferon beta-1b: experience during the first three years. Neurology 1996;47:889–94.
[76] Rudick RA, Simonian NA, Alam JA, et al. Incidence and significance of neutralizing antibodies to interferon beta-1a in multiple sclerosis. Neurology 1998;50:273.
[77] Arnason GB, Dianzani F. Correlation of the appearance of anti-interferon antibodies during treatment and diminution of efficacy: Summary of an internationl workshop on anti-interferon antibodies. J Interferon Cytokine Res 1998;18:639–44.
[78] Reder AT, Antel JP. Injecting rationale into interferon-β therapy. Neurology 2000;54: 2034–5.
[79] Polman CH, Kappos L, White RT, et al. Neutralizing antibodies during treatment of secondary-progressive MS with interferon beta-1b. Neurology 2003;60.37–43.
[80] Ross Ch, Clemmesen KM, Svensson M, et al. Immunogenicity of interferon-beta in multiple sclerosis patients: influence of preparation, dosage, dose frequency and route of administration. Ann Neurol 2000;48:706–12.
[81] Perini P, Facchinetti A, Bulian P, et al. Interferon-beta (INF-beta) antibodies in interferon-beta1a- and interferon-beta1b-treated multiple sclerosis patients. Prevalence, kinetics, cross-reactivity, and factors enhancing interferon-beta immunogenicity in vivo. Eur Cytokine Netw 2001;12:56–61.
[82] Paty DW, Goodkin D, Thompson A, et al. Guidelines for physicians withptients on IFN beta-1b: the use of an assay for neutralizing antibodies (NAB). Neurology 1996;47: 865–6.
[83] Zeger SL, Liang KY. An overview of methods for the analysis of longitudinal data. Stat Med 1992;11:1825–39.
[84] D'Vachkova Y, Petkau J, White R. Longitudinal analyses for magnetic resonance imaging outcomes in multiple sclerosis clinical trials. J Biopharm Stat 1997;7:501–31.
[85] Petkau AJ, White RA, Ebers GC, et al. Longitudinal analyses of the effects of neutralizing antibodies on interferon beta-1b in relapsing-remitting multiple sclerosis. Mult Scler 2004; 10:126–38.

[86] Rice GP, Paszner B, Oger J, et al. The evolution of neutralizing antibodies in multiple sclerosis patients treated with interferon beta-1b. Neurology 1999;52:1277–9.

[87] Goodin DS, Frohman EM, Garmany GP, et al. Disease modifying therapies in multiple sclerosis. Report of the Therapeutics and Technology Assessment Subcommittee of the American Academy of Neurology and the MS Council for Clinical Practice Guidelines. Neurology 2002;58:169–78.

[88] Wandinger KP, Stürzebecher CS, Bielekova B, et al. Complex immunomodulatory effects of Interferon beta in multiple sclerosis include the upregulation of T helper 1-associated marker genes. Ann Neurol 2001;50:349–57.

ELSEVIER
SAUNDERS

Neurol Clin 23 (2005) 215–231

NEUROLOGIC
CLINICS

Glatiramer Acetate in the Treatment of Multiple Sclerosis

Aaron E. Miller, MD[a,b]

[a]Department of Neurology, Mt. Sinai School of Medicine, New York, NY, USA
[b]Corinne Goldsmith Dickinson Center for Multiple Sclerosis, Mt. Sinai School of Medicine, New York, NY, USA

The development of glatiramer acetate (GA) was a result of the juxtaposition of unexpected serendipity with rigorous scientific investigation. Experimental autoimmune encephalomyelitis (EAE) has long served as an animal model for multiple sclerosis (MS). This inflammatory disease can be induced with injection of whole spinal cord homogenate or specific proteins, including myelin basic protein (MBP), proteolipid protein, or myelin oligodendrocyte glycoprotein. In the early 1960s, investigators at the Weitzmann Institute in Israel sought to generate a polymer that would reproduce the effects of MBP in eliciting EAE. They believed that development of a synthetic molecule that could mimic the encephalitogenic effects of EAE might provide a useful tool for further investigation of that animal model. Among the many polymers they produced, one, in particular, failed to produce EAE. Surprisingly, this compound, then referred to as copolymer 1 (Cop 1), prevented and suppressed EAE [1].

Initial experiments demonstrated a markedly suppressive effect on EAE in rabbits and guinea pigs induced with bovine and human MBP [2]. The incidence of EAE decreased from approximately 75% in the control group to approximately 20% in the Cop 1–treated animals. EAE is species specific regarding the species from which the MBP is derived and the species in which the disease is induced. Thus, the next logical step was to investigate the effects of Cop 1 in other species. The originally unexpected outcome of suppression of EAE was recapitulated in a variety of animal species, including mice [3] and subhuman primates. The experimental work in rhesus monkeys [4] and baboons [5] particularly was encouraging. In these species, MBP-induced EAE is highly lethal. Yet, administration of Cop 1 was able to reverse the condition even after symptoms had appeared, a situation

E-mail address: aaron.miller@mssm.edu

doi:10.1016/j.ncl.2004.11.002 ***neurologic.theclinics.com*** analogous to treatment of human MS. The primate results were striking. All five control rhesus monkeys succumbed to EAE within 4 to 11 days. In contrast, 4 out of 5 Cop 1–treated animals began to show improvement after 4 to 5 days of treatment and eventually recovered completely. The fifth treated monkey initially improved but relapsed 35 days later and finally died. Similarly, dramatic benefit was seen in baboons. The six control animals developed progressive paralysis and died within 4 to 11 days, whereas seven of nine baboons that received daily treatment beginning at the first symptoms of weakness recovered completely, despite progressing initially to complete paralysis. These repeated successes led to the introduction of Cop 1 into human clinical trials.

Cop 1, subsequently renamed GA, is a random assortment of L-glutamine, lysine, alanine, and tyrosine in a molar ratio of 4.2:3.4:1.4:1.0. Preparations may vary in their particular amino acid sequence and range from 40 to 90 amino acids in length, with a corresponding molecular weight ranging from 4.7 to 10 kilodaltons.

Clinical trials were initiated in Israel in three patients who had acute disseminated encephalomyelitis and in four patients in the terminal stages of MS [6]. Soon thereafter, pilot trials in the United States were initiated by Bornstein et al [7], ultimately leading to successful treatment of relapsing-remitting MS (RRMS) and approval by the United States Food and Drug Administration and regulatory agencies in many other countries.

Mechanism of action

Popular conception of the pathogenesis of MS postulates the initiation of an autoimmune process with activation of autoreactive CD4+ T cells in the peripheral blood. This may occur through a process known as molecular mimicry, in which an unknown antigen, perhaps a microbe, is presented by dendritic cells or macrophages in association with major histocompatibility complex (MHC) class II molecules. This trimolecular complex then is recognized by a T-cell receptor on a responding cell. Optimal T-cell activation also requires the activity of costimulatory molecules, including the interaction between CD40 and CD40 ligand and between B7 and CD28. These activated CD4+ Th1 cells secrete the cytokines interleukin (IL)-1, IL-12, interferon (IFN)-γ, and tumor necrosis factor α (TNF-α), which, in turn, upregulate adhesion molecules on the vascular endothelial cells. Attracted by chemokines, these Th1 cells stick to the vascular wall through the interaction of adhesion molecules on their surface and complementary receptors on the endothelium. These Th1 cells then elaborate matrix metalloproteinases, which help digest the basement membrane, thereby enabling passage of the lymphocytes through the blood-brain barrier into the central nervous system (CNS). Once in the brain and spinal cord, these cells are amplified further and activated after stimulation by antigens presented by microglial cells.

Further production of proinflammatory cytokines ensues and leads to activation of macrophages, which can strip myelin directly or produce molecules that are toxic to myelin, such as TNF-α, nitric oxide, or free radicals. These cells also may contribute to the stimulation of complement-dependent antibody-mediated damage [8–10].

In contrast to Th1 cells, Th2 cells are regarded as anti-inflammatory. They secrete cytokines, such as IL-4, IL-5, and IL-10, which tend to downregulate the proinflammatory cytokine production by Th1 cells or macrophages.

This paradigm raises the possibility that GA could exert its therapeutic activity either at the level of antigen presentation or by altering the cytokine production pattern. Evidence supports both mechanisms.

At least four potential mechanisms of action have been proposed for the therapeutic effects of GA in MS [11]: (1) competition with MBP for binding at the MHC; (2) competition of the GA/MHC with that of MBP/MHC for binding to the T-cell receptor; (3) partial activation and induction of tolerance in MBP-specific T cells; and (4) generation of GA-reactive Th2 regulatory cells.

Although in vitro studies suggest that GA competes with MBP in some manner, this does not seem to be the relevant mechanism for its therapeutic action. One reason for this belief is the fact that the stereoisomer of GA, composed exclusively of D-amino acids, binds equally effectively to MHC class II but is ineffective in suppressing EAE. Evidence for the competition of GA/MHC for binding to the antigen-specific MBP T-cell receptor is controversial. Even if this phenomenon is true in vitro, GA is unlikely to reach the sites necessary for competition with MBP.

The third proposed mechanism requires that GA act like an altered peptide ligand, by which GA/MHC binds to the T-cell receptor (TCR) of MBP-specific T cells and, in so doing, renders those pathogenic T cells anergic or altered in some other way. Although such a process could occur in the periphery at or near the GA injection sites, no direct evidence indicates if the functional properties of MBP-specific T cells have been modified.

The mechanism currently most favored is the induction of a Th1 to Th2 shift by treatment with GA. Neuhaus et al [11] suggest a scenario in which the GA-activated Th2-like cells are able to cross the blood-brain barrier. Once inside the CNS, they encounter antigens released by myelin turnover that are presented by local microglia. This stimulates the cells to release anti-inflammatory cytokines, such as IL-4, IL-6, and IL-10. Some studies postulate the release of neurotrophic factors also. This results in a decrease in the production of proinflammatory cytokines through the process of bystander suppression. Conceivably, this process also could occur in the periphery, where antigens, perhaps microbial in origin, that stimulate MBP-specific T cells through molecular mimicry, simultaneously might activate GA-specific downregulatory T cells.

Clinical trials

Preliminary studies

The first human clinical trials of what then was called Cop 1 were reported by Abramsky et al [6] in three patients who had acute disseminated encephalomyelitis and four patients who had advanced MS. The drug was tolerated well and no safety issues were raised, but no judgment about efficacy was warranted.

After that, Bornstein et al [7] conducted an open-label trial in 16 patients who had various types and severity of MS. The patients tolerated the administration of 20 mg daily of Cop 1 with no significant toxicity or other adverse experiences. Improvement was noted in five of 16 patients, encouraging the investigators to proceed with randomized clinical trials.

Pilot trial

The Bornstein investigative group reported the results of the first randomized, double-blind, placebo-controlled study of Cop 1 in patients who had RRMS in 1987 [12]. This trial is noteworthy in that it was probably the first controlled study to show the efficacy of any disease-modifying therapy (other than corticotropin or corticosteroids) in MS. The study was designed in a matched pair format with a primary endpoint of the proportion of relapse-free patients. The trial enrolled 24 pairs, matched according to age, sex, and disability, and stratified them according to the Kurtzke disability status scale (DSS) [13] into three groups: DSS 0-2, 3-4, and 5-6. Two additional patients who were unmatched also were entered into the study. Entry requirements included age between 20 and 35 years and at least two exacerbations in the prior 2 years. Patients were assessed regularly at 3-month intervals for 2 years by a blinded neurologist and also were evaluated quickly after reporting symptoms of an acute attack. Exacerbations were registered only when symptoms existed for at least 48 hours and produced objective changes on the neurologic examination resulting in at least a 1-point increase on one of the eight functional groups of the DSS or the overall DSS itself. Subjective symptoms alone did not constitute a relapse as counted in this study.

The primary endpoint was analyzed for 22 matched pairs and showed 12 discordant pairs. These included 10 pairs in which the patient receiving Cop 1 experienced no relapses, whereas the corresponding patient receiving placebo had at least one attack. In contrast, in only two pairs did the patient who was receiving placebo remain attack-free, whereas the Cop 1–treated patients experienced relapse. This result statistically significantly favored Cop 1 ($P = 0.039$).

Data from a total of 48 patients were available for unmatched analysis of relapse frequency. Only 16 exacerbations occurred among 25 patients who were treated with Cop 1, compared with 62 attacks in the 23 placebo-treated patients ($P = 0.045$). Whereas patients in the lowest disability stratum had the greatest reduction in relapse rate, those who had higher DSS scores also seemed to benefit from the drug. In addition to being less likely to remain relapse-free, placebo-treated patients also were significantly more likely to have three or more relapses. Disability progression of at least 1 point on the DSS, sustained for at least 3 months, was reduced in the Cop 1–treated group at the $P = 0.05$ level.

The treatment was tolerated well and associated with no significant laboratory abnormalities. The trial was, however, notable for the first recognized occurrence of what is now referred to as a systemic postinjection reaction. Two patients experienced episodes, within a few minutes of injection, characterized by tightness of the chest and flushing, sometimes accompanied by shortness of breath, palpitations, and a sensation of anxiety. The episodes resolved spontaneously in 5 to 30 minutes. Rechallenge in one patient was associated with urticaria and pruritus, which prompted treatment with epinephrine and corticosteroids.

Pivotal trial of relapsing-remitting multiple sclerosis

The promising results achieved in the pilot trial encouraged the undertaking of a much larger phase III randomized, double-blind, placebo-controlled study. Unfortunately, several issues, most notably those related to the consistent production of large amounts of GA, delayed the initiation of such a trial until late 1991. The trial, sponsored by Teva Pharmaceuticals, was conducted at 11 academic MS centers in the United States [14]. Originally planned as a 24-month trial, the study eventually was extended until each patient had completed the full 2 years on study. The primary endpoint of the trial was a comparison between the mean number of relapses in the GA and placebo-treated groups during the 2 years. Confirmation of relapse required patients to have symptoms, in the absence of fever, that were accompanied by objective changes on the neurologic examination, resulting either in an increase of at least a half step on the expanded disability status scale (EDSS) [15], a 2-point increase on one of the seven functional systems, or a 1-point increase on two or more of the functional systems. Predetermined secondary endpoints included proportion of relapse-free patients, time to first relapse, proportion of patients who had sustained disease progression, and mean change in EDSS and ambulation index between the GA and placebo groups from baseline to conclusion.

Eligibility for the study required a diagnosis of clinically definite or laboratory-supported definite MS by Poser criteria [16], age between 18 and 45 years, disease for at least 1 year, an EDSS of 0 to 5.0, and at least two relapses in the previous 2 years (but none in the previous 30 days). Enrollment included 251 patients, 125 assigned to GA treatment and 126 to placebo. The study employed a two-neurologist technique. The first physician served as a blinded examiner, completing the objective neurologic evaluation without discussion of symptoms or adverse experiences. The second neurologist, also blinded, functioned as the treating physician, evaluating symptoms and adverse experiences and determining the need for steroids at a time of confirmed relapse.

Results of the study (Table 1) showed a statistically significant reduction in 2-year relapse rate, the primary endpoint, of 29% for the GA-treated group compared with the placebo-treated group ($P = 0.007$). The final 2-year relapse rate was 1.19 ± 0.13 for the GA group and 1.68 ± 0.13 for the placebo group. Trends in favor of GA were seen in median time to first relapse (287 versus 198 days) and in proportion of patients who were relapse-free (33.6% versus 27.0%), which did not achieve statistical significance. Progression of disability was assessed in several ways. When patients were classified categorically as improved, unchanged, or worse (by ≥ 1 step on the EDSS at 24 months), results were statistically significant in favor of the GA-treated group on a categoric repeated-measures analysis ($P = 0.037$) and on analysis from baseline to 24 months ($P = 0.024$). Comparison of mean change in EDSS also statistically significantly favored the GA group ($P = 0.023$), although this type of analysis has been criticized because the EDSS is a nonlinear scale. No difference between the two groups occurred on the measure of sustained disability, defined as a progression of at least one step on the EDSS, maintained for at least 3 months. Mean ambulation index scores were nearly identical in the two groups.

As in the pilot trial, GA was tolerated well. Most patients developed, at least at some point, an injection-site reaction consisting of mild erythema

Table 1
Relapse experience of glatiramer acetate and placebo groups in the United States pivotal phase III trial

	Glatiramer acetate (N = 125)	Placebo (N = 126)	Reduction relative to placebo	*P* value
Primary endpoints				
Relapse rate[a]	1.19	1.68	−29%	0.007
Annualized relapse rate	0.59	0.84		
Observed relapses[b]	161	210		
Secondary endpoints				
Proportion relapse-free	33.6%	27.0%		0.098
Median days to first relapse	287	198		0.097
Relapses per patient				
0	42	34		0.023
1–2	60	55		
≥3	23	37		

[a] 24-month, covariate adjusted.
[b] More than 24 months.

and induration, sometimes persisting for several days. The transient self-limited systemic reaction (described previously) for the pilot trial occurred at least once in 15% of GA-treated patients, compared with 3% of those receiving placebo. Most of the patients experiencing such an event had only one during the trial, however, although one patient had seven episodes. These reactions led to discontinuation of therapy for four patients in the GA group and one in the placebo group. No differences in blood or urine studies were seen between the two groups at any time nor were any significant changes in ECG encountered. The withdrawal rates were similar: 15.2% in the GA group and 13.5% in the placebo group.

Phase III trial extension

In the early stages of the phase III trial, the investigative group decided to ask all patients in the study to continue in the blinded study until the last patient enrolled had completed 24 months. This resulted in a mean increase of 5.2 months for the GA group and 5.9 months for the placebo group, with an extension ranging from 1 to 11 months [17]. Of the 106 GA patients who completed 24 months, 99 continued into the extension period, with 97 completing it. Among the 109 placebo patients who completed the original 24-month period, 104 entered the extension period and 97 completed it. Among the 12 patients who completed 24 months, but elected not to enter the extension phase, most had decided to discontinue the study to begin treatment with IFN-β1b, which had become available shortly before the completion of the original 24-month trial.

The results of the double-blind trial that included the extension period showed a slightly greater relapse rate reduction of 32% ($P = 0.002$) than that achieved in the core 24-month study. Through the entire extended trial, the proportion of patients taking GA who remained relapse-free was 33.6%, statistically greater than the 24.6% of the placebo group ($P = 0.035$).

Several statistical analyses were applied to the data on progression of disability between the two treatment groups. When a categoric approach of improved, unchanged, or worsened was employed, the results reiterated those of the core study alone, with the GA group achieving superiority ($P = 0.001$) (Fig. 1). The GA group also showed less mean change from baseline to last observed EDSS score ($P = 0.006$). Using a Kaplan-Meier survival analysis for time to worsening by greater than or equal to 1.5 EDSS steps, but omitting periods of relapse, 41.6% of placebo patients progressed, compared with 21.6% of GA patients ($P = 0.001$) (Fig. 2). As in the core study, however, the difference in sustained progression between the placebo group (29.4%) and the GA group (23.2%) was not significant ($P = 0.199$).

No additional adverse experiences were encountered during the extension period. Throughout the study, no difference occurred between the groups in symptoms suggesting depression.

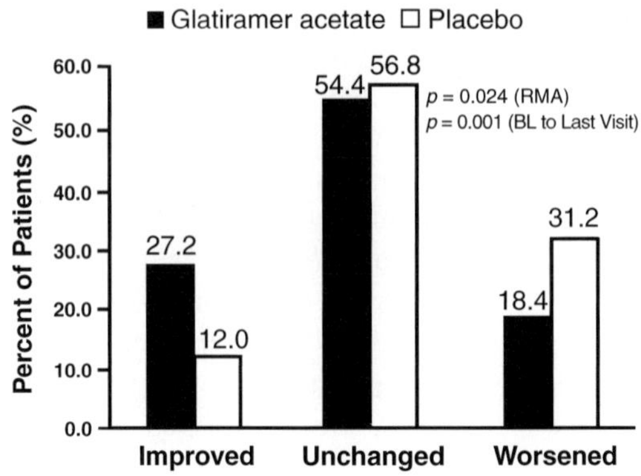

Fig. 1. Percent of patients in the extended trial who improved, were unchanged, or worsened by one or more steps on the EDSS between baseline and the last measurement. RMA, repeated measures analysis; BL, baseline.

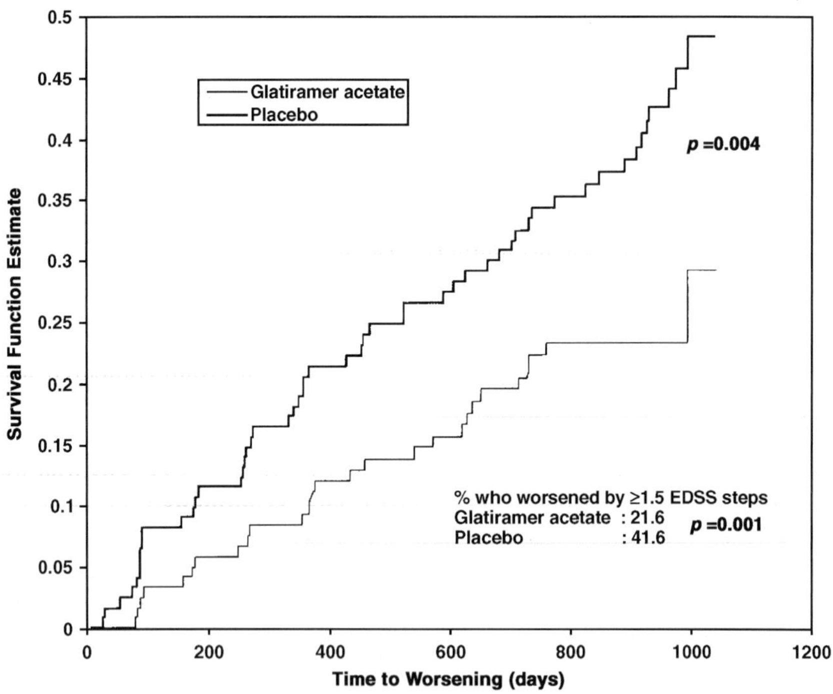

Fig. 2. Kaplan-Meier survival curve for time to increased disability of $\geq$1.5 EDSS steps during the extended trial. EDSS scores during the period of recovery from acute relapses were excluded.

After the completion of the randomized, double-blind, placebo-controlled trial, with its extension period, the investigators offered patients the opportunity to continue in an open-label study. In this study, patients originally assigned to GA continued on drug, whereas those patients originally on placebo were switched to GA. Of the 251 patients originally enrolled in the trial, 152 patients completed a total of 6 years in study [18]. In the group of patients always on GA, the relapse rate declined steadily, so that the rate was only 0.23 in year 6. The percentage of these patients progressing one or more steps on the EDSS essentially was stable from year 3 through year 6 and remained lower than that for patients who had been assigned originally to the placebo group, suggesting an advantage to starting treatment early. A similar phenomenon has been observed in extension studies using IFN-β1a (Rebif) [19]. Data reported from open-label trials must be regarded cautiously because of the potential biases inherent in such studies.

The open-label cohort of patients treated with GA continues to be followed and maintains a low relapse rate with little progression on the EDSS. Investigation of patients who failed to enroll in or dropped out of the open-label study recently has been conducted. Most patients who discontinued treatment with GA did so for personal reasons. These included pregnancy, difficulties adhering to the logistics of the study profile, or a desire to switch or combine therapies. Only 26% discontinued treatment because of perceived disease worsening. Comparison of those dropouts, who were available for evaluation after 10 years, indicated that they had significantly greater disability as a group than those patients who had continued treatment with GA throughout the observation period [20].

Trial of chronic progressive multiple sclerosis

A randomized, double blind, placebo-controlled, two-center trial of patients who had chronic progressive MS was reported in 1991 and failed to show a reduction in progression for the GA-treated group compared with the placebo group (17.6% versus 25.5%) [21]. The trial was small, however, enrolling 106 patients, and included patients who now would be described as having secondary progressive MS or primary progressive MS. The trial was unique in that it required observation and confirmation of sustained progression by the investigative team before patients could be eligible for enrollment in the treatment phase of the study. This resulted in only 106 of 169 patients meeting criteria for entry into the double-blind portion of the trial. The primary endpoint of the trial was time to confirmed progression of 1.5 steps on the EDSS for patients entering at EDSS less than or equal to 5.0 and 1.0 for patients entering at a level of greater than 5.0. This study introduced the concept of sustained progression as an endpoint for clinical trials of progressive forms of MS, which has become standard in subsequent studies. This degree of worsening is greater than that used in subsequent trials of interferons in secondary progressive MS and undoubtedly contributed to the low percentage of patients who actually met criteria for sustained progression during the double-blind randomized period of the trial. Post hoc analysis suggests that patients retrospectively classified as having primary, rather than secondary, progressive MS may have fared better on GA, an observation that prompted a subsequent large trial of primary progressive MS.

MRI studies

Small studies

The pivotal randomized clinical trial of GA in RRMS, unlike the comparable trials of IFN-β1b and IFN-β1a, failed to include a major MRI component in which all patients underwent neuroimaging procedures. The trial did include a small substudy, in which 27 patients at a single center underwent serial, frequent MRI. This study suggested a benefit for GA, compared with placebo, in reducing gadolinium enhancements and the progression of cerebral atrophy, but the results did not achieve statistical significance [22]. Another small Italian study was performed by Mancardi et al [23], in which 10 patients underwent monthly MRI for 9 to 27 months before beginning treatment with GA, followed by monthly scans for another 10 to 14 months after starting therapy. Results showed a reduction in the incidence of new gadolinium-enhancing lesions from 2.2 per month before treatment to 0.92 per month after treatment. This reduction of 57% resulted in a *P* value of 0.1, however, one below that regarded as significant.

European/Canadian MRI trial

Because the pivotal trial of GA in RRMS did not provide useful MRI information, a second large study was undertaken in Europe and Canada specifically to examine the effects of the treatment on this neuroimaging procedure [24]. The study enrolled 239 patients (119 assigned to GA and 120 to placebo) who met the entry criteria of RRMS with at least one attack in the 2 years before entry and at least one gadolinium-enhancing lesion on a screening MRI. The randomized, placebo-controlled, double-blind study had a duration of 9 months, during which patients underwent monthly MRI, with and without administration of gadolinium, and clinical assessments. The primary endpoint of the trial was the total number of gadolinium-enhanced lesions, with predetermined secondary endpoints that included the proportion of patients who had enhancing lesions, the number of new enhancing lesions and their change in volume, the number of new lesions on T2-weighted images, the change in volume of T2 lesions, and the change in volume on unenhanced T1-weighted images. In addition, clinical outcomes were compared.

Results for the primary endpoint showed a mean reduction of 10.8 total gadolinium-enhancing lesions (29%) for the GA-treated group (25.96) compared with the placebo-treated group (36.80), significant at $P = 0.003$). Statistically significant differences favoring treatment with GA occurred in most secondary endpoints also. These included number of new enhancing lesions ($P < 0.003$), cumulative monthly change in volume of enhancing lesions ($P = 0.01$), total number of new T2 lesions ($P < 0.003$), and median change in T2 lesion volume from baseline to month 9 ($P = 0.006$). The difference in change of hypointense lesion volume on T1-weighted images, although greater in the GA-treated group, was not statistically significant.

Clinical outcomes showed a reduction in observed mean relapse rate of 33% for the GA-treated group (0.51 relapses/subject) compared with the placebo group (0.76 relapses per subject) ($P = 0.012$). Expressed differently, these results convert to annualized relapse rates of 0.81 and 1.21, respectively. The number of relapse-free patients was not different between the two treatment groups, but only 6.7% of GA-treated patients experienced two or more attacks, compared with 15.8% of the placebo-treated patients. In GA- and placebo-treated groups, statistically significant correlation occurred between cumulative number of enhancing lesions and total number of relapses (Spearman rank correlation coefficient = 0.35, $P = 0.0001$ for placebo; Spearman rank correlation coefficient = 0.24, $P = 0.01$ for GA).

An unanticipated delay in the apparent benefits of GA occurred for MRI and clinical outcomes. The statistically significant difference in mean number of enhancing lesions per patient per month first became apparent at month 6 and persisted for the duration of the study. The percentage of patients who had scans free of enhancing lesions, in monthly comparisons, became significant in the third trimester of the trial, as did the cumulative median-enhancing lesion volume. Similarly, the difference in median number of new lesions on T2-weighted imaging became statistically significant beginning after month 6. The timeline for clinical results mirrored those for MRI parameters. The numbers of relapses were similar between the two treatment groups during the first two trimesters. Sharp divergence occurred in the third trimester, however, when only five relapses occurred in the GA-treated group compared with 26 among the placebo-treated patients. The investigators suggest that the time-dependent benefits of GA reflect immunologic observations indicating a delay in the induction and expansion of a protective GA-specific regulatory T-cell population.

As in previous studies, GA was tolerated well, with the principal adverse experiences consisting of injection-site reactions and immediate post-injection systemic reactions (IPISR). Skin reactions generally were mild and skin necrosis never occurred. The IPISR developed within seconds to minutes of an injection and resolved spontaneously without sequelae in 10 to 30 minutes. If the development of any of its variably occurring components—facial flushing, chest tightness, dyspnea, palpitations, tachycardia, and anxiety—was regarded as indicative of an episode, then the IPISR occurred at least once in 37.8% of GA-treated patients, compared with 13.3% of the placebo patients. Few patients, however, experienced more than one such reaction.

In a post hoc analysis, Filippi et al [25] examined the evolution of lesions into T1 "black holes." New lesions from the 239 patients in both arms of the randomized MRI trial, defined as T2 lesions in an area of previously normal white matter with gadolinium-enhancement on a corresponding T1-weighted image, were followed to determine the persistence of T1 hypointensity (ie, a black hole) and the frequency of re-enhancement over the 9 months of the double-blind phase of the study. Thus, lesions could be tracked for up to 8 months after their initial identification. Fewer lesions evolved into black holes among the GA-treated patients than among the placebo patients, at 7 months (18.9 versus 26.3%; $P = 0.04$) and at 8 months (15.6 versus 31.4%; $P = 0.002$). Black holes generally are considered to represent areas with more severe tissue damage.

In another study, MRI from patients in both treatment groups were segmented for brain volume measurements at baseline at the end of the 9-month double-blind phase and at the end of an additional 9-month open-label treatment period. No statistically significant treatment effect on the progression of brain atrophy was detected in this study [26].

Trial of primary progressive multiple sclerosis

No treatment has been demonstrated to have a statistically significant benefit in patients who have primary progressive MS. After a suggestion of a possible effect of GA in this patient population in a two-center trial of chronic progressive MS [21], the largest MS trial ever undertaken as of that time was initiated. The PROMiSe trial enrolled 943 patients internationally. Unfortunately, the trial was terminated slightly prematurely as a result of recommendations by the data and safety monitoring committee because of futility. With approximately 85% of the planned data available, the committee concluded that GA could not achieve its primary efficacy endpoint of reduction in time to confirmed disease progression, defined as a change of greater than or equal to 1 EDSS point for patients entering at 3.0 to 5.0 or greater than or equal to 0.5 point for those entering at 5.5 to 6.5, sustained for 3 months. Although a trend was observed for less worsening in the GA-treated group and for changes on MRI, statistical significance was not achieved for the primary endpoint. A post hoc analysis did show statistically significant slowing of progression in the subset of 455 men enrolled. The placebo-treated group in the study did not progress at the anticipated rate, resulting in a loss of power for the study [27].

Oral glatiramer acetate

As discussed previously, injectable GA was introduced into human clinical trials because of its marked efficacy in EAE. Spurred by similar success in the EAE animal model of oral administration of GA, a large randomized, placebo-controlled, double-blind trial of RRMS was undertaken, using 5-mg and 50-mg oral doses. The extremely rapid recruitment for this 1-year study underscores the potential value of an orally effective therapy. Although as yet unpublished, the results in both GA-treated groups were virtually identical to those in the placebo-treated patients, disappointing participants and investigators alike. Additional laboratory investigation is continuing, with the possibility of additional human trials.

Combination therapy

Glatiramer acetate and interferon

Many investigators believe that combination therapy is a potentially useful strategy for clinical therapeutics in MS, analogous to the approach often successfully employed in the treatment of cancer. Along those lines, many potential combinations exist. Perhaps most intriguing is the possibility of using GA and an interferon together in hopes of achieving results superior to treatment with either agent alone. Experimental investigations in vitro show conflicting effects. Milo and Panitch [28] found additive effects of GA and IFN-β1b on the suppression of proliferation of MBP-specific T-cell lines. In contrast, Zang et al, found that IFN-β antagonized the effects of GA on the induction of activation and cytokine production of T cells [29]. Furthermore, in a murine EAE study, disease was suppressed by GA or IFN-α but not by the combination of the two drugs [30]. To ascertain the safety of the combination of IFN-β and GA in humans, Lublin et al [31] conducted a serial frequent MRI study in patients treated previously with IFN-β1a (Avonex, Biogen IDEC, Cambridge, Massachusetts) who then received the addition of GA or placebo while continuing interferon therapy. No increment in MRI activity occurred among the patients treated with combination therapy, suggesting that the two agents could be used together safely. In addition, neither an increase in adverse experiences nor the emergence of unexpected side effects was detected. Enrollment recently began in a large (1000 patient) study, funded by the National Institutes of Health, that will randomize patients who have RRMS into three arms. One group (50% of patients) will receive GA and IFN-β1a (Avonex); a second group (25%) will receive GA alone; and the third group (25%) will receive IFN-β1a alone. Patients will be followed for 3 years with a primary endpoint comparing relapse rates in the three treatment groups.

Glatiramer acetate and natalizumab

Natalizumab (Tysabri, Cambridge, Massachusetts) is a humanized monoclonal antibody directed against an adhesion molecule (α4β1 integrin or VLA4) on the surface of T lymphocytes. By blocking the interaction of this adhesion molecule with its complementary receptor on the surface of the vascular endothelial cell, natalizumab presumably prevents the entry of immunogenic T cells into the CNS. A phase II, double-blind, randomized, placebo-controlled trial of natalizumab showed striking reduction of MRI activity and a statistically significant reduction in clinical relapses [32]. Phase III trials of natalizumab alone versus placebo and natalizumab or placebo added to IFN-β1a (Avonex) are nearing completion. A 6-month phase II trial in which natalizumab or placebo was added to GA in patients continuing to experience attacks, however, has been finished and results are pending.

Neuroprotection

Results of several recent studies have prompted the suggestion that GA may have a neuroprotective role in MS. Kipnis et al [33] used a rat model of optic nerve crush injury in which secondary degeneration of optic nerve axons develops in untreated animals after the original trauma. Both active immunization with GA, administered in adjuvant, and adoptive transfer of T cells reactive to GA are able to markedly attenuate the progression of secondary degeneration. Similarly, in another study, the passive transfer of GA-reactive T cells protected retinal ganglion cells from the damaging effects of glutamate-induced ocular hypertension [34]. Kipnis and Schwartz [35] suggest the possibility that GA treatment induces "protective autoimmunity," which might be mediated through the production of neurotrophic factors. Subsequently, the adoptive transfer of GA-specific T cells into normal mice and those with EAE resulted in prominent expression of brain-derived neurotrophic factor, IL-10, and transforming growth factor β on these cells in the CNS [36]. In addition, in vitro studies show that some GA-reactive T-cell lines, derived from MS patients treated with GA, produced high levels of brain-derived neurotrophic factor [37].

Other lines of evidence, from work in animal models, suggest the possibility that GA conveys neuroprotection. In a mouse model of amyotrophic lateral sclerosis, "vaccination" with GA improves survival and motor function [38]. Mice who had EAE also were demonstrated to have reduced axonal damage [39]. Although these findings are intriguing, more definitive evidence in humans is needed before a neuroprotective role of GA in patients who have MS can be established.

Summary

The use of GA for treatment of MS highlights the importance of animal models in the development of human therapeutic agents. GA has gained wide acceptance as one option for the treatment of RRMS and its use is not accompanied by some of the undesirable adverse experiences, such as flu-like symptoms, associated with the interferons. Although its precise immunologic mechanisms continue to be investigated, current views suggest that its principal effect may be mediated by a shift from a proinflammatory Th1-cell bias to an anti-inflammatory Th2-cell bias. Ongoing studies are exploring the possibility that GA confers neuroprotection and are seeking novel ways to use the agent alone or in combination with other medications.

References

[1] Arnon R. The development of Cop 1 (Copaxone), an innovative drug for the treatment of multiple sclerosis: personal reflections. Immunol Lett 1996;50:1–15.
[2] Teitelbaum D, Webb C, Meshorer A, et al. Suppression by several synthetic polypeptides of experimental allergic encephalomyelitis induced in guinea pigs and rabbits with bovine and human basic encephalitogen. Eur J Immunol 1973;3:273–9.
[3] Lando Z, Teitelbaum D, Arnon R. Genetic control of susceptibility to experimental allergic encephalomyelitis in mice. Immunogenetics 1979;9:435–42.
[4] Teitelbaum D, Webb C, Bree M, et al. Suppression of experimental allergic encephalomyelitis in rhesus monkeys by a synthetic basic copolymer. Clin Immunol Immunopathol 1974; 3:256–62.
[5] Teitelbaum D, Meshorer A, Arnon R. Suppression of experimental allergic encephalomyelitis in baboons by Cop 1. Isr J Med Sci 1977;13:1038.
[6] Abramsky O, Teitelbaum D, Arnon R. Effect of a synthetic polypeptide (Cop 1) on patients with multiple sclerosis and with acute disseminated encephalomyelitis. J Neurol Sci 1977;31: 433–8.
[7] Bornstein MB, Miller AI, Teitelbaum D, et al. Multiple sclerosis: trial of a synthetic polypeptide. Ann Neurol 1982;11:317–9.
[8] Martin R, Sturzebecher CS, McFarland HF. Immunotherapy of multiple sclerosis: where are we? Where should we go? Nat Immunol 2001;2:785–8.
[9] O'Connor KC, Bar-Or A, Hafler DA. The neuroimmunology of multiple sclerosis: possible roles of T and B lymphocytes in immunopathogenesis. J Clin Immunol 2001;21:81–92.
[10] Dhib-Jalbut S. Glatiramer acetate (Copaxone®) therapy for multiple sclerosis. Pharmacol Ther 2003;98:245–55.
[11] Neuhaus O, Farina C, Wekerle H, et al. Mechanisms of action of glatiramer acetate in multiple sclerosis. Neurology 2001;56:702–8.
[12] Bornstein MB, Miller AI, Slagle S, et al. A pilot trial of Cop 1 in exacerbating-remitting multiple sclerosis. N Engl J Med 1987;317:408–14.
[13] Kurtzke JF. A new scale for evaluating disability in multiple sclerosis. Neurology 1955;5: 580–3.
[14] Johnson KP, Brooks BR, Cohen JA. Copolymer 1 Multiple Sclerosis Research Group. Copolymer 1 reduces relapse rate and improves disability in relapsing-remitting multiple sclerosis: results of a phase III multicenter, double-blind, placebo-controlled trial. Neurology 1995;45:1268–76.
[15] Kurtzke JF. Rating neurologic impairment in multiple sclerosis: an expanded disability status scale (EDSS). Neurology 1983;33:1444–52.
[16] Poser C, Paty D, Scheinberg L, et al. New diagnostic criteria for multiple sclerosis: guidelines for research protocols. Ann Neurol 1983;13:227–31.
[17] Johnson KP, Brooks BR, Cohen JA. Copolymer 1 Multiple Sclerosis Research Group. Extended use of glatiramer acetate (Copaxone) is well-tolerated and maintains its clinical effect on multiple sclerosis relapse rate and degree of disability. Neurology 1998;50:701–8.
[18] Johnson KP, Brooks BR, Ford CC, et al. Sustained clinical benefits of glatiramer acetate in relapsing multiple sclerosis patients observed for 6 years. Copolymer 1 Multiple Sclerosis Study Group. Mult Scler 2000;6:255–66.

[19] The PRISMS Study Group, University of British Columbia MS/MRI Analysis Group. PRISMS-4: long-term efficacy of interferon-beta-1a in relapsing MS. Neurology 2001;56: 1628–36.
[20] Johnson KP, Panitch HS, Ford CC, et al. Long-term slowing of disability progression in patients receiving continuous Glatiramer acetate compared with those withdrawing from therapy: 10 year results from an ongoing trial. Neurology 2004;62(7 Suppl 5):A180.
[21] Bornstein MB, Miller AI, Slagle S, et al. A placebo-controlled, double-blind, randomized, two-center, pilot trial of Cop 1 in chronic progressive multiple sclerosis. Neurology 1991;41: 533–9.
[22] Ge Y, Grossman RI, Udupa JK, et al. Glatiramer acetate (Copaxone) treatment in relapsing-remitting MS: quantitative MR assessment. Neurology 2000;54:813–7.
[23] Mancardi GL, Sardanelli F, Parodi RC. Effect of copolymer-1 on serial gadolinium-enhanced MRI in relapsing-remitting multiple sclerosis. Neurology 1998;50:1127–33.
[24] Comi G, Filippi M, Wolinsky JS, et al. European/Canadian multicenter, double-blind, randomized, placebo-controlled study of the effects of glatiramer acetate on magnetic resonance imaging-measured disease activity and burden in patients with relapsing multiple sclerosis. European/Canadian Glatiramer Acetate Study Group. Ann Neurol 2001;49: 290–7.
[25] Filippi M, Rovaris M, Rocca MA, et al. Glatiramer acetate reduces the proportion of new MS lesions evolving into 'black holes'. Neurology 2001;57:731–3.
[26] Rovaris M, Comi G, Rocca MA, et al. Short-term brain volume change in relapsing-remitting multiple sclerosis: effect of glatiramer acetate and implications. Brain 2001;124: 1803–12.
[27] Wolinsky JS, Pardo L, Stark Y, et al. Effect of Glatiramer acetate on primary progressive multiple sclerosis: initial analysis of the complete PROMiSe trial. Neurology 2004;62(7 Suppl 5):A97.
[28] Milo R, Panitch H. Additive effects of copolymer-1 and interferon beta-1b on the immune response to myelin basic protein. J Neuroimmunol 1995;61:185–93.
[29] Zang Y, Hong J, Robinson R, et al. Immune regulatory properities and interactions of copolymer-I and beta-interferon 1a in multiple sclerosis. J Neuroimmunol 2003;137:144–53.
[30] Brod SA, Lindsey JW, Wolinsky JS. Combination therapy with glatiramer acetate (copolymer-1) and a type I interferon (IFN-alpha) does not improve experimental autoimmune encephalomyelitis. Ann Neurol 2000;47:127–31.
[31] Lublin F, Baier M, Cutter G, et al. Results of the extension of a trial to assess the longer term safety of combining interferon beta-1a and Glatiramer acetate. Neurology 2002;(7 Suppl): A85.
[32] Miller DH, Khan OA, Sheremata WA, et al. A controlled trial of natalizumab for relapsing multiple sclerosis. N Engl J Med 2003;348:15–23.
[33] Kipnis J, Yoles E, Porat Z, et al. T cell immunity to copolymer 1 confers neuroprotection on the damaged optic nerve: possible therapy for optic neuropathies. Proc Natl Acad Sci USA 2000;97:7446–51.
[34] Schori H, Kipnis J, Yoles E, et al. Vaccination for protection of retinal ganglion cells against death from glutamate cytotoxicity and ocular hypertension: implications for glaucoma. Proc Natl Acad Sci USA 2001;98:3398–403.
[35] Kipnis J, Schwartz M. Dual action of glatiramer acetate (Cop-1) in the treatment of CNS autoimmune and neurodegerative disorders. Trends Mol Med 2002;8:319–23.
[36] Aharoni R, Kayhan B, Eilam R, et al. Glatiramer acetate-specific T cells in the brain express T helper 2/3 cytokines and brain-derived neurotrophic factor in situ. Proc Natl Acad Sci USA 2003;100:14157–62.
[37] Chen M, Valenzuela M, Dhib-Jalbut S. Glatiramer acetate-reactive T cells produce brain-derived neurotrophic factor. J Neurol Sci 2003;214:37–44.

[38] Angelov DN, Waibel S, Guntinas-Lichius O, et al. Therapeutic vaccine for acute and chronic motor neuron diseases: Implications for amyotrophic lateral sclerosis. Proc Natl Acad Sci USA 2003;100:4790–5.

[39] Gilgun-Sherki Y, Panet H, Holdengreber V, et al. Axonal damage is reduced following glatiramer acetate treatment in C57/bl mice with chronic-induced experimental autoimmune encephalomyelitis. Neurosci Res 2003;47:201–7.

ELSEVIER
SAUNDERS

Neurol Clin 23 (2005) 233–246

NEUROLOGIC
CLINICS

Natalizumab and Other Monoclonal Antibodies

Melanie R. Ursell, MSc, MD[a,b],
Paul W. O'Connor, MSc, MD[a,b,*]

[a]*University of Toronto, Toronto, Ontario, Canada*
[b]*Division of Neurology, St. Michael's Hospital, Toronto, Ontario, Canada*

T lymphocytes respond to pathogens only after direct contact with their antigens in the context of major histocompatibility complex molecules and costimulatory signals [1]. Immune cells, therefore, must gain entry to sites where antigens reside. In multiple sclerosis (MS), these antigens are localized, at least initially, in central nervous system (CNS) myelin.

The blood-brain barrier, across which lymphocytes migrate to gain access to myelin antigens, is unique compared with other blood-tissue interfaces. This partly is because of the anatomic structure of the barrier, which is composed of an organized array of intercellular tight junctions, perivascular spaces, and astroglial and microglial processes interdigitating with one another to form the characteristic glia limitans. In addition to this structural barrier, the entry of leukocytes into CNS tissue is regulated by complex interactions of adhesion molecules with their ligands, expressed and presented on vascular endothelial cells and circulating leukocytes.

Knowledge of the mechanism of action of adhesion molecules is important in understanding the initial events that lead to MS lesion development and in designing therapies to inhibit this process. During the past decade, details of these interactions have been partially delineated and now are being exploited toward the development of more specific and possibly more effective therapies for MS.

This article reviews the basis of antiadhesion molecule therapy for MS in general and then focuses on natalizumab (Antegren; Elan Corporation,

Dr. P. O'Connor has participated in and played a leadership role in the phase 2 and 3 and acute relapse trials with the Biogen Idec Elan Corporation.

* Corresponding author. Divison of Neurology, St. Michael's Hospital, University of Toronto, 30 Bond Street, Room 3-007, Shuter Wing, Toronto, ON M5B 1W8, Canada.
E-mail address: oconnorp@smh.toronto.on.ca (P.W. O'Connor).

doi:10.1016/j.ncl.2004.09.005

Cambridge, Massachusetts Biogen Idec, Cambridge, Massachusetts), a humanized monoclonal antibody (mAb) that blocks the binding of adhesion molecules on the surface of activated lymphocytes and monocytes with their endothelial ligands, thereby inhibiting the trafficking of leukocytes across the blood-brain barrier and reducing disease activity in animal and human demyelinating diseases.

Immune trafficking

Leukocytes circulate rapidly in the bloodstream. Physiologically, lymphocytes home toward lymphoid tissue, where they are collected, presented to antigen, and redistributed by a selective process involving high endothelial vessels located in lymph tissue [1]. This homing behavior does not, however, preclude the interaction of leukocytes with the vascular endothelium of other organs, including the CNS.

Leukocytes transiently roll and bump over CNS vessel endothelium before they are forcefully taken up again into the circulation. These weak and transient interactions between the leukocyte and the vessel endothelium are mediated by the presence of low-affinity adhesion molecules called selectins. The selectins are a family of adhesion molecules produced and presented on the surface of vessel endothelial cells (P-selectin and E-selectin) and lymphocytes (L-selectin). For T lymphocytes, the expression of selectin ligands is driven primarily by the cytokine interleukin 12 (IL-12) [2]. These low-affinity interactions contribute to the transient tethering of leukocytes to the surface endothelium, but they are insufficient to allow for leukocyte arrest and transmigration [2].

This situation changes when there is local inflammation at the site of lymphocyte-endothelial contact. The release of inflammatory cytokines and chemokines from the site of tissue injury results in the rapid mobilization of P-selectin and E-selectin reservoirs from secretory granules of the endothelial cells, which then are transported to the endothelial plasma membrane for presentation [3]. The P-selectins interact with L-selectin on circulating lymphocytes, and with specific receptor ligands, called P-selectin glycoprotein ligand–1 (PSGL-1), that are present on the leukocyte cell surface [4]. The expression of selectins by endothelial cells in the brain seems to be an inducible event, triggered by tissue inflammation. In the MS mouse model, experimental allergic encephalomyelitis (EAE), noninflamed vascular endothelium is almost entirely devoid of selectin molecule expression until after disease induction has taken place. In contrast, PSGL-1 is expressed constitutively by all circulating leukocytes, so that even naive lymphocytes have the potential to be captured by inflamed vascular endothelium and recruited into CNS tissue, provided appropriate endothelial signals are presented [4].

Integrins

The massive infiltration of leukocytes that occurs into the early MS lesion likely is mediated by more specific interactions. This is orchestrated primarily by the expression of secondary adhesion molecules on the lymphocyte cell surface, called integrins [3]. The integrins are a family of cell surface transmembrane heterodimer receptors that play a physiologic role in immune responses against invading pathogens [5]. Integrins involved in the adhesion of leukocytes to CNS vascular endothelium include leukocyte function-associated integrin type-1 (LFA-1, $\alpha_L\beta_2$), macrophage antigen–1 ($\alpha_M\beta_2$), the alpha-9 integrin $\alpha_9\beta_7$, and two alpha-4 integrins ($\alpha_4\beta_1$ and $\alpha_4\beta_7$) called very late antigen–4 (VLA-4) [3].

The receptor ligands expressed on endothelial cell surfaces to which these integrin molecules bind are members of the immunoglobulin gene superfamily (IgSF) [3]. The integrin-ligand interactions most important in transmigration of lymphocytes across the blood-brain barrier seem to be between LFA-1 and VLA-4 on lymphocytes with their endothelial receptor ligands, intercellular adhesion molecule-1 and -2 (ICAM-1 and ICAM-2), and vascular cell adhesion molecule-1 (VCAM-1), (Fig. 1) [4]. Thus, although initial interactions between leukocytes and endothelial selectin molecules contribute to the slowing and transient tethering of leukocytes to the endothelial surface, arrest and transmigration are dependent on the activity of integrin receptor-endothelial ligand interactions. Furthermore, the expression of LFA-1 and VLA-4 on the lymphocyte surface is an inducible event and is dependent on the level of activation of the lymphocyte itself. Memory T lymphocytes show two to three times' increased expression of LFA-1 and VLA-4 compared with resting T lymphocytes, and the surface expression of these molecules is increased after T-cell activation [4]. Therefore, although antigen presentation is not in itself a prerequisite for the migration of T lymphocytes across the blood-brain barrier, activated or previously activated (memory) T lymphocytes are favored highly over resting T lymphocytes for transmigration.

Direct evidence of leukocyte attachment to endothelium and transmigration into the CNS tissue in humans is still unavailable because of the constraints involved in sampling human tissue, yet acute lesions isolated from MS lesion autopsy material show high levels of expression of VLA-4 and its endothelial ligand, VCAM-1 [6]. Human serum levels of soluble endothelial ligands ICAM-1 also are increased in patients who have MS compared with control patients, and these levels are shown to coincide with the presence of active gadolinium-enhancing lesions on MRI of the brain [7]. Furthermore, levels of adhesion molecules in the serum of patients who have MS are shown to fluctuate with clinical worsening of disease [8].

Extrapolations from the EAE model have played a large role in understanding lymphocyte trafficking steps in human MS. Acutely inflamed lesions

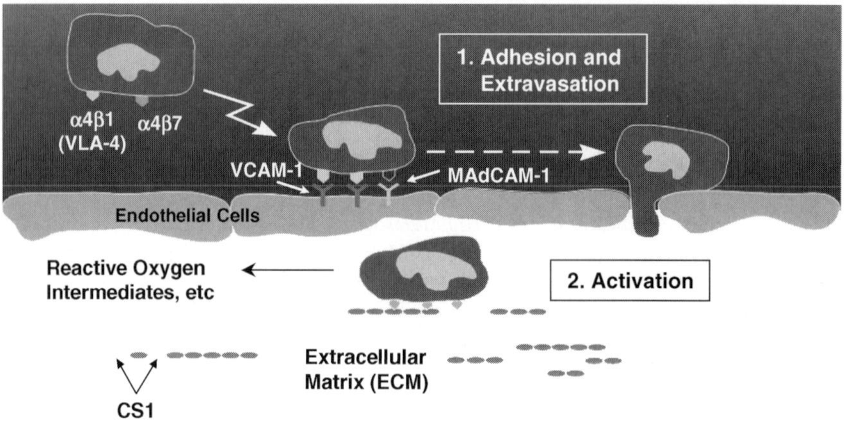

Fig. 1. Molecular pathways involved in leukocyte trafficking. (Courtesy of Biogen Incorporated and Elan Corporation, Cambridge, Massachusetts.)

in the EAE model show high levels of expression of VLA-4 and VCAM-1 compared with nondiseased animal controls, and VLA-4 expression on Myelin Basic Protein (MBP)-specific T cells is a prerequisite for lymphocyte trafficking into the CNS and for the induction of disease in this model [9].

Lymphocytes attached to endothelial cells proceed to pass through the endothelial cell cytoplasm into Virchow-Robin spaces after migrating at parajunctional areas close to endothelial tight junctions. This trafficking process, or diapedesis, occurs in response to chemotactic signals supplied by chemokine molecular gradients. Chemokines, like cytokines, are secreted polypeptides that can induce increased production of integrin molecules by lymphocytes and switch these integrin molecules into a higher affinity state that allows them to transmigrate more effectively across CNS endothelium [10]. Once within inflamed CNS tissue, T lymphocytes likely encounter antigen, producing a cascade of inflammatory events, including further release of cytokines and chemokines. Cytokine production, including tumor necrosis factor α (TNF-α), interferon-γ (IFN-γ), and interleukin 6 (IL-6), provides signals for further expression of integrin adhesion molecules on lymphocytes and the recruitment of additional T cells and other immune-active cells in an escalating inflammatory response [9].

Immune cell migration across the blood-brain barrier therefore is dependent on a multistep process characterized by selectin-dependent tethering followed by integrin-dependent arrest and transmigration. Lymphocytes are recruited into CNS tissue only if each of these steps occurs successfully.

Anti-inflammatory T lymphocytes (Th2 cells) also can enter the CNS by these mechanisms and likely contribute to the suppression and ultimate resolution of inflammation. The importance of this process in relation to other anti-inflammatory or remyelinative repair processes in demyelinating disease is unclear.

Overview of antiadhesion molecule therapy

The large number of adhesion ligands, endothelial counter-receptors, chemokines, and chemokine receptors involved in leukocyte migration translates into hundreds of possible combinations by which lymphocytes can diapedese through the blood-brain barrier. This offers many potential targets for the development of antiadhesion therapies. An MS-specific homing adhesion molecule expressed on the surface of activated CNS T cells or CNS endothelium has not been identified [11]. Furthermore, the expression of adhesion molecules in MS tissue is shown to be widespread, and lesion and nonlesion areas of MS brains exhibit increased expression of selectin and integrin molecules [11].

The clinical benefit of IFN-β treatment of MS may be at least in part the result of an inhibitory effect on lymphocyte trafficking, making it the first MS treatment to target T-cell trafficking. In vitro assays show that T lymphocytes isolated from patients treated with IFN-β for less than 2 years have decreased migration capability compared with untreated control patients [12]. VLA-4 expression is shown to be decreased on the surface of lymphocytes isolated from fresh whole blood from patients who have MS during the initial stages of interferon therapy, particularly on T cells of the memory cell phenotype [13].

Increased levels of soluble, circulating VCAM-1 also are demonstrated in patients treated with IFN-β, with the corresponding hypothesis that circulating VCAM-1 molecules antagonize the binding of T lymphocytes to endothelial-anchored VCAM-1, decreasing the number of T cells transmigrating into inflamed tissue. In support of this hypothesis, increased VCAM-1 levels in patients after treatment with IFN-β are associated with reduced gadolinium enhancement on MRI [14]. Unfortunately, this effect seems to decrease over time, and lymphocytes from patients who received interferon treatment for more than 3.5 years demonstrate migration patterns similar to those of patients who never have been treated with IFN-β [12]. The cause of this waning effect of interferon on leukocyte migration is unclear, although two possible explanations are the use of alternative adhesion-transmigration pathways by activated lymphocytes and the overexpression of adhesion molecules on lymphocytes that overwhelm the effect of the drug [12].

Targeting proteases, such as the matrix metalloproteinases, with inhibitors is another approach being tested to block inflammatory cell entry into the CNS [12]. Several cytokines have known regulatory effects on adhesion molecule synthesis, including TNF-α and -β, and are the targets of treatment protocols designed to interfere with the availability of these molecules. Early studies of EAE have shown profound effects on the binding and transmigration of T cells into the CNS with these therapies [11].

Chemokines, and chemokine receptor molecules expressed on the surface of activated leukocytes contribute to firming the adhesion of lymphocytes to vascular endothelium for transmigration, probably through enhancement of integrin-ligand binding affinities [2]. These molecules already have been targeted in animal models for several autoimmune diseases with varying success [1]. They also are in the early stages of human trials of MS.

The most direct approach for targeting lymphocyte trafficking, however, is the direct blockade of receptor-ligand (ie, integrin-IgSF) interactions. The development of antagonists toward integrin molecules and their endothelial ligands currently is one of the most actively pursued areas in pharmaceutical research. The prototype for these therapies has been the mAb, which is target specific, metabolically stable, and already studied extensively in animal disease models. All such antibodies must be administered parenterally.

For most clinical applications, these antibodies are humanized to avoid the development of immune responses against murine protein structures [3]. Disease models in which direct mAb blockade of adhesion molecule pathways has been exploited (in preclinical and, in selected cases, human clinical trials) include MS, renal allograft rejection, rheumatoid arthritis, inflammatory bowel disease, stroke/reperfusion injury, and psoriasis [15]. For MS, mAbs to VLA-4 and its endothelial binding ligand VCAM-1 and to ICAM-1 on the endothelial surface have shown profound inhibition of T-lymphocyte binding to CNS vessel endothelium in EAE [15].

Synthetic small molecule inhibitors, which can be given orally and which could one day replace prototypic mAb therapies, are being developed actively and could overcome difficulties arising from the immunogenicity and the expense of recombinant, humanized antibody production [5]. There already have been varying successes with small molecule antagonists directed against interactions between VLA-4 and VCAM-1 and between LFA-1 and ICAM-1 [16]. Finally, antagonist peptides, which simulate the binding regions of VLA-4 to VCAM-1 and theoretically could compete with biologic interactions on vessel endothelium, are being developed and tested in animal models [17].

Antiadhesion therapies have been tested in phase II and phase III trials in several autoimmune diseases, including rheumatoid arthritis, Crohn's disease, ischemic/reperfusion injury, psoriasis, and MS. Positive trials have been completed for mAb therapies directed against VLA-4 in Crohn's disease and in MS and for anti–LFA-1 mAb therapy for the treatment of psoriasis [3]. Others, unfortunately, including a humanized mAb designed to block macrophage antigen–1 in EAE, have produced negative results [2]. The reasons for the disparity in the effectiveness of these treatments, which presumably target the same pathway in the earliest events preceding lesion development, are unknown. Nevertheless, the initial etiologic insult in MS is itself obscure and with improved understanding of the complex trafficking mechanisms generated by these proof-of-concept trials, more specific and intelligent approaches to immune therapy may be designed.

Natalizumab

Although originally used for assay tools and diagnosis, mAbs now are used as legitimate drug treatments. This has been made possible by recombinant technologies and by the ability to humanize murine mAbs by grafting a murine antibody clone onto a human IgG4 framework at the complementary determining region (Fig. 2). MAbs are also stable metabolically and have the advantage of high target specificity [5]. Because adhesion molecules, such as VLA-4, are expressed on the leukocyte cell surface and circulate in the blood stream, they are accessed easily by mAb infusions given intravenously.

The integrins are heterodimers of noncovalently associated glycoproteins composed of two subunits, designated alpha and beta (Fig. 3). They are expressed on every type of immune cell except for neutrophils [18], and at least 24 different noncovalent associations of the subunits may be presented on the cell surface [5]. VLA-4 is an alpha-4 integrin composed of 4 alpha subunits and 1 beta subunit ($\alpha_4\beta_1$). The interaction of VLA-4 on the surface of activated lymphocytes with VCAM-1 on brain vessel endothelial cells is considered crucial for the recruitment of immune cells into the CNS (see Fig. 1) [19].

More than a dozen anti–alpha-4 integrin mAbs have been tested in animal models of autoimmune and inflammatory diseases [5]. Two of these antibodies have entered human clinical trials, including an mAb directed against integrin $\alpha_4\beta_7$ for ulcerative colitis (Mellennium Pharmaceuticals, Cambridge, Massachusetts) and natalizumab directed against VLA-4 ($\alpha_4\beta_1$, Antegren; Elan and Biogen Idec) for Crohn's Disease and MS. Because natalizumab binds the alpha subunit of the VLA-4 molecule regardless of its associated beta chain, it targets $\alpha_4\beta_7$ (the integrin receptor for mucosal addressin cell adhesion molecule expressed on gut vasculature) and VLA-4 on brain endothelium, and, therefore, has been tested with some success in clinical trials for both diseases. Natalizumab is infused intravenously once per month. It has a half-life of 90 to 170 hours. Serum concentrations are detectable 3 to 8 weeks after infusions at doses of 6 mg/kg [20].

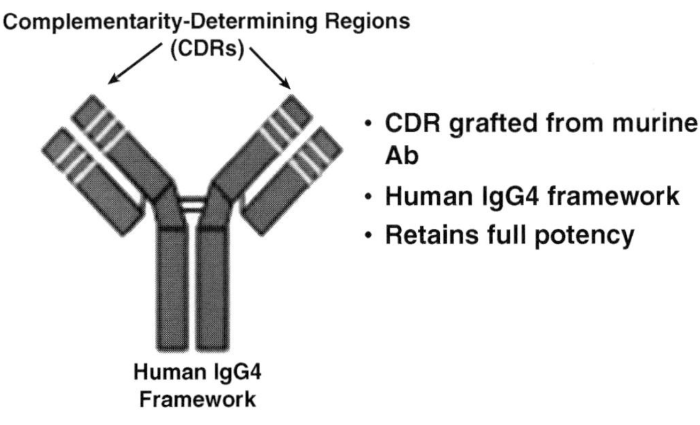

Fig. 2. Natalizumab. (Courtesy of Biogen Incorporated and Elan Corporation, Cambridge, Massachusetts 2004.)

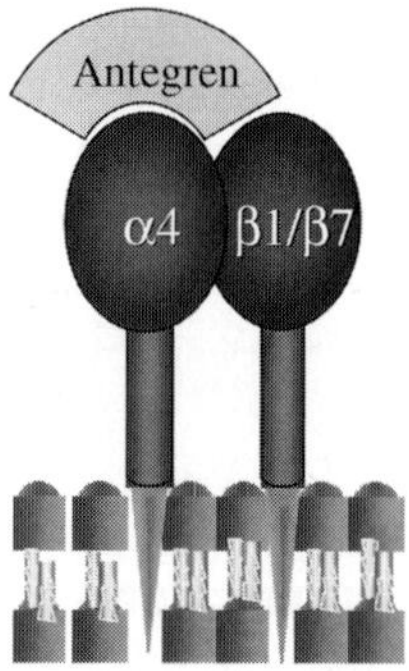

- Humanized mouse-derived monoclonal IgG4 antibody to human α4 integrin
- Blocks adhesion of α4+ lymphocytes to VCAM1 and MAdCAM *in vitro.*

Fig. 3. Interaction of natalizumab (Antegren) with the alpha-4 subunit of VLA-4. (Courtesy of Biogen Incorporated and Elan Cooporation, Cambridge, Massachusetts 2004.)

It has been proposed that natalizumab may work by mechanisms other than adhesion cell molecule antagonism. That natalizumab should work at all in Crohn's disease is somewhat surprising given that Crohn's disease primarily is a neutrophil-mediated disease and VLA-4 is not expressed on neutrophils. In addition, the antagonism of VLA-4 is significantly more effective than antagonist therapy directed to its endothelial ligand, VCAM-1 [20]. Alpha-4 integrins also interact with fibronectin in the extracellular matrix via a separate binding site, and interaction with VCAM-1 molecules on nonendothelial cells, including bone marrow and lymphoid tissue, has been demonstrated, suggesting that interactions at these sites may result in additional modulatory effects on the immune system through mechanisms independent of immune cell migration [5]. That natalizumab may exert effects beyond mechanisms of T lymphocyte migration may be advantageous in the treatment of an immunologically heterogeneous disease, such as MS.

Clinical trials

The first animal studies assessing the efficacy of a mAb to alpha-4 integrin were performed in a primate model of inflammatory bowel disease [21]. In 1992, Yednock et al reported an anti–alpha-4 integrin mAb that recognized an activated confirmation of VLA-4 in murine EAE and successfully prevented the accumulation of leukocytes within the CNS, suppressing the development of EAE in 75% of the animals [22]. In a second EAE model in the guinea pig, anti–alpha-4 integrin antibody was found equally effective in reversing clinical symptoms of disease after disease development [23]. This seemed to correlate with the clearing of leukocytes out of CNS inflammatory lesions after lesions were established, suggesting that therapy could be used not only for the prevention of recurrent relapses but also as an acute treatment similar to corticosteroids. An acute relapse trial of MS comparing therapy with a single dose of natalizumab versus placebo has been completed [24].

Phase I clinical trials using a five-level dose escalation protocol in 28 patients who had MS diminished concerns about safety and tolerability; the most frequently reported side effect was headache [25]. In 1999, Turbridy et al published the results of an exploratory, randomized, double-blind, placebo-controlled study of humanized anti–VLA-4 antibody, demonstrating that two injections of natalizumab separated by 4 weeks reduced the number of active lesions (new or enlarging T2 lesions or enhancing lesions) on MRI in 37 patients who had relapsing-remitting or secondary progressive MS at 12 weeks [26]. The two injections had no effect on relapse rates during the 12 weeks of the trial and in the following 12 weeks a trend toward more relapses was seen in the group that was treated. The small size and limited duration of the study, however, reduced its power to demonstrate significant effects on secondary clinical outcome measures. It was the observed MRI effect that prompted the initiation of a larger phase 2 trial.

In the phase 2 trial reported by Miller et al, 213 patients who had relapsing-remitting and relapsing progressive MS were assigned randomly to 6 monthly infusions of low-dose (3 mg/kg/mo) or high-dose (6 mg/kg/mo) natalizumab versus placebo [27]. Those who were receiving treatment demonstrated a robust 90% reduction in gadolinium-enhancing lesions on MRI, confirming results reported in the initial exploratory study. In addition, although the trial was powered to investigate only a treatment effect on MRI activity, there was a significant reduction in relapses (approximately 50%) during the 6-month treatment period. Treated patients reported improved quality of life compared with those who were taking placebo, as measured on a visual-analog scale. Adverse events did not differ significantly between the natalizumab and placebo groups, although there was a trend toward a higher incidence of infections, in particular pharyngitis, in the treated groups. The most common adverse events were headache, asthenia, and urinary tract infection. Presumed allergic reactions mostly were mild (flushing or hives) and infrequent in the treated patients, although one patient who received 3 mg/kg natalizumab experienced anaphylaxis, which responded readily to therapy. In addition, absolute circulating lymphocyte numbers increased marginally, confirming that T-cell lysis was not occurring.

Of concern, 15 of the 142 patients (11%) assigned to treatment developed anti-idiotypic antibodies despite the short treatment course, with 13 developing these during treatment and the remaining 2 developing them during the post-treatment follow-up period. The clinical importance of these antibodies remains to be determined. Furthermore, after cessation of treatment with natalizumab, lesion enhancement and clinical attacks returned to baseline, suggesting there is neither a persistent treatment effect nor a tendency for relapse/enhancement rebound after discontinuation of therapy. Although a direct comparison cannot be made, the magnitude of the treatment effect demonstrated during the 6-month treatment period seems greater than that seen with currently available therapies (including IFN-β and glatiramer acetate).

Because of the small number of patients and short duration of the trial, definite conclusions about natalizumab safety and long-term efficacy cannot be made until larger phase 3 studies are completed. Two larger (>900 patients each) and longer-term (2 years or more) phase 3 studies are ongoing. The AFFIRM (Natalizumab safety and efficacy in relapsing-remitting MS) study is comparing natalizumab to placebo in patients who have relapsing-remitting MS, with primary endpoints at year 1 of relapse rate and at year 2 of sustained disability progression. As of this writing, the year 1 relapse data has been filed with the Food and Drug Administration, reportedly to accelerate the drug review and approval process; results remain strictly confidential. The SENTINEL (safety and efficacy of natalizumab in combination with AVONEX(R)interferon beta-1a) study has enrolled patients who have relapsing-remitting MS and who have

Table 1
Ongoing human clinical trials using monoclonal antibody therapies

Target	Drug (company)	Phase
CD52 (antibody-dependent cell-mediated T lymphocyte lysis)	Alemtuzumab (CAMPATH-1H; ILEX Pharmaceuticals Boston, Massachusetts)	II/III (open label)
B7/CD28 (cytotoxic T-lymphocyte–associated antigen)	CTLA-4 (Bristol Meyers Squib New Brunswick, New Jersey)	II (terminated)
CD20 (B lymphocyte surface cytolytic molecule)	Rituximab (Rituxin; Genentech, San Francisco, California)	II/III
IL-12 (inflammatory cytokine-activating T lymphocytes)	CNTO 1275 (Centocor and, separately Abbott Pharmaceuticals, Abbott Park, Illinois) daclizumab (Zenapex; Roche)	II
CD25 (IL-2) (receptor of activated lymphocytes)		II (open label)
CD40 (CD154) (activation of B cells)	IDEC-131 (IDEC Pharmaceuticals, Cambridge, Massachusetts)	Safety, open label
VLA-4 ($\alpha_4\beta_1$) (+ IFNβ1a) (blocks lymphocyte migration)	Natalizumab (Antegren) IFNβ1a (Avonex) (Biogen Idec and Elan, Cambridge, Massachusetts)	III (SENTINEL)
VLA-4 ($\alpha_4\beta_1$)	Natalizumab (Antegren; Biogen Idec and Elan, Cambridge, Massachusetts)	III (AFFIRM)
VLA-4 ($\alpha_4\beta_1$) + (glatiramer acetate)	Natalizumab (Antegren; Biogen IDEC and Elan) Glatiramer acetate (Copaxone; Teva Pharmaceuticals, Petach Tikva, Israel)	I (safety)

experienced a relapse while on weekly intramuscular IFN-β1a (Avonex, Biogen Idec) and randomized them to natalizumab or placebo while continuing the IFN-β therapy (Table 1).

Conclusions about long-term safety and efficacy of natalizumab require more data from human trials, although results to date are encouraging. Of possible but unproven relevance are the observations of Theien et al [28], who note that in the SJL mouse, chronic EAE model treatment with an antibody directed toward VLA-4 was helpful when administered before disease onset and worsened disease when given during relapses or remissions. The phase 2 data do not suggest that this happens in humans.

Other monoclonal antibodies

Other mAbs are being developed, with several being tested in phase II human clinical trials. Development of these therapies bears reminding of the complex role that certain mediators play in human immune responses, which may be contradictory to those observed in EAE models. This is illustrated, for example, in clinical trials of an anti–TNF-α mAb, one of the first mAb therapies tested in human MS. Although this molecule reversed paralysis in the animal model, it worsened disease activity in patients who had MS [29]. Similarly, a clinical trial assessing the efficacy of a humanized mAb to macrophage antigen–1 (CD18), a leukocyte integrin similar to in many ways VLA-4, also was negative, failing to demonstrate either a clinical or MRI benefit in patients who had MS [30].

Antibodies against other adhesion molecules, including LFA-1 and MAC-1, were ineffective in inhibiting clinical symptoms and leukocyte infiltration in EAE animal models [31,32]. Similarly, although anti ICAM mAbs seemed to have a modest clinical benefit in a virally induced relapsing model of EAE, the treatment resulted in CNS hemorrhages [33]. Alternate adhesion molecule antagonists directed to ICAMs and the selectins are being investigated in animal models [33].

Another potential target for mAb antagonist therapy is the chemokine receptors, of which CCR5 and CXCR3 seem to be relevant because of their role in enhancing integrin-binding affinity to vascular endothelium [34]. CD4+ T-cell receptor molecules have presented an attractive target to scientific researchers for many years; if this target is successful, it overcome limitations of achieving immune specificity. Unfortunately, the development of these agents has been confounded by challenges of antigenic epitope spreading in T-cell responses. Cytokines, including IL-6 and IL-12, also are being targeted [2]. CD52, a leukocyte surface signal antigen, has been antagonized successfully by the humanized mAb alemtuzumab (Campath-1H, Schering, Germany), resulting in potent T-lymphocyte suppression via an antibody-dependent cell-mediated lysis mechanism in the presence of human complement [35]. Unfortunately, one third of participants in phase II clinical trials using alemtuzumab developed autoimmune thyroiditis (Graves' disease), believed to be the result of redirection of Th1-cell populations to antibody-producing Th2 responses [36]. Despite this setback, alemtuzumab continues to be studied in phase III trials and, more recently, in a phase II randomized and open-label three-arm study comparing low and high doses of mAb with high-dose IFN-β1a in early relapsing-remitting MS [37]. Other active human trials of mAbs are summarized in Table 1. Of these, the phase II trial assessing the clinical efficacy of CTLA-4 (Bristol Myers Squibb, New York), a humanized mAb directed to the costimulatory interaction between T lymphocytes and antigen-presenting macrophages (B7/CD28), has been terminated prematurely, for as yet undisclosed reasons. Other trials listed are ongoing.

Future directions

Antiadhesion therapies targeting lymphocyte trafficking show promise in the treatment of MS. Other mAbs with different targets are in various stages of clinical development and suggest promising treatment options. Whether or not these types of mAb therapies will be more effective in relapsing versus progressive forms of the illness is unknown and needs to be investigated. It is possible that all peripherally administered immune modifiers will be ineffective in progressive disease when the condition is well established in the CNS.

These therapies share the advantage of being more immune specific than those currently available. As they do not interfere with the responses of memory, T cells, and B cells, they are not globally immunosuppressive while possessing potentially superior efficacy and comparable or better safety and patient acceptability than current disease modulating agents, such as mitoxantrone and cyclophosphamide. Because VLA-4 is not expressed on neutrophils, the ability to combat serious bacterial and fungal infections does not seem to be impaired, as it is for more potent broad-spectrum chemotherapeutic agents, such as mitoxantrone and cyclophosphamide [28].

Further issues need to be addressed, however, including the possibility of efficacy-reducing antibody induction, the acceptability of intravenous administration to patients who have MS, and issues of long-term efficacy and safety [38,39].

Summary

The evolution of hypothesis-driven and proof-of-concept clinical trials, exemplified by the development of natalizumab, has led to a more complete understanding of early immune mechanisms in lesion development and has provided fertile ground for the design of additional biologically plausible therapies. The hope is that one or many of these therapies will show major short- and long-term efficacy with an acceptable safety profile, cost, and patient convenience. Perhaps this is asking a lot, but certainly it is not more than patients deserve.

References

[1] Von Andrian U, Mackay CR. T cell function and migration: two sides of the same coin. N Engl J Med 2000;343:1020–34.

[2] Steinman L. Assessment of animal models for MS and demyelinating disease in the design of rational therapy. Neuron 1999;24:511–4.

[3] Harlan JM. Leukocyte-endothelial interactions: clinical trials of anti-adhesion therapy. Crit Care Med 2002;30(5, Suppl):S214–9.

[4] Van Noort JM, Amor S. Cell biology of autoimmune diseases. Int Rev Cytol 1998;178: 127–206.

[5] Jackson DY. Alpha 4 integrin antagonists. Curr Pharm Dis 2002;8:1229–53.

[6] Cannella B, Raine CS. The adhesion molecule and cytokine profile of multiple sclerosis lesions. Ann Neurol 1995;37:424–35.

[7] Hartung HP, Michels M, Reiners K, et al. Soluble ICAM-1 serum levels in multiple sclerosis and viral encephalitis. Neurology 1993;43:2331–5.

[8] Cannella B, Cross AH, Raine CS. Upregulation and co-expression of adhesion molecules correlate with relapsing autoimmune demyelination in the central nervous system. J Exp Med 1990;172:1521–4.

[9] Al-Omaishi J, Bashir R, Gendelman HE. The cellular immunology of multiple sclerosis. J Leukoc Biol 1999;65:444–52.

[10] Xie JH, Nomura N, Lu M, et al. Antibody-mediated blockade of the CXCR3 chemokine receptor results in diminished recruitment of T helper 1 cells into sites of inflammation. J Leukoc Biol 2003;73:771–80.

[11] Raine CS. The Dale E. McFarlin Memorial Lecture: the immunology of the multiple sclerosis lesion. Ann Neurol 1994;36:S61–72.

[12] Uhm JH, Dooley NP, Stuve O, et al. Migratory behavior of lymphocytes isolated from multiple sclerosis patients: effects of interferon beta-1b therapy. Ann Neurol 1999;46: 319–24.

[13] Muraro PA, Leist T, Bielekova B, et al. VLA-4/CD49d downregulated on primed T lymphocytes during interferon-beta therapy in multiple sclerosis. J Neuroimmunol 2000;111: 186–94.

[14] Calabresi PA, Tranquill LR, Damborosia JM, et al. Increases in soluble VCAM-1 correlate with a decrease in MRI lesions in multiple sclerosis treated with interferon beta-1b. Ann Neurol 1997;41:669–74.

[15] Merril JE, Benveniste N. Cytokines in inflammatory brain lesions: helpful and harmful. Trends Neurosci 1996;19:331–8.

[16] Lin K, Ateeq HS, Hsiung SH, et al. Selective, tight-binding inhibition of integrin alpha4beta1that inhibit allergic airway hyperresponsiveness. J Med Chem 1999;42: 920–34.

[17] Van der Laan LJ, Van der Goes A, Wauben MH, et al. Beneficial effect of modified peptide inhibitor of alpha4 integrins on experimental allergic encephalomyelitis in Lewis rats. J Neurosci Res 2003;67:191–9.

[18] Fong S, Jones S, Renz ME, et al. Mucosal addressin adhesion molecule-1 (MAdCAM-1). Its binding motif for alpha-4 beta-1 and the role in experimental colitis. Immunol Res 1997;16: 299.

[19] Shimizu Y, Newman W, Tanaka Y, et al. Lymphocyte interactions with endothelial cells. Immunol Today 1992;13:106–12.

[20] Von Andrian UH, Engelhardt B. Alpha-4 integrins as therapeutic targets in autoimmune disease. N Engl J Med 2003;348:68–72.

[21] Podolsky DK, Lobb RR, King N, et al. Attenuation of colitis in the cotton-top tamarin by anti-alpha 4 integrin monoclonal antibody. J Clin Invest 1993;92:372.

[22] Yednock TA, Cannon C, Fritz LC, et al. Prevention of experimental autoimmune encephalomyelitis by antibodies against alpha4beta1. Nature 1992;356:63–6.

[23] Kent SJ, Karlik SJ, Cannon C, et al. A monoclonal antibody to alpha-4 integrin suppresses and reverses active experimental allergic encephalomyelitis. J Neuroimmunol 1995;58: 1–10.

[24] O' Connor PW, Goodman A, Willmer-Hume AJ, et al. (Natalizumab Multiple Sclerosis Trial Group). Randomized multicenter trial of natalizumab in acute MS relapse: clinical and MRI effects. Neurology 2004;62(11):2038–43.

[25] Sheremata WA, Vollmer TL, Stone LS, Willmer-Hume AJ, Koller M. A safety and pharmacokinetic study of intravenous natalizumab in patients with MS. Neurology 1999;52: 1072–4.

[26] Tubridy N, Behan PO, Capildeo R, et al. The effect of anti-alpha-4 integrin antibody on brain lesion activity in MS. Neurology 1999;53:466–72.

[27] Miller DH, Khan OA, Sheremata WA, et al, for the International Natalizumab Multiple Sclerosis Trial Group. A controlled trial of natalizumab for relapsing multiple sclerosis. N Engl J Med 2003;348:15–23.

[28] Theien BE, Vanderlugt CL, Eagar TN, et al. Discordant effects of anti-VLA-4 treatment before and after onset of relapsing experimental autoimmune encephalomyelitis. J Clin Invest 2001;107:995–1006.

[29] Hartung HP, Gonsette R, Konig N, et al, and the Mitoxantrone in Multiple Sclerosis Study Group (MIMS). Mitoxantrone in progressive multiple sclerosis: a placebo-controlled, double-blind, randomized, multicentre trial. Lancet 2002;360:2018–25.

[30] Van Oosten BW, Barkhof F, et al. Increased MRI activity and immune activation in two multiple sclerosis patients treated with the monoclonal anti-tumour necrosis factor antibody c A2. Neurology 1996;47:1531–4.

[31] Dow Jones Newswires. Icos Corporation will not study LeukArrest as chronic MS treatment. Available at: http://www.btinternet.com/-ms_pages/LeukArrestStudyStopped.html. Accessed September 29, 1999.

[32] Cannella B, Cross AH, Raine CS. Anti-adhesion molecule therapy in experimental autoimmune encephalomyelitis. J Neuroimmunol 1993;46:43–56.

[33] Lublin, FD and the Hu 23F2G MS Study Group (1999). A phase II trial of anti-CD11/CD18 monoclonal antibody in acute exacerbations of multiple sclerosis. Neurology 1999;52: A290–1.

[34] Huitinga I, Damoiseaux JG, Dopp EA, et al. Treatment with anti-CR3 antibodies ED7 and ED8 suppresses experimental allergic encephalomyelitis in Lewis rats. Eur J Immunol 1993; 23:709–15.

[35] Soilu-Hanninen M, Roytta M, Salmi A, et al. Therapy with antibody against leukocyte integrin VLA-4 (CD49d) is effective and safe in virus-facilitated experimental allergic encephalomyelitis. J Neuroimmunol 1997;72(1):95–105.

[36] Trebst C, Staugaitis SM, Tucky B, et al. Chemokine receptors on infiltrating leukocytes in inflammatory pathologies of the central nervous system (CNS). Neuropathol Appl Neurobiol 2003;29:584–91.

[37] Paolillo A, Coles AJ, Molyneux PD, et al. Quantitative MRI in patients with secondary progressive MS treated with monoclonal antibody Campath 1H. Neurology 1999;53:751–7.

[38] Coles AJ, Wing M, Smith S, et al. Pulsed monoclonal antibody treatment and autoimmune thyroid disease in multiple sclerosis. Lancet 1999;354:L1691–5.

[39] Polman CH, Uitdehaag MJ. New and emerging treatment options for multiple sclerosis. Lancet Neurol 2003;2:563–6.

ELSEVIER
SAUNDERS

Neurol Clin 23 (2005) 247–272

NEUROLOGIC
CLINICS

Immunosuppressive Therapy for Multiple Sclerosis

Susan A. Gauthier, DO, Guy J. Buckle, MD,
Howard L. Weiner, MD*

*Partners Multiple Sclerosis Center, Brigham and Women's Hospital,
333 Longwood Avenue, Boston, MA 02115, USA*

The rationale for treating multiple sclerosis (MS) with immunosuppressive therapy rests on the hypothesis that MS is an inflammatory, cell-mediated, autoimmune disease, affecting the central nervous system [1–3]. Elevation of interferon-γ (IFN-γ), endothelial-cell activation with increased expression of major histocompatibility complex (MHC) class II antigens and adhesion molecules, and macrophage-mediated destruction of myelin via receptor-mediated endocytosis provide evidence that MS is an inflammatory disease [4]. Further evidence for a Th1- or cell-mediated autoimmune process includes interleukin 2 (IL-2) expression and B7-1 upregulation within active lesions [5]. Therapy with drugs that have pronounced anti-inflammatory and immunosuppressive effects has been used for the treatment of non-neoplastic diseases in which autoimmune mechanisms are considered important in the pathogenesis [6,7].

The current categories of therapy used to treat MS, which include anti-inflammatory, immunomodulatory, and immunosupressive therapies, have overlapping immunologic effects and, therefore, are not absolutely distinct. In general, therapies considered immunosuppressive have directed intracellular mechanisms that involve DNA synthesis or immune-cell activation, targeted primarily within the bone marrow and other lymphoid organs. Cyclophosphamide and mitoxantrone interfere with cellular DNA and RNA synthesis within organs in which there are rapidly dividing cells, including gastrointestinal and bladder epithelium, and bone marrow derived cells, thus accounting for a variety of toxicities. Other immunosupressive drugs target metabolic properties specific to dividing immune cells and have

* Corresponding author.
E-mail address: hweiner@rics.bwh.harvard.edu (H.L. Weiner).

doi:10.1016/j.ncl.2004.09.007 *neurologic.theclinics.com*

been used widely in tissue transplantation. These include oral agents, such as methotrexate, azathioprine, and mycophenylate mofetil, all inhibitors of the de novo purine synthesis pathway upon which B cells and T cells depend for DNA replication. Older immunophylins, such as cyclosporine, are being replaced for use in transplantation by newer xenobiotic agents, such as sirolimus (rapamycin) and tacrolimus (FK506), largely because of their favorable toxicity profiles and currently are undergoing evaluation in small-scale clinical trials of MS. These agents interfere with specific intracellular steps in the activation of T cells, such as disruption of the IL-2 signaling process or, as with sirolimus, disruption of the CD28-dependent costimulatory pathways, both believed required for T-cell activation. These agents are targeted specifically to the cellular arm of the immune response. Immunosuppressive therapy for MS recently has involved monoclonal antibody therapy, which has become an area of active investigation in MS and differs from standard immunosuppressive therapy because it uses agents that bind to specific extracellularly expressed molecules. Specific monoclonal antibodies with immunosuppressive effects that are in early-stage trials of MS include daclizumab and rituximab.

This article will review published trials, mechanistic studies, and long-term safety data for immunosuppressive agents used in the treatment of MS and will focus specifically on cyclophosphamide and mitoxantrone. These agents serve as a paradigm for the use of newer agents that have less toxic side effects in the treatment of patients who have an inadequate response to immunomodulatory therapy with interferon-β (IFN-β) and glatiramer acetate (GA).

Cyclophosphamide

Cyclophosphamide (Cytoxan) is an alkylating agent used to treat malignancy and was first tested in MS in 1966 [8]. During the past 30 years, cyclophosphamide has been used for the treatment of selected patients with MS and for other nonmalignant immune-mediated inflammatory processes, including immune-mediated neuropathies and lupus nephritis, for which it is standard therapy. There are more than 40 published reports on the clinical and immunologic effects of cyclophosphamide in MS, many of which found positive effects, although not all studies found it efficacious [9]. The results of these studies initially led to conflicting opinions regarding the use of cyclophosphamide in MS. Recently, with improved knowledge of the inflammatory and degenerative processes ongoing in MS, and with the advent of MRI, there is a better understanding of how to use cyclophosphamide in a manner that is both efficacious and safe. Because cyclophosphamide is not a drug under patent, as is mitoxantrone, which has Food and Drug Administration (FDA) approval for patients who have worsening MS, there is no expectation that pharmaceutical support for large-scale testing of cyclophosphamide required for FDA approval is forthcoming. Thus, physicians must determine which patients who have MS are appropriate to be treated with cyclophosphamide based on the studies of its clinical and immunologic effects published to date.

Initial clinical studies of cyclophosphamide

In 1966, Aimard et al described the successful arrest of a progressive case of MS using cyclophosphamide [8]. This led to an open-label, uncontrolled clinical trial by Girard et al in which 30 patients who had MS were treated with 200 mg/d of intravenous (IV) cyclophosphamide for 4 to 6 weeks, with a total dose ranging from 4 to 9 g. At the 2-year follow-up, 50% of the patients were improved or stable [10]. After a series of small studies [11–15], larger studies of cyclophosphamide in MS were conducted by Gonsette and Hommes. Hommes et al reported stabilization or improvement in 15 of 25 progressive patients 6 to 33 months after treatment with a short course of cyclophosphamide (400 mg/d) and prednisone (100 mg/d) for a 20-day period for a total of 8 g [16]. In a second report of 39 progressive patients by Hommes et al, 69% of the patients had disease stabilization during a period of 1 to 5 years [17,18]. Factors predictive of treatment response included disease onset before age 28, short duration of disease before treatment, rapid progression of disease, low initial disability, and being HLA-DRw2 positive. Similarly, Gonsette et al reported 62% stabilization in a study of 110 patients who had relapsing-remitting MS during a 2- to 4-year follow-up using a 2-week induction protocol of cyclophosphamide [19,20]. Consistent with previous studies, the effect was most dramatic in patients who had the shortest disease duration and was relatively ineffective in patients who were severely handicapped at baseline. The positive results reported by Hommes and Gonsette led to further investigation of cyclophosphamide in larger randomized trials.

Randomized clinical trials of cyclophosphamide in multiple sclerosis

In 1983, a randomized controlled study of the use cyclophosphamide in patients who had progressive MS was reported by Hauser et al [21]. Fifty-eight patients were randomized to receive one of three treatments: a 2- to 3-week course of IV cyclophosphamide at 400 to 500 mg/d to achieve a leukopenia of 2000/μl and ACTH; ACTH alone; or plasma exchange with ACTH and oral cyclophosphamide. This was not a blinded or a placebo-controlled trial. The results revealed that 80% (16/20) of the patients treated with cyclophosphamide were improved or stabilized at 1 year compared with 50% (9/18) in the plasma exchange group and only 20% (2/20) in the group treated with ACTH alone. In a subsequent report by Carter et al of 164 patients treated with the same protocol of cyclophosphamide induction and ACTH as used by Hauser et al, after initial period of stabilization, virtually all the patients began to progress again by 30 months after induction [22]. Thus, it was apparent that a strategy to prolong the beneficial effect of cyclophosphamide therapy was required. Goodkin et al randomized 27 progressive patients to receive either every 2-month boosters of 700 mg/m^2 cyclophosphamide after induction versus no maintenance therapy; both were compared to control group of 24 nonrandomized untreated patients [23]. There was a significant benefit in both cyclophosphamide groups compared with the control patients and a trend in favor of boosters over induction only. Soon after, the Northeast Cooperative Multiple Sclerosis Treatment Group studied the effect of pulse cyclophosphamide therapy and a modified induction regimen with a fixed dose compared with a previous published induction regimen based on white blood cell (WBC) counts [24]. The patients were randomized into one of four groups and were evaluated in a single-blind fashion. Treatment failure or improvement was defined as a change of 1 point on the Kurtzke disability status scale (DSS) sustained during a 2-month period. There were 261 patients who had progressive MS and were randomized to receive the published or modified induction followed by an every 2-month booster (700 mg/m^2) during a 2-year period or no pulse therapy. There was no placebo group. There was no difference between the published versus the modified induction regimen either by stabilization at 12 and 24 months or subsequent progression by the time-to-failure analysis. A modest, although significant, benefit of delayed progression at 24 and 30 months (P = 0.04) was found in patients who received booster therapy. There was, however, a significant age effect with booster therapy: 40% of patients ages 18 to 40 were stabilized or improved at 30 months (P = 0.01) compared with only 14% of older patients (P = 0.27). Time-to-failure analysis revealed similar results: a significant delay in treatment failure in patients ages 18 to 40 years (P = 0.003) compared with patients ages 41 to 55 (P = 0.97). Subgroup analysis revealed that patients who had primary progressive MS had a poorer prognosis with more than 55% failing at 12 months compared with 41% of secondary progressive patients failing. In addition, patients who had recent onset of progression responded better to boosters (P = 0.02) than patients who had progressive disease longer than 7 years (P = 0.58).

In summary, the Northeast Cooperative Multiple Sclerosis Treatment Group was the first large randomized trial that demonstrated the benefit of booster IV cyclophosphamide therapy and led the way to currently used protocols, in which treatment is given as outpatient pulses similar to lupus nephritis treatment. Subsequently, the authors' group has developed an outpatient induction protocol with 5 consecutive days of 1 g IV methylprednisolone (MP) with a single dose (800 mg/m^2) of cyclophosphamide given on day 5. Monthly pulses of cyclophosphamide/MP are given at increasing cyclophosphamide doses until the dose is reached that produces a midmonth nadir of 1500 to 2000 total WBC/μl or a maximum dose of 1600 mg/m^2. Pulses are given monthly for the first year, every 6 weeks during the second year, and every 2 months during the third year. A retrolective study (a retrospective review of prospectively collected data) identified factors associated with clinical response in 95 patients who had progressive MS and were treated with this protocol [25]. A shorter length of time within the progressive stage was found to be linked to a positive clinical response and there was a suggestion that primary progressive patients were a non-responsive subgroup. This confirmed findings from the Northeast Co-operative Multiple Sclerosis Treatment Group and the earlier European studies that cyclophosphamide therapy may benefit progressive MS, particularly if patients are treated earlier. Currently, the authors' group treats most patients only with pulse doses of cyclophosphamide/MP therapy, reserving induction therapy for patients who have very active inflammatory disease requiring immediate stabilization. Some centers continue to study the effect of large doses of induction therapy with cyclophosphamide in patients who have aggressive disease.

There have been two randomized placebo-controlled studies using a 2-week cyclophosphamide treatment regimen that did not demonstrate a positive clinical response [26,27]. The Kaiser study was a single-blind study of 43 patients who had chronic progressive MS and were randomized to receive outpatient induction of IV cyclophosphamide or IV folic acid [26]. In the Canadian Cooperative Trial, 55 patients who had progressive MS received either 1 g IV cyclophosphamide on alternate days until the WBC fell below 4500/μl or a total dose of 9 g plus 40 mg prednisone orally for 10 days [27]. This study was randomized, placebo controlled, and single masked and included a third treatment group that received plasma exchange with oral cyclophosphamide and prednisone.

The failure of the Kaiser and Canadian studies to find a benefit of cyclophosphamide therapy led to controversy in the literature over its use; this debate occurred before our current understanding of anti-inflammatory therapy in MS and the use of MRI to measure inflammatory lesions with contrast-enhanced images [9,19,28–30]. A strict comparison of the trials is impractical because of differing trial designs, patient selection, and treatment regimens. Additionally, in the Kaiser and Canadian studies, there was a lack of progression in the placebo groups at 1 and 2 years; therefore, both potentially were subject to type-II (false negative) error. Stabilization of the placebo group in the Kaiser study was 70% and 63% at 1 and 2 years, respectively, and 75% and 67%, respectively, in the Canadian study. Furthermore, as established in multiple studies [17–20,24,25], it is clear now that there are patient subgroups that are more likely to respond to cyclophosphamide, specifically younger patients who have a shorter duration of progressive disease and have an inflammatory component to their disease, as evidenced by MRI imaging or clinical attacks. The Kaiser and Canadian studies seem to have identified subsets of progressive patients who were not responsive to induction therapy with cyclophosphamide. This may explain the differing results between various studies, especially when considering that the patients treated by Hauser et al were younger and had a shorter duration of disease before treatment than the patients from the Canadian and Kaiser studies. Regarding treatment regimens, Carter et al established that patients require pulse therapy, because without it, the majority of patients again progress. There followed a series of small open-label studies that observed a clinical benefit of intermittent pulse IV cyclophosphamide therapy in relapsing-remitting and progressive MS [31–34]. The results from these pre-MRI cyclophosphamide studies are consistent with the current theory regarding the pathophysiology of the disease: treating MS aggressively and earlier, during the inflammatory stage, leads to the greatest benefit of cyclophosphamide therapy.

Recent studies of cyclophosphamide in multiple sclerosis and MRI

With the advent of MRI and approval of immunomodulatory therapy, the effective use of pulse cyclophosphamide therapy has been defined better in studies of patients who have continued disease activity while on IFN-β or GA. Gobbini et al reported the first MRI-based study of cyclophosphamide [35]. Five relapsing patients refractory to immunomodulatory therapy were treated with monthly pulses of 1000 mg/m^2 and were followed with monthly MRI and clinical evaluations for a mean of 28 months. All patients showed a rapid reduction in contrast-enhancing lesion frequency and three patients had a decrease in T2 lesion load within the first 5 months of starting therapy. This was a crucial study that introduced the use of cyclophosphamide in patients who were failing IFN-β and demonstrated a dramatic effect on MRI. Patti et al reported an open-label study of pulse IV cyclophosphamide (500–1500 mg/m^2) monthly for 12 months, then bimonthly for an additional 6 months, in combination with IFN-β [36]. Ten patients who had relapsing-remitting MS were selected for study based on the presence of frequent and severe attacks, and an accumulation of disability on IFN-β alone. There was a significant decrease in relapse rate ($P < 0.0001$), a decrease in expanded disability status scale (EDSS) ($P < 0.0001$), and a decrease in T2 lesion burden on MRI ($P < 0.001$). Additionally, Perini et al reported an open-label trial of monthly pulse cyclophosphamide with 1 g IV MP, followed by bimonthly pulses for a second year, that stabilized 16 patients who had rapidly deteriorating secondary progressive MS compared with a control group treated with only IV MP for relapses [37]. Patients treated with cyclophosphamide/MP had a significant decrease in EDSS at the first and second years when compared with entry ($P < 0.0001$) and remained without new contrast-enhancing lesions or a significant increase in the T2 lesion load. Although these studies were small, they demonstrated an effect of pulse cyclophosphamide therapy on clinical stabilization of actively deteriorating patients and a marked effect on MRI inflammatory activity.

Recently, Zephir et al reported on an open-label, retrospective study of 490 progressive patients treated with monthly pulse cyclophosphamide therapy (700 mg/m^2/mo) with 1 g IV MP and defined factors that predicted response at 12 months [38]. Stabilization by EDSS at 12 months was found in 78.6% of patients who had secondary progressive MS (n = 362) and 73.5% of patients who had primary progressive MS (n = 128). Furthermore, there was a significant decrease in relapse rate in the patients who had secondary progressive MS ($P < 0.0001$). A response to therapy at 12 months was found in patients who had a progressive phase of 5.1 years compared with a progressive phase of 7.1 years and in patients who had a response to pulse cyclophosphamide within 6 months of treatment. Again, the main distinguishing factor associated with a treatment response to cyclophosphamide was use within the early stage of progressive disease. Unique to this study was the predictive value of a 6-month response and an observed benefit in patients who had primary progressive MS. Although this was a retrospective analysis, it involved one of the largest cohorts treated with cyclophosphamide and contributed to a better understanding of patient selection for immunosuppressive therapy.

The authors' group, in a recent MRI-based, single-blind study, randomized 59 patients who had relapsing-remitting MS and continued disease activity while on IFN-β to receive 3 days of 1 g IV MP followed by 6 monthly treatments with 1 g IV MP or cyclophosphamide (800 mg/m^2) plus 1 g IV MP while remaining on IFN-β [39]. Patients were followed for an additional 18-month postinfusion phase, in which all patients received IFN-β alone. There was a significant decrease in number of contrast-enhancing lesions in the group that received cyclophosphamide versus the IV MP group at 3 ($P = 0.01$), 6 ($P = 0.04$), and 12 ($P = 0.02$) months. The clinical endpoint, time-to-treatment failure, also was delayed significantly ($P = 0.02$) compared with the MP group. This study confirms the effect of pulse cyclophosphamide therapy for clinical stabilization of active relapsing-remitting MS and its ability to significantly reduce MRI inflammatory lesions compared with monthly IV MP.

Immunologic effects of cyclophosphamide

Cyclophosphamide was one of the first drugs found effective in experimental allergic encephalitis (EAE), the animal model of MS [40]. In studies of the immunologic effects of cyclophosphamide, the authors have found that although cyclophosphamide has been believed a general immunosuppressant, selective effects on the immune system occur and seem to be related to its beneficial effects in MS (Table 1). Several studies show the pronounced suppression of CD4+ cells with cyclophosphamide therapy [41–44]; however, further studies demonstrate specific evidence of increased Th2 activity with increased levels of IL-4, IL-5, IL-10, and transforming growth TGF-β, an associated eosinophilia, and a decrease in IFN-γ [45,46]. Additionally, cyclophosphamide normalized elevated levels of IL-12, which is a cytokine that drives a Th1 response, and correlates with disease activity [46].

Table 1
Immunosuppressive effects of cyclophosphamide

Cell type			Immunologic effect
CD4	Th1	↓	↓IFN-γ (46)
	Th2	↑	↑IL-4 (45) ↑IL-5 (45) ↑IL-10 (45) ↑TGF-β (46) Eosinophils (45)
CD8		↓	↓IFN-γ (48)
B cells		↓	↓IgG (51)
Monocytes		↓	↓IL-12(46)
		↑	↑TGF-β(46)

In terms of antigen-specific mechanisms, Takashima et al found that cyclophosphamide preferentially deviates myelin reactive cells to those secreting IL-4 [47]. The authors report an increased frequency of myelin basic protein (MBP) and proteolipid protein (PLP) cells secreting IL-4 in patients treated with cyclophosphamide. This increase was found neither in tetanus-toxoid–secreting cells nor in patients treated with IV MP. Thus, cyclophosphamide therapy preferentially induces antigen-specific Th2 responses to myelin autoantigens. Furthermore, the authors' group recently found that cyclophosphamide reverses increased IFN-γ production of CD8+ T cells in secondary progressive MS [48]. Additionally, cyclophosphamide increased the percentage of CCR4+ T cells that produce high levels of IL-4 and reverses the increase in the percentage of IFN-γ–producing CCR5+ and CXCR3+ CD8+ T cells [48]. Thus, according to the immunologic paradigm of MS, the effect of cyclophosphamide can be demonstrated in the peripheral blood not only through decreasing INF-γ but also from causing a pronounced Th2/Th3 immune deviation. Furthermore, cyclophosphamide crosses the blood-brain barrier and may have local central nervous system anti-inflammatory effects [49–52].

Safety profile of cyclophosphamide

The adverse effects of cyclophosphamide are well known, as the drug has been used for more than 30 years (Box 1). Tolerability of pulse cyclophosphamide therapy was reported by Portaccio et al in a series of

Box 1. Side effects of cyclophosphamide

Nausea
Alopecia
Menstrual disorders and infertility
Leukopenia and infection
Bladder toxicity
Risk of cancer

112 patients who had MS and were treated with 700 mg/m^2 monthly for 12 months, then bimonthly for an additional 12 months [53]. Approximately 77 patients (68.9%) had their overall tolerability to cyclophosphamide measured with a visual analog scale and 53.2% rated the treatment as acceptable or very well tolerated; 28.6% reported a relative tolerability. This data is consistent with most investigators' and with the authors' experience that pulse cyclophosphamide generally is well tolerated [34–38].

Infertility occurs in men and women receiving alkylating agents, such as cyclophosphamide. Boumpas et al reported on the risk of amenorrhea in patients who had lupus and were treated with pulse cyclophosphamide therapy; 12% of patients receiving 7 doses and 39% of patients receiving 15 or more doses developed sustained amenorrhea [54,55]. Gourley et al reported 23 of 46 women (50%) developed amenorrhea after receiving cyclophosphamide for a 6-month course then quarterly for at least an additional 2 years [55]. Lastly, Portaccio et al, in the study described previously, reported 8 of 24 fertile women developed sustained amenorrhea; all of the affected women were older than age 34 [53]. There is little data concerning the frequency of infertility in men treated with cyclophosphamide for immune-mediated diseases.

Long-term oral cyclophosphamide has been established as associated with substantial bladder toxicity, including hemorrhagic cystitis, bladder cancer, and other secondary malignancies; therefore, oral therapy has been avoided in MS [56–58]. Radis et al published a 20-year follow-up study in a cohort of 119 patients who had rheumatoid arthritis (RA) and were treated with oral cyclophosphamide; the mean dose of cyclophosphamide in patients who developed malignancy was 79.0 g [57]. The magnitude of increased risk of malignancy seems to increase as a function of total dose, and care must be taken when the cumulative dose exceeds 80 to 100 g [56–58]. Based on this, at a dose of 1000 mg/m^2, patients may receive approximately 50 doses of cyclophosphamide in their lifetime. Long-term safety data on pulse cyclophosphamide therapy, as it is used in immune-mediated diseases, has yet to be reported. At the authors' center, patients are hydrated with 3 L of fluid on the day of the treatment and the day after treatment. Additionally, urine cytology is obtained at yearly intervals and patients undergo a yearly cystoscopy after 3 years of treatment.

Current clinical use of cyclophosphamide

Cyclophosphamide has been studied extensively in MS and its use has evolved over 3 decades toward the administration of intermittent pulse therapy given during a 1- to 3-year period. The pulse IV cyclophosphamide/MP combined regimens used in MS are analogous to the lupus nephritis protocols and are summarized in Table 2. This combination was developed after studies of lupus nephritis suggested the addition of steroids may enhance the effects of cyclophosphamide [55]. Based on published studies (discussed previously) and experience, the authors consider cyclophosphamide an established therapeutic option for patients who fail standard immunotherapy and remain with a strong inflammatory component to their disease; the authors consider these patients as having active relapsing-remitting or early progressive MS.

Mitoxantrone

Mitoxantrone (Novantrone) is a synthetically produced anthraquinone with known antineoplastic effects in advanced breast cancer, lymphoma, and leukemia [59]. Mitoxantrone has been shown to block DNA synthesis by inducing DNA strand-breaks and interstrand crosslinks, while also interfering with RNA synthesis and inhibiting the enzyme topoisomerase II, which is involved in DNA repair [60–63]. Because of the reduced incidence of serious side effects of mitoxantrone compared with the related anthracyclines that have similar antitumor activity, mitoxantrone was considered a promising new chemotherapy agent [64]. In addition to its antineoplastic activity, mitoxantrone was highly suppressive in the acute and relapsing forms of EAE; as a result, mitoxantrone became a candidate for clinical study in MS [65–68]. Recently, on the basis of an early phase II trial [69] and a subsequent phase III clinical trial [70], mitoxantrone was approved by the FDA for treatment of patients who have secondary progressive MS, progressive relapsing MS, or relapsing-remitting MS.

Initial clinical studies of mitoxantrone in multiple sclerosis

Gonsette and Demonty presented the original open-label pilot study of mitoxantrone and reported stabilization of 15 of 22 patients who had relapsing-remitting MS or progressive MS. Patients were treated with 14 mg/m^2 every 3 weeks with mitoxantrone until lymphopenia was equal to or below 1000/μL and were followed for a mean of 12 months [71]. In 8 of 12 patients who had a high pretreatment relapse rate, there was a marked decline in relapses after treatment. At the same time, Kappos et al presented preliminary data from a pilot MRI study in 14 patients who had rapidly progressive MS and were treated with 10 mg/ m^2 of mitoxantrone every

3 weeks for 3 to 5 cycles resulting in a mean decrease in contrast-enhancing lesions from 9 to 1 at 6 months' follow-up [72]. A subsequent small phase II pilot study by Mauch et al reported on 10 rapidly deteriorating MS patients treated with 12 mg/m^2 of mitoxantrone every 3 months over a 12-month period [73]. There were 6 patients who had relapsing-remitting MS and 4 patients who had secondary progressive MS fulfilling the criteria of rapidly deteriorating MS by a progression of at least 1.0 on the DSS during the preceding 12 months. During the 12-month treatment period, 5 patients remained clinically stable and 4 patients improved; MRI results revealed that a total of 169 pretreatment contrast-enhancing lesions decreased to 10. Krapf et al published a subsequent MRI report on these patients extending the follow-up to 24 months [74]. Because of the favorable results in the first year, 8 of 9 of the remaining patients received an additional 18 cycles of mitoxantrone (2.2 cycles/patient) and had continued suppression of contrast-enhancing activity. Conversely, a study by Noseworthy et al of 13 patients who had progressive MS and were treated with 8 mg/m^2 of mitoxantrone every 3 weeks for a total of 7 infusions failed to reveal a benefit similar to that seen in the previous studies did [75].

Randomized clinical trials of mitoxantrone

Bastianello et al reported the first randomized, doubled-blind, placebo-controlled trial of low-dose mitoxantrone in 25 patients who had relapsing-remitting MS [76]. Inclusion criteria required patients to have had 2 attacks within the previous 24 months and an EDSS between 2 and 5. Patients were randomized to receive either mitoxantrone, 8 mg/m^2 monthly infusions for 1 year, versus placebo, both delivered in a black IV bag and tubing for blinding. Clinical outcomes included relapse rate and 12-month EDSS, with clinical worsening defined as a change of greater than 1 point on EDSS. There was a significant decrease in relapse rate in the mitoxantrone group compared with the placebo group at 12 months ($P = 0.014$); however, the mean change in EDSS between the two groups was not significantly different. Serial MRI measurements that included the mean number of new, enlarging, or contrast-enhancing lesions between the two groups were not significantly different, although there was a trend toward a reduction of these in the mitoxantrone group.

Edan et al published results of a randomized trial of 42 patients who had active MS and were treated with 6 monthly doses of mitoxantrone (20 mg IV) and IV MP (1g) verses IV MP (1 g) alone [69]. Patients had either relapsing-remitting or secondary progressive MS with clinical inclusion criteria requiring 2 relapses or progression by at least 2 points on EDSS within the previous 12 months. An MRI criterion of at least one contrast-enhancing lesion on one of three serial MRIs during a period of 2 months was a requirement of all patients who met the clinical criteria. The primary outcome was the proportion of patients that developed new

Table 2
Treatment protocols of immunosuppressive therapy in multiple sclerosis

Treatment regimen	Safety monitoring
1. Cyclophosphamide (Cytoxan)	
Pulse therapy: 800 mg/m^2 with dose escalation to produce leukopenia of 2000/µL; every 4 weeks × 1 year, every 6 weeks × 1 year, every 8 weeks × 1 year. 1 g IV MP with each dose. Maximum dose 1600 mg/m^2.	WBC prior to each dose at mid-month (nadir). Urinalysis and cytology yearly during treatment.
Fixed dose pulse therapy: CTX pulses given at 800–1000 mg/m^2 every 4–8 weeks for 12–24 months; given with or without MP.	Cystoscopy if abnormal cytology and yearly after third year of CTX. Maximum lifetime dose: 80–100 g.
Inpatient induction: 600 mg/m^2 CTX given on days 1, 2, 4, 6, 8 plus 1 g MP given daily for 8 days.	
Outpatient induction: 1 g MP given daily for 5 days and CTX 800 mg/m^2 is given on day 5.	
Combination therapy: IV pulse CTX therapy given concomitantly with IFN-β or GA in nonresponders for various time periods.	
Patients are instructed to drink 3 litres of fluid the day of and after CTX treatment. If oral intake is not possible, fluids must be given IV.	
2. Mitoxantrone (Novantrone)	
Pulse therapy: 8–12 mg/m^2 given every 3 months; next dose held if leukopenia <1500/µL 2 weeks after infusion.	WBC prior to each dose and 2 weeks post infusion. 2D echocardiogram at baseline and every 6 months to monitor ejection fraction.
Induction therapy: 8–12 mg/m^2 given monthly × 3, followed by every 3-month infusions.	When dose reaches 100 mg/m^2, 2D echocardiogram prior to each dose. Baseline EF must be >50% and if decrease of 10%; discontinue therapy. Maximum lifetime dose: 140 mg/m^2
3. Methotrexate	
Dose range 7.5–20 mg once per week (subcutaneous injection or oral).	Baseline and routine WBC, liver, and renal function tests. Avoidance of sulfa-containing medications. Avoidance of alcohol.
4. *Mycophenolate* mofetil (CellCept)	
Dose 2 g per oral daily (1g bid). Titration to maximum dose for 1 month	Baseline and routine WBC and liver function monitoring.
5. Azathioprine (Imuran)	
Dose range 1–2 mg/kg daily	Baseline CBC, renal and liver function, and routine monitoring of WBC.

Table 2 *(continued)*

Treatment regimen	Safety monitoring
6. Pulse methylprednisolone 1000 mg IV every 4 weeks. *Alternatives:* 500 mg IV every 2 weeks; 1000 mg IV × 3–5 days every 3–4 months *Typically, oral tapers are not used at the authors' center.*	Yearly bone densitometry. Calcium (1000–1500 mg/d). Vitamin D (400–800 units/d).

Abbreviation: CTX, cyclophosphamide.

contrast-enhancing lesions, and this was the only blinded component to the study. Five patients within the MP group discontinued the study because of deterioration. At 6 months, there was a highly significant difference in the percentage of patients who did not have new contrast-enhancing lesions in the mitoxantrone/MP group (90.5%) compared with the group that had MP alone (31.3%, $P < 0.001$). The mean EDSS of the mitoxantrone/MP group compared with MP alone was only significantly different at month 4; however, within the mitoxantrone/MP patients, there was a significant improvement in EDSS between baseline and months 2 to 6. The beneficial effect of mitoxantrone on MRI activity demonstrated in this study was used to obtain FDA approval for mitoxantrone. Consistent with these findings, Millefiorini et al published a randomized study of 51 patients who had active relapsing-remitting MS and were treated with monthly infusions of mitoxantrone (8 mg/m^2) for 12 months and followed for 24 months [77]. The primary clinical endpoint, the proportion of patients that had confirmed progression, demonstrated by an increase of greater than 1 point on EDSS, tended to favor mitoxantrone in the first year and became significant in the second year, with 2 of 27 (7%) of the mitoxantrone patients and 9 of 24 (37%) of the placebo patients progressing ($P < 0.02$). Although fewer patients who were treated with mitoxantrone met the primary outcome, there was no difference in the mean EDSS between the two groups in either year of the study. Secondary outcome measures resulted in a significant decrease in the mean number of exacerbations in the treated group versus the placebo group at 12 ($P = 0.001$) and 24 months ($P = 0.005$), and a reduction of new T2 lesions on MRI ($P < 0.05$). Additionally, Van de Wyngaert et al reported a clinical and MRI benefit of mitoxantrone verses IV MP in patients who had secondary progressive MS; 51% of the patients, however, discontinued the study; therefore, interpretation of this study is limited significantly [78]. These trials demonstrated that mitoxantrone has a marked effect on MRI inflammatory lesions; in addition, clinical stabilization seemed to be achieved with mitoxantrone in patients who had active MS.

FDA approval of mitoxantrone for the treatment of MS was based on a randomized, double-blind, placebo-controlled trial, reported by Hartung et al [70], of 194 patients who had worsening relapsing-remitting or secondary progressive MS. Patients enrolled had a 1-point decline on EDSS within 18 months before randomization to either mitoxantrone 12 mg/m^2 or 5 mg/m^2 or an infusion of 3 mg of methylene blue every 3 months for a 2-year period. Forty five percent of the patients had relapsing-remitting MS and 55% of the patients had secondary progressive MS with a combined baseline mean EDSS of 4.69. The primary outcome measure was a composite of five clinical measures: change in EDSS, change in ambulation index (AI), number of relapses treated with corticosteroids, time to first relapse, and change in standardized neurologic status. Blinding was not complete because the treating physician monitoring relapses was not blinded. A significant treatment effect was determined by the composite outcome measure when the 12-mg/m^2 group was compared with the placebo group. More importantly, the results of all the individual components of the composite revealed a significant difference in favor of higher-dose mitoxantrone compared with placebo. The 5-mg/m^2 group failed to reveal a difference regarding AI; therefore, further analysis was not completed. The proportion of patients that deteriorated by 1 point on EDSS was reduced significantly in the high-dose group (8%) compared with the placebo group (25%) ($P = 0.013$). Regarding the MRI data, there was a significant reduction of new T2 lesions ($P = 0.03$) and there were fewer patients who had new contrast-enhancing lesions at 24 months ($P = 0.022$) in the higher-dose mitoxantrone group compared with the placebo group.

Immunologic effects of mitoxantrone

Mitoxantrone has a profound effect on the humoral immune system, including direct suppression of the B-lymphocyte population, macrophage-mediated inhibition of B cells, and suppression of antimyelin immunoglobulin G (IgG) production [61,79]. The effect of mitoxantrone on T-lymphocyte function was demonstrated through macrophage-mediated inhibition of T-helper cells and enhancement of T-suppressor cells [62]. Additionally, Mustafa et al demonstrated mitoxantrone suppression of the spontaneous production of IFN-γ–secreting T cells and those primed by myelin antigens [79]. Consistent with an effect on cell-mediated immunity were studies of mitoxantrone in EAE that revealed suppression of acute and relapsing models [65–67]. The effect of mitoxantrone on demyelination was demonstrated by suppression of leukocyte- and macrophage-mediated myelin degradation in the EAE model [68]. Additional studies by these investigators demonstrated that mitoxantrone inhibited the development of EAE after 12 days of immunization and prevented the incidence of subsequent relapses when given in the recovery phase of a paralytic episode. These results indicate that mitoxantrone exerts a broad spectrum of immunosuppression affecting T cells, B cells, and macrophages, all of which are believed influential in the ongoing immune process in MS.

Safety profile of mitoxantrone

In general, most groups believed that mitoxantrone generally is well tolerated, with the expected side effects common to anthraquinone antineoplastic agents (Box 2) [69,70,77,80,81]. As with cyclophosphamide, amenorrhea is a potential serious side effect of mitoxantrone. Hartung et al report that 7 of 25 patients treated in the higher-dose mitoxantrone group had amenorrhea during treatment, which was sustained in 5 patients 1 year after cessation of therapy. Conversely, patients treated with a lower dose of mitoxantrone (5 mg/m^2) had a lower rate of amenorrhea (2 of 27 during treatment and none 1 year afterwards), and it has been suggested that this effect is related to treatment schedule verses total cumulative dose [70,82]. Edan et al report that in seven women who had transient amenorrhea and were treated for 6 months with mitoxantrone (20 mg), the amenorrhea was persistent in only one patient, who was 44 years old [69].

A major concern with the use of mitoxantrone is the potential for cardiac toxicity. The cardiotoxic effect of mitoxantrone, although less than related compounds doxyrubicin and epirubicin, has been studied and established within the oncology literature [64,83–86]. Potential cardiac events include the development of arrhythmias, asymptomatic decrease in left ventricular ejection fraction (LVEF), or symptomatic congestive heart failure (CHF). The risk factors reported in the oncology literature for developing cardiac toxicity are related to cumulative mitoxantrone dose and prior exposure to doxyrubicin. Ghalie et al published the largest report of cardiac events in patients who had MS and were treated with mitoxantrone [80]. Data from three mitoxantrone clinical trials, which included data from 1378 patients, were used for the analysis. Baseline and follow-up LVEF was available for 779 of these patients, with a mean duration of 29 months. The cumulative dose ranged from 2 to 183 mg/m^2, with a mean of 60.5 mg/m^2, and 141 patients received more than 100 mg/m^2. All patients had baseline LVEF greater than 50%. Of 1398 patients, two patients died (<0.2%) from CHF; one patient received a cumulative dose of 162 mg/m^2; and the other patient had received one dose of 9 mg/m^2. Seventeen of 779 patients developed asymptomatic decreased LVEF less than 50%; an incidence rate of 1.8%

Box 2. Side effects of mitoxantrone

Nausea
Alopecia
Menstrual disorders and infertility
Leukopenia and infection
Cardiac toxicity
Risk of leukemia

was determined for a cumulative dose below 100 mg/m^2 compared with 5.0% for a cumulative dose of 100 mg/m^2 or higher. Additionally, Avasarala et al reported on 47 patients prospectively treated with mitoxantrone 12.5 mg/m^2 every 3 months and determined that 5 of 28 patients who received a minimum of 3 doses had a significant decrease in mean LVEF (13.4%) [87]. These investigators proposed that LVEF monitoring should start early and be repeated on a routine basis during treatment with mitoxantrone. This challenges the current recommended guidelines that suggest routine monitoring of LVEF only after cumulative dose reaches 100 mg/m^2, at which time it should be completed before every additional dose. Because of concerns for potential cardiac toxicity, the package insert for mitoxantrone recommends a maximum cumulative dose of 140 mg/m^2, which allows a patient potentially to receive 2 to 3 years of mitoxantrone at 8–12 mg/m^2 administered every 3 months.

Topoisomerase inhibitors, such as mitoxantrone, are known to be associated with therapy-related leukemias, with an incidence ranging from 2% to 12% [88]. The risk of mitoxantrone as a single agent, as it is used in MS, is difficult to determine from the oncology literature where it typically is used in combination with other chemotherapy agents. Ghalie et al published a second report evaluating the risk of therapy-related leukemia after mitoxantrone treatment in MS on the same 1378 patients used to evaluate the risk of cardiac toxicity [81]. The mean cumulative dose of mitoxantrone was 60.5 mg/m^2 with a mean follow-up of 36 months; only one case of leukemia was found; therefore, an incidence proportion of 0.07% was calculated. The patient was part of the French cohort and was diagnosed with acute promyelocytic leukemia 13 months after the sixth monthly dose of mitoxantrone (20 mg/m^2) [89]. Subsequently, three additional reports of therapy-related leukemia have been diagnosed in patients treated with mitoxantrone for MS [90,91]. The long-term risk of leukemia from mitoxantrone used to treat MS, therefore, needs to be defined.

Current clinical use of mitoxantrone

Mitoxantrone obtained FDA approval in the fall of 2000, primarily based on the phase III data reported by Hartung et al [70]. In general, mitoxantrone is considered to have the potential to provide a beneficial effect similar to pulse cyclophosphamide therapy in patients who are selected properly (ie, those who have a strong inflammatory component to their disease). As with cyclophosphamide, the most consistent finding with mitoxantrone in the published trials is the improvement in relapse rate and suppression of inflammatory lesions seen on MRI. The protocol widely used for mitoxantrone is 12 mg/m^2 every 3 months for 24 months (see Table 2). Alternatively, protocols are proposed that include an induction period of 12 mg/m^2 monthly for 3 months, followed by a maintenance phase with infusions every 3 months for a total of 2 years or a maximum cumulative dose of 120 mg/m^2 [82]. At the authors' center, a lower dose of 8 mg/m^2 of mitoxantrone is used for the induction and for the every 3-month infusions in an attempt to extend the duration of therapy. Marked immunosuppression has been achieved after 3 to 4 monthly infusions of mitoxantrone followed by a maintenance period; therefore, an induction regimen potentially may maximize the immunosuppressive effect of mitoxantrone for active patients who have a prominent inflammatory component to their disease [82].

Methotrexate

In a randomized placebo-controlled trial of 60 patients who had primary or secondary progressive MS, conducted during a 3-year follow-up period before the widespread use of IFN-β and GA, weekly low-dose (7.5 mg) oral methotrexate (MTX) was shown to reduce the rate of progression of upper extremity functional impairment significantly ($P = 0.007$), as measured by a 9-hole peg test [92]. More recently, Calabresi et al reported a 44% reduction in the number of MRI contrast-enhanced lesions ($P = 0.02$) in 15 relapsing patients treated with weekly doses of 20 mg of oral MTX in combination with weekly IM injections of IFN-β1a (30 μg IM) for a 6-month period [93]. This combination likewise is considered relatively safe and well tolerated, with nausea the primary side effect. The combination of MTX (20 mg oral) and IFN-β1a (30 μg IM) with or without monthly pulse MP in patients who have breakthrough disease activity on IFN-β1a is currently being studied in a randomized multicenter study.

Azathioprine

Azathioprine (Imuran) is a purine analog used widely in Europe for the treatment of MS and in the United States as a steroid-sparing agent in a variety of rheumatic and autoimmune diseases. A 1991 meta-analysis of 793 patients from seven controlled clinical trials, including patients who had relapsing-remitting and secondary progressive MS, concluded that there was a modest effect on EDSS by the second year of treatment that was sustained into the third year [94]. Small studies of combination therapy with various IFN preparations, especially in treatment refractory MS, have shown modest positive results in clinical [95,96] and MRI [97] parameters.

Mycophenolate mofetil

This newer antimetabolite, mycophenolate mofetil (MMF; CellCept), blocks de novo purine metabolism in B and T lymphocytes and has gained wide acceptance in the transplantation community as a less toxic replacement of azathioprine. In a small, open-label trial of MMF of seven patients who had chronic progressive or relapsing-remitting MS, five patients stabilized after a treatment duration of 1 to 18 months [98]. Two abstracts presented at the 2004 American Academy of Neurology annual meeting reported preliminary data on the safety and efficacy of MMF in patients who had MS. The first of these studies reported on 42 patients who had relapsing-remitting or progressive MS and who received 2 g/d of MMF as monotherapy for a 3-year duration and found it safe and well tolerated [99]. The second was an open-label study of 30 patients who had relapsing-remitting MS who received MMF in combination with weekly IFN-β1a (30 μg IM) during a 6-month period and reported that 25 of 28 patients had clinical stabilization by EDSS and a decrease in contrast-enhancing lesions, suggesting a potential clinical and MRI benefit to this combination [100].

Methylprednisolone

Despite its widespread use in the treatment of relapses and as add-on therapy in worsening MS, controlled clinical trials of high-dose MP as a primary immunosuppressant therapy in MS are few. Goodkin et al reported a significant delay in time-to-treatment progression in patients who had secondary progressive MS and were treated with 3 days of high-dose MP (500 mg/d), compared with low-dose MP (10 mg/d), followed by an oral prednisone taper given every 8 weeks for 2 years [101]. Zivadinov et al randomized 88 patients who had relapsing-remitting MS to receive 5 days of 1000 mg/d MP pulse therapy with an oral prednisone taper or treatment with the same regimen of MP for acute relapses only [102]. Pulse MP therapy was given every 4 months for 3 years and then every 6 months for the subsequent 2 years. There was a significant delay of sustained progression on EDSS in the pulse therapy group and a significant improvement in MRI measures, including T1 black hole volume and brain parenchymal volume. There was no significant difference between treatment arms regarding change in T2 lesion volume or annualized relapse rate. These two studies suggest an effectiveness of MP in the treatment of MS, as indicated by clinical and MRI parameters, in addition to a large body of accumulated clinical experience in the MS community suggesting that regular pulses of high-dose (eg, 500–1000 mg) IV MP generally are well tolerated and may be effective in the slowing of disability in MS.

Summary

Based on the review of the literature and the authors' experience, immunosuppressive therapy plays an important role in the treatment of MS. Furthermore, given the understanding of the pathologic processes involved, the beneficial effect of immunosuppressive therapy is assumed to

Box 3. Factors associated with a response to cyclophosphamide

1. Rapidly progressive course
2. Gadolinium-positive lesions on MRI
3. Relapses in the year prior to therapy
4. Fewer than 2 years in progressive phase
5. Younger age

be greater in the earlier stages of the illness and relatively ineffective in the later stages, or in patients who have primary progressive disease. This concept is exemplified by the factors predictive of a response to cyclophosphamide, which correlate more with the inflammatory components of the disease and less with the degenerative processes (Box 3). Presumably, these factors can be applied to all immunosuppressive agents used to treat patients who are not responding to standard immunomodulatory therapy.

Characteristics of patients who have active MS and are not responding to standard immunomodulatory therapy with IFN-β or GA have yet to be clearly established; however, there are typical characteristics used to define treatment failures in clinical trials (Box 4). The authors use these definitions as a guide for selecting patients for immunosuppressive therapy; however, clinical judgment based on the individual clinical situation prevails. Certainly, the severity of clinical progression, and MRI activity, as well as the severity and frequency of relapses will influence the decision to change therapy. Nevertheless, the definitions of a nonresponder from clinical trials resemble the predictive factors for a response to immunosuppressive therapy. Therefore, nonresponders potentially represent ideal candidates for this type of therapy. The authors have created an algorithm as a general guide for selecting appropriate patients and the manner in which to use each type of immunosuppressive therapy (Fig. 1). Although oral immunosuppressants and pulse MP lack the profound immunosuppressive and anti-inflammatory activity demonstrated by cyclophosphamide and mitoxantrone, studies

Box 4. Definition of nonresponders to interferon-β or glatiramer acetate from clinical trials

All occurring within a 1-year period:

1. Progression > 1 point on EDSS if baseline EDSS > 0 or >1.5 points if baseline EDSS = 0
2. At least 2 relapses with objective change on neurologic examination
3. Increased MRI activity: at least 2 contrast-enhancing lesions or two new T2 lesions

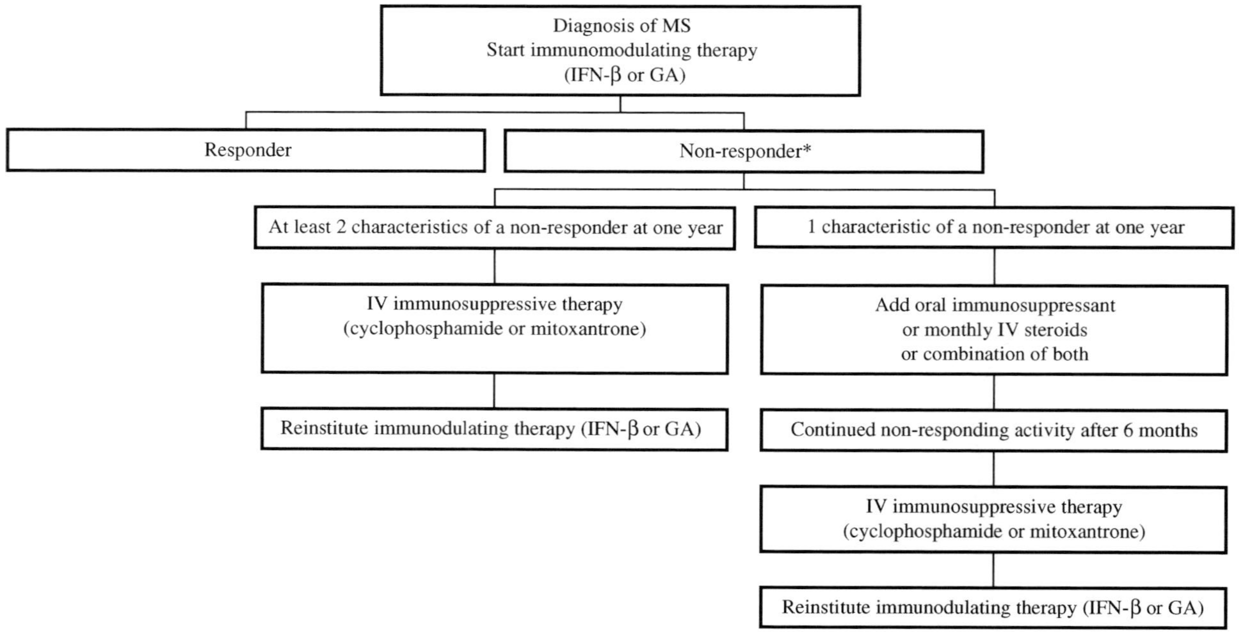

Fig. 1. Algorithm for the use of immunosuppressant therapy in nonresponders to IFN-β or GA. *May consider switching to a different immunomodulator if considered to have mild clinical or MRI activity.

show a beneficial effect of both and the authors believe they are used best in combination with IFN-β or GA in patients who have less severe disease activity. Based on the published literature, patients who are failing standard therapy and patients who have very active relapsing-remitting or early progressive MS, as represented by multiple characteristics of continued disease activity, should be considered candidates for either cyclophosphamide or mitoxantrone treatment. The treatment regimens and proper safety monitoring for all the immunosuppressants reviewed are outlined in Table 2. As discussed previously, induction therapy with cyclophosphamide is limited to selected cases of fulminant MS and must be used judiciously with special regard to monitoring for toxicity.

Given that early inflammatory events seem to correlate with later disability, a major question is whether or not strong anti-inflammatory drugs, such as cyclophosphamide or mitoxantrone, will have an impact on later degenerative changes if given early in the disease to halt inflammation. Because standard immunomodulatory therapy is known to be only partially effective, immunosuppressive therapy plays an important role in early treatment of the inflammatory stage of the disease. The time of intervention and duration of treatment requires further study and the degree to which these agents are synergistic with IFN-β or GA is unknown. Nonetheless, cyclophosphamide and mitoxantrone are limited by their toxicity for widespread use in the early stages of MS, and testing the hypothesis that a strong anti-inflammatory or immunomodulatory regimen has a greater impact if given earlier in the disease requires less toxic immune specific agents. Additionally, because of the risk of long-term toxic effects of cyclophosphamide and mitoxantrone, there is a limited duration for their use and patients eventually need an alternative therapy. Currently, the authors reinstitute treatment with IFN-β or GA after completion of treatment with either cyclophosphamide or mitoxantrone. The role of immunosuppressive therapy is expected to change with the potential approval of natalizumab (Antegren), which may occur in 2005. Because of the safety profile and the effect on inflammatory MRI lesions demonstrated in the phase II trial of natalizumab, it might be considered first-line therapy for patients who are failing IFN-β and GA [103]. Immunosuppressive therapy then would be considered in patients who are not responding to natalizumab.

References

[1] Martin R, McFarland H, McFarlin D. Immunological aspects of demyelinating diseases. Annu Rev Immunol 1992;10:153–87.

[2] Hafler D, Weiner H. Immunologic mechanisms and therapy in multiple sclerosis. Immunol Rev 1995;144:75–107.

[3] Conlon P, Oksenberg J, Zhang J, et al. The immunobiology of multiple sclerosis: an autoimmune disease of the central nervous system. Neurobiol Dis 1999;6:149–66.

[4] Weiner HL. A 21 point unifying hypothesis on the etiology and treatment of multiple sclerosis. Can J Neurol Sci 1998;25:93–101.
[5] Windhagen A, Newcombe J, Dangond F, et al. Expression of co-stimulatory molecules B7–1(CD80), B7–2 (CD86),and interleukin 12 cytokine in multiple sclerosis lesions. Exp Med 1995;182:1985–96.
[6] Langford C, Klippel J, Balow J, et al. Use of cytotoxic agents and cyclosporine in the treatment of autoimmune disease: part 1. Rheumatologic and renal diseases. Ann Intern Med 1998;128:1021–8.
[7] Langford C, Klippel J, Balow J, et al. Use of cytotoxic agents and cyclosporine in the treatment of autoimmune disease: part 2. Inflammatory bowel disease, systemic vasculitis, and therapeutic toxicity. Ann Intern Med 1998;129:49–58.
[8] Aimard G, Girard P, Raveau J. Multiple slerosis and autoimmunization process. Treatment by antimitotics. Lyons Med 1966;215:345–52.
[9] Weiner H, Cohen J. Treatment of multiple sclerosis with cyclophosphamide: critical review of clinical and immunologic effects. Mult Scler 2002;8:142–54.
[10] Girard P, Pellet H. Therapeutique immuno-depressive en neurogie. Presse Med 1967;75: 967–8.
[11] Millac P, Miller H. Cyclophosphamide in multiple sclerosis. Lancet 1967;1:783.
[12] Weiczorek VL, Brodkorb W. Erfahrungen mit der immunosuppressive behandlung der multiplen sklerose mit cyclophamid und imuran. Disch Ges Wesen 1971;26:1791–4.
[13] Gopel W, Benkenstein H, Banzhaf M. Immunosuppressive therapy of multiple sclerosis using cyclophosphamide and imuran. Report on 57 cases. Dtsch Gesundheitsw 1972;27: 1955–61.
[14] Cendrowski W. Combined therapeutic trial in multiple sclerosis: hydrocortisone hemisuccinate with cyclophosphamide or cytosine arabinoside. Acta Neurol Belg 1973;73: 209–19.
[15] Drachman D, Paterson P, Schmidt R, et al. Cyclophosphamide in exacerbations of multiple sclerosis. Therapeutic trial and a strategy for pilot drug studies. J Neurol Neurosurg Psychiatry 1975;38:592–7.
[16] Hommes O, Prick J, Lamers K. Treatment of the chronic progressive form of multiple sclerosis with a combination of cyclophosphamide and prednisone. Clin Neurol Neurosurg 1975;78:59–72.
[17] Hommes O, Lamers K, Reekers P. Effect of intensive immunosuppression on the course of chronic progressive multiple sclerosis. J Neurol 1980;223:177–90.
[18] Hommes O, Lamers K, Reekers P. Prognostic factors in intensive immunosuppression on the course of chronic progressive multiple sclerosis. Berlin: Springer-Verlag; 1980. p. 396–400.
[19] Gonsette RE, Demonty L, Delmotte P. Intensive immunosuppression with cyclophosphamide in multiple sclerosis. Follow up of 110 patients for 2–6 years. J Neurol 1977;214: 173–81.
[20] Gonsette RE, Demonty L, Delmotte P. Intensive immunosuppression with cyclophosphamide in remittent forms of multiple sclerosis: follow-up of 134 patients for 2–10 years. In: Bauer HJ, editor. Progress in multiple sclerosis research. Berlin (Germany): Springer-Verlag; 1980.
[21] Hauser S, Dawson D, Lehrich J, et al. Intensive immunosuppression in progressive multiple sclerosis. A randomized, three-arm study of high-dose intravenous cyclophosphamide, plasma exchange, and ACTH. N Engl J Med 1983;308:173–80.
[22] Carter JL, Hafler DA, Dawson DM, et al. Immunosuppression with high-dose i.v. cyclophosphamide and ACTH in progressive multiple sclerosis: cumulative 6-year experience in 164 patients. Neurology 1988;38:9–14.
[23] Goodkin D, Plencner S, Palmer-Saxerud J, et al. Cyclophosphamide in chronic progressive multiple sclerosis. Maintenance vs nonmaintenance therapy. Arch Neurol 1987;44:823–7.

[24] Weiner HL, Mackin GA, Orav EJ, et al. Intermittent cyclophosphamide pulse therapy in progressive multiple sclerosis: final report of the Northeast Cooperative Multiple Sclerosis Treatment Group. Neurology 1993;43:910–8.
[25] Hohol M, Olek M, Orav E, et al. Treatment of progressive multiple sclerosis with pulse cyclophosphamide/methylprednisolone: response to therapy is linked to the duration of progressive disease. Mult Scler 1999;5:403–9.
[26] Likosky W, Fireman B, Elmore R, et al. Intense immunosuppression in chronic progressive multiple sclerosis: the Kaiser study. J Neurol Neurosurg Psychiatry 1991;54: 1055–60.
[27] The Canadian Cooperative Trial of Cyclophosphamide and Plasma Exchange in Progressive Multiple Sclerosis. Lancet 1991;337:441–6.
[28] Noseworthy J, Ebers G, Roberts R. Cyclophosphamide and MS. Neurology 1994;44: 579–81.
[29] Weiner HL, Dawson DM, Hafler DA, et al. Cyclophosphamide and plasma exchange in multiple sclerosi. Lancet 1991;337:1033–4.
[30] Noseworthy J, Vandervourt MK, Penman M, et al. Cyclophosphamide and plasma exchange in multiple sclerosis. Lancet 1991;337:1540–1.
[31] Killian J, Bressler R, Armstrong R, et al. Controlled pilot trial of monthly intravenous cyclophosphamide in multiple sclerosis. Arch Neurol 1988;45:27–30.
[32] D'Andrea F, D'Aurizio C, Marini C, et al. Cyclophosphamide in relapsing remitting multiple sclerosis. Ital J Neurol Sci 1990;11:271–4.
[33] Millefiorini E, Di Giovanni M, Bernardi S, et al. 24-month follow-up of multiple sclerosis patients treated with cyclophosphamide. Ital J Neurol Sci 1990;11:605–7.
[34] Khan O, Zvartau-Hind M, Caon C, et al. Effect of monthly intravenous cyclophosphamide in rapidly deteriorating multiple sclerosis patients resistant to conventional therapy. Mult Scler 2001;7:185–8.
[35] Gobbini M, Smith M, Richert N, et al. Effect of open label pulse cyclophosphamide therapy on MRI measures of disease activity in five patients with refractory relapsing-remitting multiple sclerosis. J Neuroimmunol 1999;99:142–9.
[36] Patti F, Cataldi M, Nicoletti F, et al. Combination of cyclophosphamide and interferon-beta halts progression in patients with rapidly transitional multiple sclerosis. J Neurol Neurosurg Psychiatry 2001;71:404–7.
[37] Perini P, Gallo P. Cyclophosphamide is effective in stabilizing rapidly deteriorating secondary progressive multiple sclerosis. J Neurol 2003;250:834–8.
[38] Zephir H, De Seze J, Duhamel A, et al. Treatment of progressive forms of multiple sclerosis by cyclophosphamide: a cohort study of 490 patients. J Neurol Sci 2004;218:73–7.
[39] Smith DR, Weinstock-Guttman B, Cohen JA, et al. Randomized trial of pulse cyclophosphamide therapy and interferon beta 1a in patients with active MS [abstract]. Presented at the annual meeting of the American Academy of Neurology. Hawaii, 2003.
[40] Paterson P, Drobish D. Cyclophosphamide:effect on experimental allergic encephalomyelitis in Lewis rats. Science 1969;165:191–2.
[41] Moody D, Fahey J, Grable E, et al. Administration of monthly pulses of cyclophosphamide in multiple sclerosis patients. Delayed recovery of several immune parameters following discontinuation of long-term cyclophosphamide treatment. J Neuroimmunol 1987;14: 175–82.
[42] Moody D, Kagan J, Liao D, et al. Administration of monthly-pulse cyclophosphamide in multiple sclerosis patients. Effects of long-term treatment on immunologic parameters. J Neuroimmunol 1987;14:161–73.
[43] Hafler D, Orav J, Gertz R, et al. Immunologic effects of cyclophosphamide/ACTH in patients with chronic progressive multiple sclerosis. J Neuroimmunol 1991;32:149–58.
[44] Mickey M, Ellison G, Fahey J, et al. Correlation of clinical and immunological states in multiple sclerosis. Arch Neurol 1987;44:371–5.

[45] Smith D, Balashov KE, Hafler DA, et al. Immune deviation following pulse cyclophosphamide/methylprednisolone treatment of multiple sclerosis: increased interleukin-4 production and associated eosinophilia. Ann Neurol 1997;42:313–8.
[46] Comabella M, Balashov K, Issazadeh S, et al. Elevated interleukin-12 in progressive multiple sclerosis correlates with disease activity and is normalized by pulse cyclophosphamide therapy. J Clin Invest 1998;102:671–8.
[47] Takashima H, Smith DR, Fukaura H, et al. Pulse cyclophosphamide plus methylprednisolone induces myelin-antigen-specific IL-4-secreting T cells in multiple sclerosis patients. Clin Immunol Immunopathol 1998;88:28–34.
[48] Karni A, Balashov K, Hancock W, et al. Cyclophosphamide modulates CD4(+) T cells into a T helper type 2 phenotype and reverses increased IFN-gamma production of CD8(+) T cells in secondary progressive multiple sclerosis. J Neuroimmunol 2004;146:189–98.
[49] Hommes O, Aerts F, Bahr U, Schulten H. Cyclophosphamide levels in serum and spinal fluid of multiple sclerosis patients treated with immunosuppression. J Neurol Sci 1983;58:297–303.
[50] Bahr U, Hommes O, Aerts F. Determination of cyclophosphamide in urine, serum, and cerebrospinal fluid of multiple sclerosis patients by field desorption spectrometry. Clin Chim Acta 1980;103:183–92.
[51] Wender M, Tokarz E, Michalowska G, Wajgt A. Therapeutic trials of multiple sclerosis and intrathecal IgG production. Ital J Neurol Sci 1986;7:205–8.
[52] Lamers K, Uitdehaag B, Hommes O, et al. The short-term effect of an immunosuppressive treatment on CSF myelin basic protein in chronic progressive multiple sclerosis. J Neurol Neurosurg Psychiatry 1988;51:1334–7.
[53] Portaccio E, Zipoli V, Siracusa G, et al. Safety and tolerability of cyclophosphamide 'pulses' in multiple sclerosis: a prospective study in a clinical cohort. Mult Scler 2003;9:446–50.
[54] Boumpas D, Austin H, Vaughan E, et al. Risk for sustained amenorrhea in patients with systemic lupus erythematosus receiving intermittent pulse cyclophosphamide therapy. Ann Intern Med 1993;119:366–9.
[55] Gourley M, Austin H, Scott D, et al. Methylprednisolone and cyclophosphamide, alone or in combination, in patients with lupus nephritis. A randomized, controlled trial. Ann Intern Med 1996;125:549–71.
[56] Moore MJ. Clinical pharmacokinetics of cyclophosphamide. Clin Pharmacokinet 1991;20:194–208.
[57] Radis C, Kahl L, Baker G, et al. Effects of cyclophosphamide on the development of malignancy and on long-term survival of patients with rheumatoid arthritis. A 20-year followup study. Arthritis Rheum 1995;38:1120–7.
[58] Talar-Williams C, Hijazi YM, Walther MM, et al. Cyclophosphamide-induced cystitis and bladder cancer in patients with Wegener granulomatosis. Ann Intern Med 1996;124:477–84.
[59] Ehninger G, Proksch B, Heinzel G, et al. Clinical pharmacology of mitoxantrone. Cancer Treat Rep 1986;70:1373–8.
[60] Crespi M, Ivanier S, Genovese J, et al. Mitoxantrone affects topoisomerase activities in human breast cancer cells. Biochem Biophys Res Commun 1986;136:521–8.
[61] Fidler J, DeJoy S, Gibbons JJ. Selective immunomodulation by the antineoplastic agent mitoxantrone. I. Suppression of B lymphocyte function. J Immunol 1986;137:727–32.
[62] Fidler J, DeJoy S, Smith FR, et al. Selective immunomodulation by the antineoplastic agent mitoxantrone. II. Nonspecific adherent suppressor cells derived from mitoxantrone-treated mice. J Immunol 1986;136:2747–54.
[63] Rosenberg LS, Carvlin MJ, Krugh T. The antitumor agent mitoxantrone binds cooperatively to DNA: evidence for heterogeneity in DNA conformation. Biochemistry 1986;25:1002–8.

[64] Posner L, Dukart G, Goldberg J, et al. Mitoxantrone: an overview of safety and toxicity. Invest New Drugs 1985;3:123–32.
[65] Levine S, Saltzman A. Regional suppression, therapy after onset and prevention of relapses in experimental allergic encephalomyelitis by mitoxantrone. J Neuroimmunol 1986;13: 175–81.
[66] Ridge SC, Sloboda A, McReynolds R, et al. Suppression of experimental allergic encephalomyelitis by mitoxantrone. Clin Immunol Immunopathol 1985;35:35–42.
[67] Lublin F, Lavasa M, Viti C, Knobler R. Suppression of acute and relapsing experimental allergic encephalomyelitis with mitoxantrone. Clin Immunol Immunopathol 1987;45: 122–8.
[68] Watson CM, Davison AN, Baker D, et al. Suppression of demyelination by mitoxantrone. Int J Immunopharmacol 1991;13:923–30.
[69] Edan G, Miller D, Clanet M, et al. Therapeutic effect of mitoxantrone combined with methylprednisolone in multiple sclerosis: a randomised multicentre study of active disease using MRI and clinical criteria. J Neurol Neurosurg Psychiatry 1997;62: 112–8.
[70] Hartung H, Gonsette R, Konig N, et al. Mitoxantrone in progressive multiple sclerosis: a placebo-controlled, double-blind, randomised, multicentre trial. Lancet 2002;360: 2018–25.
[71] Gonsette R, Demonty L. Immunosuppression with mitoxantrone in multiple sclerosis: a pilot study for 2 years in 22 patients. Neurology 1990;40(Suppl 1):261.
[72] Kappos L, Gold R, Künstler E, et al. Mitoxantrone (Mx) in the treatment of rapidly progressive MS: a pilot study with serial gadolinium (Gd)-Enhanced MRI. Neurology 1990;40(Suppl 1):261.
[73] Mauch E, Kornhuber H, Krapf H, et al. Treatment of multiple sclerosis with mitoxantrone. Eur Arch Psychiatry Clin Neurosci 1992;242:96–102.
[74] Krapf H, Mauch E, Fetzer U, et al. Serial gadolinium-enhanced magnetic resonance imaging in patients with multiple sclerosis treated with mitoxantrone. Neuroradiology 1995;37:113–9.
[75] Noseworthy J, Hopkins M, Vandervoort M, et al. An open-trial evaluation of mitoxantrone in the treatment of progressive MS. Neurology 1993;43:1401–6.
[76] Bastianello S, Pozzilli C, D'Andrea F, et al. A controlled trial of mitoxantrone in multiple sclerosis: serial MRI evaluation at one year. Can J Neurol Sci 1994;21:266–70.
[77] Millefiorini E, Gasperini C, Pozzilli C, et al. Randomized placebo-controlled trial of mitoxantrone in relapsing-remitting multiple sclerosis: 24-month clinical and MRI outcome. J Neurol Sci 1997;244:153–9.
[78] Van de Wyngaert FA, Beguin C, D'Hooghe MB, et al. A double-blind clinical trial of mitoxantrone versus methylprednisolone in relapsing, secondary progressive multiple sclerosis. Acta Neurol Belg 2001;101:210–6.
[79] Mustafa M, Diener P, Sun J, et al. Immunopharmacologic modulation of experimental allergic encephalomyelitis: low-dose cyclosporin-A treatment causes disease relapse and increased systemic T and B cell-mediated myelin-directed autoimmunity. Scand J Immunol 1993;38:499–507.
[80] Ghalie R, Edan G, Laurent M, et al. Cardiac adverse effects associated with mitoxantrone (Novantrone) therapy in patients with MS. Neurology 2002;59:909–13.
[81] Ghalie R, Mauch E, Edan G, et al. A study of therapy-related acute leukemia after mitoxantrone therapy for multiple sclerosis. Mult Scler 2002;8:441–5.
[82] Gonsette RE. Mitoxantrone in progressive multiple sclerosis: when and how to treat? J Neurol Sci 2003;206:203–8.
[83] Dukart G, Barone J. An overview of cardiac episodes following mitoxantrone administration. Cancer Treat Symp 1984;3:35–41.
[84] Foster B, Lev L, Bermann C, et al. Cardiac events in Phase II trials with mitoxantrone. Cancer Treat Symp 1984;3:43–6.

[85] Mather F, Simon R, Clark G, Von Hoff D. Cardiotoxicity in patients treated with mitoxantrone: Southwest Oncology Group phase II studies. Cancer Treat Rep 1987;71: 609–13.

[86] Aviles A, Arevila N, Diaz Maqueo J, et al. Late cardiac toxicity of doxorubicin, epirubicin, and mitoxantrone therapy for Hodgkin's disease in adults. Leuk Lymphoma 1993;11: 275–9.

[87] Avasarala J, Cross A, Clifford D, et al. Rapid onset mitoxantrone-induced cardiotoxicity in secondary progressive multiple sclerosis. Mult Scler 2003;9:59–62.

[88] Felix CA. Secondary leukemias induced by topoisomerase-targeted drugs. Biochem Biophys Acta 1998;1400:233–55.

[89] Brassat D, Recher C, Waubant E, et al. Therapy-related acute myeloblastic leukemia after mitoxantrone treatment in a patient with MS. Neurology 2002;59:954–5.

[90] Goodkin DE. Therapy-related leukemia in mitozantrone treated patients. Mult Scler 2003; 9:426.

[91] Cattaneo C, Almici C, Borlenghi E, et al. A case of acute promyelocytic leukaemia following mitoxantrone treatment of multiple sclerosis. Leukemia 2003;17:985–6.

[92] Goodkin D, Rudick R, VanderBrug-Medendorp S, et al. Low-dose (7.5 mg) oral methotrexate reduces the rate of progression in chronic progressive multiple sclerosis. Ann Neurol 1995;37:30–40.

[93] Calabresi P, Wilterdink J, Rogg J, et al. An open-label trial of combination therapy with interferon beta-1a and oral methotrexate in MS. Neurology 2002;58:314–7.

[94] Yudkin PL, Ellison GW, Ghezzi AG, et al. Overview of azathioprine treatment in multiple sclerosis. Lancet 1991;338:1051–5.

[95] Lus G, Romano F, Scuotto A, et al. Azathioprine and interferon beta (1a) in relapsing-remitting multiple sclerosis patients: increasing efficacy of combined treatment. Eur Neurol 2004;51:15–20.

[96] Fernandez O, Guerrero M, Mayorga C, et al. Combination therapy with interferon beta-1b and azathioprine in secondary progressive multiple sclerosis. A two-year pilot study. J Neurol 2002;249:1058–62.

[97] Markovic-Plese S, Bielekova B, Kadom N, et al. Longitudinal MRI study: the effects of azathioprine in MS patients refractory to interferon beta-1b. Neurology 2003;60:1849–51.

[98] Ahrens N, Salama A, Haas J. Mycophenolate-mofetil in the treatment of refractory multiple sclerosis. J Neurol 2001;248:713–4.

[99] Vukusic S, Ducray F, Gignoux L, et al. Mycophenolate mofetil: an open-label study in 42 MS patients [abstract]. Presented at the annual meeting of the American Academy of Neurology. San Francisco, 2004.

[100] Vermersch P, Waucquier N, Bourteel H, et al. Treatment of multiple sclerosis with a combination of interferon beta-1a (Avonex) and mycophenolate mofetil (CellCept): results of a phase II clinical trial [abstract]. Presented at the annual meeting of the American Academy of Neurology. San Francisco 2004.

[101] Goodkin D, Kinkel R, Weinstock-Guttman B, et al. A phase II study of i.v. methylprednisolone in secondary-progressive multiple sclerosis. Neurology 1998;51: 239–45.

[102] Zivadinov R, Rudick RA, De Masi R, et al. Effects of IV methylprednisolone on brain atrophy in relapsing-remitting MS. Neurology 2001;57:1239–47.

[103] Miller D, Khan O, Sheremata W, et al. A controlled trial of natalizumab for relapsing multiple sclerosis. N Engl J Med 2003;348:15–23.

NEUROLOGIC CLINICS

Neurol Clin 23 (2005) 273–300

Immunoablative Therapy as a Treatment for Aggressive Multiple Sclerosis

Harold Atkins, MD[a], Mark Freedman, MD[b,*]

[a]*Ottawa Hospital Blood and Marrow Transplant Program, Ottawa, Ontario, Canada*
[b]*Ottawa Hospital Multiple Sclerosis Clinic, Ottawa, Ontario, Canada*

In the majority of patients, multiple sclerosis (MS) begins with a course of clinical relapses and remissions. The relapses often are accompanied by activity on MRI that has been correlated to evidence of localized inflammation in the central nervous system (CNS). These inflammatory lesions are characterized pathologically by infiltrates of immune cells. In later stages of disease, the relapses and remissions and the MRI activity seem to become less prominent and are replaced by a slowly progressive clinical course. Magnetic resonance spectroscopy studies show a reduction in neuronal expression markers, such as n-acetylaspartate, supporting the concept that the pathologic basis of progression is the destruction of neurons and axons [1,2]. The seminal observations of Trapp and colleagues [3] show that axonal transections are most numerous in lesions that are the most inflammatory. Kuhlmann et al [4] demonstrate the expression of early death markers in neurons at the initial stages of relapsing-remitting disease. These and other studies strongly support the hypothesis that early inflammatory events lead to the eventual loss of axons and neurons [5]

Current disease-modifying agents that either down-regulate or stem the flow of inflammatory immune cells into the brain reduce clinical and MRI-linked inflammatory events and slow, at least in the short-term, observed clinical progression. When these agents seem unable to control disease progression, the introduction of therapy that is more immunosuppressive often slows down the destructive neurologic disease process again. Inevitably, disease progression continues because incomplete suppression of inflammation fails to prevent the damage of axons and neurons. Complete abrogation of the inflammatory response at an early stage of MS,

* Corresponding author. University of Ottawa, Ottawa Hospital–General Campus, 501 Smyth Road, Ottawa, ON K1H 8L6, Canada.

E-mail address: mfreedman@ottawahospital.on.ca (M. Freedman).

doi:10.1016/j.ncl.2004.09.004

when the nervous system has not sustained permanent damage, is more likely to be successful at staving off the inevitable progression and even may allow more restorative repair processes.

Immunology of multiple sclerosis

Virtually all elements of the immune system, cellular and humoral, are implicated in some fashion in the pathogenesis of MS [6,7]. The triggers of autoimmunity in MS, as with so many other autoimmune diseases, are unknown. Evidence suggests that a sequence of environmental triggers upsets the delicate balance between tolerance and nontolerance of "self" antigens, possibly through the mechanism of molecular mimicry. Although the exact etiopathogenesis of MS is unknown, the leading theory suggests that T cells are the conductors of a misdirected immune response that targets myelin in the CNS. T-helper cells gaining entry to the CNS recruit B cells, monocytes, macrophages, and CNS microglia through the release of cytokines. All these elements have been demonstrated in MS lesions.

Once an immune attack commences against a "self" antigen, such as CNS myelin, it is perpetuated by immune memory. Furthermore, with time, the autoimmune attack initiated against a single myelin epitope, such as myelin basic protein, myelin oligodendroglial protein, and proteolipid protein, among others, spreads and becomes directed against additional epitopes within the same myelin protein and then to other myelin proteins, a phenomenon called epitope spreading [8]. Immune memory and epitope spreading are mechanisms believed to underlie the chronicity of the disease.

Clinical studies with low-dose immunosuppression in multiple sclerosis

Immunosuppressive therapy that leads to the overall reduction of lymphocytes is associated with some degree of benefit in MS (for more detailed discussion see the article in this issue by Gauthier, Buckle and Weiner). There are several studies aimed at either mild immunosuppression or selective reduction of lymphocyte subsets. Mild chemotherapy, with oral doses of azathioprine [9] or methotrexate [10], has shown only modest if any benefit. Total lymphoid irradiation demonstrated a transient slowing of MS disease progression but repeated treatments were not possible for resurgent disease [11]. Cyclophosphamide (CTX), a cytotoxic alkylating chemotherapeutic drug, given usually as an induction treatment followed by some degree of maintenance therapy, has shown some benefit in various regimens [12]. The purine analog, 2-chlorodeoxyadenosine, a somewhat selective lymphocytotoxic agent, seemed to reduce MRI activity and relapses but failed to prevent progression [13,14]. More recently, novel widespread immunosuppression using a monoclonal antibody to a general leukocyte marker (campath-1H) showed good suppression of MRI disease activity, a reduction in relapses, and some slowing of progression [15]. This treatment was complicated, however, by an unprecedented increase in autoimmune thyroid disease [16]. Combination therapies directed against T and B cells, such as CTX and plasma exchange, have shown only limited benefit [17,18]. The most successful immunosuppressive regimen has been mitoxantrone. This anthracycline not only suppressed MRI activity and reduced clinical relapses but also was shown to have a measurable effect at slowing progression [19]. Mitoxantrone is the only formally approved immunosuppressive drug for advancing MS.

With all of these immunosuppressive treatments, disease inevitably returns because such therapies have failed to remove the elements of the immune system involved in the CNS inflammation or have failed to remove the "memory" of myelin attack. Intensive immunosuppression using high-dose chemotherapy with or without additional total body radiation (TBI) therapy has been performed for many years in the setting of allogeneic bone marrow transplantation for leukemia [20]. Adapting the profound immunosuppression associated with the treatment of hematologic cancer to patients who have autoimmune diseases has allowed researchers to test the importance of immune ablation in the treatment of MS.

Transplantation overview

In general usage, hematopoietic stem cell transplantation (HSCT) is a colloquialism referring to a complex medical procedure (Fig. 1) that includes:

1. Collection of a graft containing hematopoietic stem cells (HSC)
2. Treatment of the underlying disease with dose-intensive therapy—the preparative regimen
3. Infusion of the HSC graft

Each component of the procedure can be performed in several ways and the exact procedure influences the expected outcome and toxicity.

High-dose cytotoxic therapy results in the ablation of the bone marrow and immune system. Patients become aplastic and immunologically crippled without replacement of the HSC. Stem cell transplantation reseeds the marrow, moderating the myelotoxicity and providing for immune recovery, thereby reducing morbidity and mortality in the immediate post-transplant period.

Reconstitution of the immune system can be accomplished with lymphocytes derived from pluripotential HSC. The adult HSC give rise to progeny responsible for endothelial, myeloid blood cell, and lymphocyte development. The progeny of the common lymphocyte precursor differentiate into the various lymphocyte lineages and give rise to a naive polyclonal immune system with a diverse protective repertoire. T-cell receptor rearrangement and B-cell immunoglobulin gene rearrangement occur at the time of or just after commitment to the specific lymphocyte lineage. Clonal

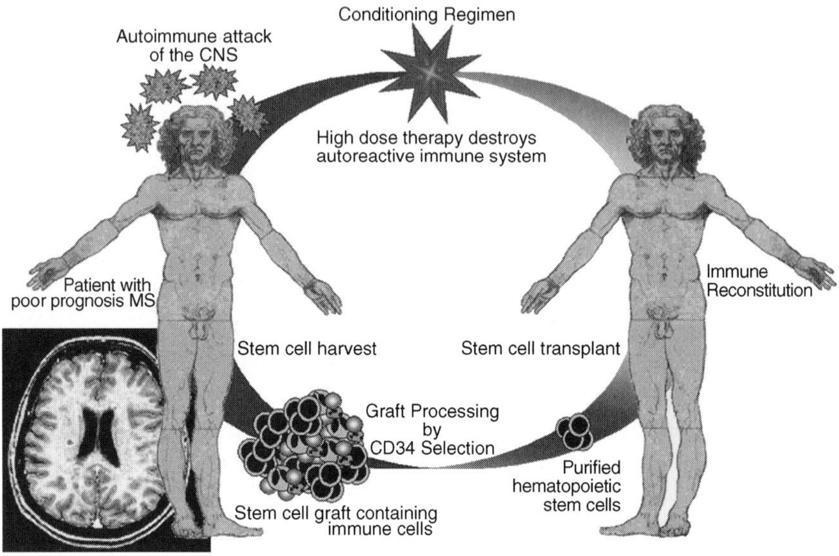

Fig. 1. Patients who have aggressive MS have HSC harvested after their mobilization from the bone marrow into the circulation by a combination of chemotherapy and cytokine. The stem cell graft is processed to remove contaminating immune cells, thereby avoiding reintroduction of autoreactive memory cells after transplantation. The conditioning regimen, consisting of intensive cytotoxic therapy, is administered to destroy the autoreactive immune system responsible for chronic CNS inflammation. The purified stem cells are transplanted into the patient to regenerate the blood organ and a naive, presumably tolerant, immune system.

expansion follows activation of the immune receptor by antigen binding with some of the cells becoming memory cells (Fig. 2). Primitive HSC do not carry the immunologic memory of previous exposures; thus, the regenerated immune system does not have a memory of its previous reactivity (and autoreactivity). Given that the exact sequence of environmental triggers is unlikely to be repeated as the new immune system evolves, a reappearance of autoimmunity is improbable.

It is estimated that more than 45,000 transplants were performed worldwide in 2002 for a variety of malignant and nonmalignant diseases [21]. The increased use of transplantation parallels the drop in mortality and improvements in morbidity associated with the use of high-dose chemotherapy and radiation. In some registries, mortality associated with the use of high-dose cytotoxic therapy with autologous stem cell rescue is as low as 3% [22]. The risk of regimen-related mortality is related to several factors, including the source of the stem cells; the intensity of the chemotherapeutic regimen employed; and patient factors, such as previous exposure to cytotoxic chemotherapy, age, and preexisting organ dysfunction. Allogeneic stem cell transplantation is associated with mortality in the 20% to 30% range, higher than autologous transplantation because of graft-versus-host disease (GVHD) and the need for post-transplant immunosuppression, which

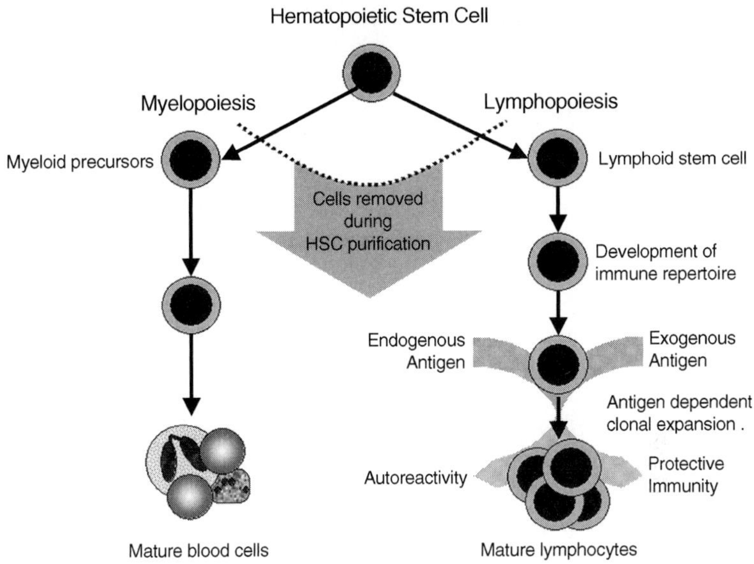

Fig. 2. The immune system's complex repertoire forms during lymphoid growth and development. Antigen exposure triggers an immune response and persistent immunologic memory. Intensive cytotoxic therapy kills the HSC and all its progeny, including the mature memory lymphocytes. Purified HSC do not have immunologic memory. After transplantation, their daughter cells grow and mature into all the cells of the blood and immune systems without recollection of pretransplantation antigen exposures.

increases the risk of opportunistic infections. Although most transplants are performed in patients under the age of 50 years, it is not uncommon for patients in their 60s to undergo autologous transplantation. Normal or near-normal cardiac, pulmonary, renal, and hepatic functions are necessary to help the patient cope with the complications of high-dose chemotherapy or TBI. The improved supportive care currently available has helped to change the resource use required. Currently, several programs perform transplants in a day hospital setting [23].

Several lines of evidence support a role for immunoablative therapy in the treatment of severe MS. These include:

- Animal studies
- Studies of humans who have autoimmune diseases and are undergoing transplantation for a malignancy
- Autologous stem cell transplantation for other autoimmune states

Animal studies of transplantation

Experimental autoimmune encephalitis (EAE) is an MS-like disease induced in susceptible rodents by immunization with spinal cord homogenates or myelin proteins. There are two phases of the disease, an acute relapsing-remitting phase and a chronic phase. As the disease moves from one phase to the next, epitope spreading occurs and the immune system responds to a greater variety of endogenous myelin antigens. In the acute phase, paresis of EAE animals resolves more rapidly after treatment with TBI or CTX and transplantation of marrow from a healthy littermate donor [24]. The remissions are durable with less than a third of animals progressing to the chronic relapsing phase, a lower incidence than in untreated affected animals [25]. Timing of the transplant is important; if the transplant is performed in the chronic phase of the illness, there is little recovery of neurologic function. Transplantation at an early time point has been shown to prevent glial scarring, whereas late transplantation may moderate but not prevent glial scarring [26]. These experiments demonstrate the effectiveness of immunoablative therapy in an MS-like illness and highlight the benefit of early intervention, before the illness undergoes a transition from primarily an inflammatory disease to a more progressive neurodegenerative disease.

This model supports the use of autologous HSC grafts, because marrow transplantation of EAE animals from donors who have active EAE is as effective as using marrow from healthy animals.The marrow used in these animal models, however, contains relatively few lymphocytes. Indeed, the reinfusion of marrow and splenocytes from an animal that has EAE, a rich source of myelin-reactive lymphocytes, increases the incidence of post-transplantation relapses [27]. Furthermore, lymphocyte transfusions, specifically myelin-reactive CD4 lymphocytes, can transfer EAE from an affected animal to a nonimmunized animal supporting the immune nature of this disease. These results argue for lymphocyte depletion of human autologous HSC grafts, as these grafts are heavily contaminated with lymphocytes.

Although EAE resolves after autologous marrow transplantation, this is not the case for all animal models of autoimmunity. The relative contribution of genetic and environmental susceptibility factors to the autoimmune process has an impact on the outcome of HSCT. Some animal models of autoimmunity have a predominant genetic predisposition, such as the MRL/lpr (fas deletion) mice that spontaneously develop a lupus-like illness [28]. But even in mice that have a single gene mutation, there are other genetic loci that influence the development of autoimmunity [29]. In other models, such as adjuvant-induced arthritis (AIA) or experimental autoimmune myasthenia gravis [30], rodents require antigenic exposure before they develop autoimmunity. Again, differences in susceptibility to autoimmune disease induction among rodent strains reveal that additional genetic susceptibility factors are required for the development of autoimmunity [31]. Autoimmunity does not recur after transplantation of HSC from isogenetic animals (pseudoautologous transplants) in models that require experimental antigenic exposure to induce the illness, such as AIA and EAE. In models of autoimmunity with a strong genetic predisposition, however, the autoimmunity tends to recur after HSCT from isogenetic animals. Allogeneic transplantation from a genetically normal donor is required to prevent the reappearance of the autoimmunity [32]. Autologous HSCT would be beneficial to patients afflicted with an autoimmune disease that requires a strong environmental trigger, whereas allogeneic transplantation may be required for prolonged disease remission in autoimmune diseases with a strong genetic basis. Unlike in animal models, where these susceptibility factors are understood, interpatient and disease heterogeneity of the genetic and environmental influences impact the outcome of human transplantation studies for autoimmune diseases in a manner that might be difficult to predict without careful clinical trials.

Human transplantation studies for coincident autoimmune diseases

Allogeneic HSCT has been used successfully for the treatment of severe aplastic anemia, an illness frequently caused by marrow-directed autoimmunity [33]. The impetus to study the role of transplantation came from the successful treatment of autoimmune diseases in case reports of patients who had malignancy and a concurrent autoimmune disease [34], including MS [35–37], and had undergone HSCT for the malignancy. The grafts were obtained from a healthy HLA-matched (allogeneic) donor. Recurrent synovitis has been reported in two patients who had a history of rheumatoid arthritis after allogeneic transplantation for gold-induced aplastic anemia, despite establishing that all the blood cells after transplantation were donor derived [38,39]. Psoriasis and an associated arthropathy recurred in a patient who had received an allogeneic transplant for chronic myelogenous leukemia [40]. Although occasional relapses have been reported, most patients had significant and lasting documented remissions of their autoimmune disease [34].

Experience in other autoimmune diseases

During the past 15 years, anecdotal case reports have suggested that high-dose chemotherapy with or without radiotherapy followed by autologous HSC support can result in long-term remissions of several autoimmune diseases. Reports to the European Bone Marrow Transplant Registry (EBMTR) and the International Bone Marrow Transplant Registry document more than 500 autologous stem cell transplants for a variety of autoimmune diseases [41]. Encouraging results emerged from phase I-II studies of patients who had advanced and refractory systemic lupus erythematosis, scleroderma, rheumatoid arthritis, and juvenile rheumatoid arthritis. Overall mortality for patients undergoing transplantation for autoimmune diseases remains in the 7% to 8% range, however. This varies by disease, with scleroderma patients, perhaps not surprisingly, having the highest treatment-related mortality. Research in this field is best illustrated by three registry-based randomized trials of autologous stem cell transplantation performed by the European Group for Blood and Marrow Transplantation in patients who had scleroderma, MS, and rheumatoid arthritis.

Transplant studies in multiple sclerosis

Nearly 150 patients have undergone autologous stem cell transplantation for MS with the procedures and outcomes reported in the literature as summarized in Tables 1 and 2. All were treated with cytotoxic chemotherapy. In some studies, TBI or an antibody preparation was added to the preparative regimen for further immune depletion. Sometimes the stem cell grafts were depleted of lymphocytes. Although these initial trials concentrated on studying the safety of the procedure for patients who had MS, some data were generated on the effectiveness of the procedure. More importantly, as patients who had various disease characteristics underwent treatment with differing transplant regimens, these studies provide clues about which factors are most important in determining positive treatment outcomes.

The impact of patient selection

Patient selection is critical when interpreting the outcomes of immune ablation and stem cell transplantation in MS. Those who have less accumulated disability have a greater chance of responding to treatments directed at modifying the immune system, given that inflammatory events are most prominent in this disease phase. Yet, given the significant risk of morbidity and mortality, treating young, less disabled patients with this procedure may be too aggressive. Alternatively, waiting until patients are too disabled would mean that the inflammation already has contributed to a significant amount of irreversible CNS damage. Such patients are more likely to have a neurodegenerative process and less likely to stabilize with a treatment directed at the detrimental effects of the immune system.

Early studies of transplantation tended to select patients who had advanced disease. In most, the median expanded disability status scale (EDSS) score before transplantation was 6.5 to 7.0. Approximately three quarters of the patients had secondary progressive MS (SPMS), whereas approximately two thirds of the remainder had a primary progressive (PPMS) course of MS; less than 10% had a purely relapsing-remitting course. Almost all patients were considered for transplantation after failing interferon therapy.

Table 1
Characteristics of patients with MS that have undergone autologous HSC transplantation

		Number of patients					EDSS		Duration (months)		Number of patients with Gd+ lesions on baseline MRI
Study	Reference	Total	PP	RR	PR	SP	Median	Range	Median	Range	
Nash et al	[43]	26	8	1	—	17	7.0	5.0–8.0	84	10–277	7
Burt et al	[50]	21	—	1	6	14	7.0	3.0–8.5	84	9–216	9
Carreras et al	[44]										
Saiz et al	[81,84]	15	—	9	—	6	6.0	4.5–6.5	96	12–228	5
Rossiev et al	[108]	23	3	3	—	17	n.a.	n.a.	—	26–144	—
Kozak et al	[46,47]	11	—	—	—	11	6.5	6.5–7.5	84	48–168	3
Openshaw et al	[45]	5	—	—	—	5	6.5	5.5–7.5	60	60–108	3
Fassas et al	[42]	24	8	—	3	13	6.0	4.5–8.0	126	24–336	6
Mancardi et al	[65,82]	10	—	—	4	6	6.5	5.5–8.0	144	72–228	7
Sun et al	[83]	4	1	—	—	3	6.0	6.0–7.0	138	84–228	—
Canadian MS-BMT	(Atkin HA, Freedman M, personal communication, 2004)	10	—	—	—	10	6.0	4.0–6.0	80	43–125	10
Total		149	20	14	13	102					50

Abbreviations: na, data not available; PP, primary progressive MS course; RR, relapsing-remitting MS course; PR, progressive-remitting MS course; SP, secondary progressive MS course.

Table 2
Treatment variables and outcomes of patients with MS that have undergone autologous HST transplantation

Study	Reference	Number of Patients	Mobilization		Graft selection	Conditioning regimen		Follow-up (months)		Outcome: number of patients positive/total number of patients		
			Cytokine	Chemotherapy		Regimen	ATG	Median	Range	Progression	Relapses	MRI activity
Nash et al	[43]	26	Yes	No	Yes	CTX/TBI	Yes	24	15–47	6/25	—	4/25
Burt et al	[50]	21	Yes	Yes	Yes	CTX/TBI	No	24	6–60	8/21	0	11/18
Carreras et al	[44]											
Saiz et al	[81,84]	15	Yes	Yes	Yes	BCNU/CTX	Yes	36	19–55	2/14	4/12	0/5
Rossiev et al	[108]	23	Yes	No	No	BEAM	Yes	—	—	—	—	—
Rossiev et al				Yes	No	No	Flud/mel	Yes				
Kozak et al	[46]	7	Yes	Yes	Yes	BEAM	Yes	9	1–18	1/10	—	1/6
Kozak et al	[47]	3	Yes	Yes	No	BEAM	Yes					
Openshaw et al	[45]	4	Yes	No	Yes	Bu/CTX	Yes	20	17–30	1/4	—	0/4
Openshaw et al		1	Yes	Yes	Yes	BEAM	Yes					
Fassas et al	[42]	15	Yes	Yes	No	BEAM	Yes	40	21–51	5/23	4/23	2/23
Fassas et al		9	Yes	Yes	Yes	BEAM	Yes					
Mancardi et al	[65,82]	10	Yes	Yes	No	BEAM	Yes	15	4–30	0/10	—	1/10
Su et al	[83]	4	Yes	No	Yes	CTX/TBI	Yes	12	6–12	0/12	—	1/3
Canadian MS-BMT	[75]	10	Yes	Yes	Yes	Bu/CTX	Yes	25	1–34	0	0	—

Abbreviations: BCNU, carmustine; BEAM, BCNU, etoposide, cytarabine and melphalan; Flud, fludarabine; Mel, melphalan.

There is some evidence that the course of MS has an impact on the outcome after transplantation. The 3-year post-transplant MS progression–free survival was reported as 92% for patients who had SPMS but was only 39% for those who had PPMS in the study by Fassas et al [42]. Although the follow-up was shorter, the incidence of continued disease activity by clinical phenotype was similar in the study by Nash et al [43]; two of 8 patients who had PPMS had sustained deterioration, whereas 4 of 17 who had SPMS progressed after transplantation. Although 2 of 9 patients who had SPMS continued to progress after transplantation in the study by Carreras et al [44], ongoing clinical evidence of disease activity was seen in 4 of the 6 patients who had relapsing-remitting MS.

Baseline disability seems to strongly influence outcome. None of the 9 patients who had EDSS less than or equal to 6.0 had significant sustained disease progression after transplantation, whereas 8 of the 12 patients who had a pretransplant EDSS greater than or equal to 6.5 had continued disease activity. Indeed, two patients in the latter group died between 12 and 18 months after transplantation from progressive MS. Similarly, in the study by Nash et al [43], 1 of 5 patients who had an EDSS less than or equal to 6.0 had sustained disease progression after transplantation, whereas 5 of the 20 patients who had a pretransplant EDSS greater than or equal to 6.5 remained active, and one patient who had a pretransplant EDSS of 7.5 died of progressive MS 23 months after the procedure. In another study, 2 of 7 patients who had an EDSS less than or equal to 6.0 had evidence of disease activity after transplantation, whereas 4 of the 7 patients who had a pretransplant EDSS greater than 6.5 manifested continued activity [44]. In a smaller study [45], 1 of 2 patients who had a baseline EDSS of 6.5 progressed after treatment, whereas disease was controlled in the two patients with EDSS less than or equal to 6.0. All 11 patients in the study by Kozak et al [46,47] had baseline EDSS scores greater than 6.5, but the patient who had the highest baseline disability progressed within 12 months of the transplant.

The applicability of the procedure is hindered by justified concern for transplant-related mortality. Transplantation is accepted in the treatment of malignancy because the illness has a substantial impact on survival; in contrast, MS generally does not have notable disease-associated mortality. Therefore, most trials were designed for patients who had advanced MS, where the impact on quality of life produced by the severe disabilities was believed to justify accepting the risks of the procedure [48,49]. In two studies that enrolled patients who had the most advanced disabilities [43,50], 3 of 47 patients died within 24 months of the transplant from progressive MS; only one patient died of transplant-related complications. These patients may be more likely to succumb to advancing MS than to transplantation complications. Procedures that control the disease may improve disease-related mortality but, ultimately, treating patients who have less advanced disabilities seems to be the most logical next step.

Stem cell mobilization

At steady state, the number of circulating HSC is low. This can be augmented by their mobilization from the bone marrow. HSC are mobilized from the bone marrow by disruption of their homing mechanisms using chemotherapy, cytokines, or both. Recombinant granulocyte colony-stimulating factor (G-CSF), administered once or twice daily by subcutaneous injection, is the most commonly used cytokine for HSC mobilization, effecting a dose-dependent mobilization of HSC. Doses of 5 μg/kg/d to 16 μg/kg/d of G-CSF have been used for stem cell mobilization of patients who have MS [51,52]. The drug is tolerated well but may cause headache, fatigue, and bone pain, which reverse with its discontinuation. G-CSF causes leukocytosis and splenic enlargement [53]. Anecdotally, this has resulted in splenic rupture in a small number of healthy donors [54–57]. G-CSF interacts with the hemostatic system and is associated with thrombosis in case reports [58,59].

G-CSF use is associated with dose-dependent flares of autoimmunity in some patients [60]. Burt et al [50] used G-CSF alone to mobilize HSC in patients who had MS until one of the first four patients had a flare of MS activity. Subsequent patients received CTX followed 72 hours later with G-CSF for HSC mobilization, and no further episodes of MS reactivation were noted. Nash et al [43] also reported a flare of MS in one of the first four patients who had MS and was treated with G-CSF mobilization. Subsequent patients received a 10-day course of prednisone (1 mg/kg) with the G-CSF and no other case of disease reactivation was reported. Openshaw et al [45] reported a patient who had MS who developed transient right hemiplegia during mobilization with G-CSF. A second attempt at HSC mobilization with chemotherapy followed by G-CSF was not complicated by flare of MS activity. Although most flares have been transient and reversible, one instance of a severe and treatment refractory flare of MS has occurred. A patient who had a cervical cord plaque developed respiratory failure after stem cell mobilization with G-CSF as a result of a flare of disease activity in the lesion [61]. Because of the recognized risk of MS flares when G-CSF is used alone, only 11% of patients reported to the EBMTR received single agent mobilization with G-CSF [62] Investigators have abandoned the use of cytokines alone for mobilization of stem cells for patients who have autoimmune diseases.

The use of chemotherapy and a hematopoietic growth factor for stem cell mobilization does not appear to be associated with activation of the autoimmune disease process. Most centers added CTX, a drug that has immune suppressing properties, to the G-CSF. Granulocyte-macrophage colony-stimulating factor is used in combination with CTX in a small proportion of patients who have MS and has not been reported to cause disease flares [46,62]. HSC are spared the cytotoxic effects of CTX because they contain a drug-inactivating enzyme, aldehyde dehydrogenase [63]. In addition to mobilizing stem cells, CTX may have a therapeutic benefit for patients who have autoimmune processes that are refractory to conventional therapy [64]. Mancardi et al [65] and Kozak et al [46,47], using CTX and G-CSF, did not report any change in MS activity associated with the mobilization protocol. In the authors' own series, an MRI scan performed 7 days after chemotherapy, but during G-CSF administration, showed a diminution of gadolinium (Gd) activity compared with baseline scans [66].

Chemotherapy increases the toxicity of the mobilization procedure. This includes transient syndrome of inappropriate antiduretic hormone secretion (SIADH), gastrointestinal upset, moderate alopecia, and transient pancytopenia, with an attendant risk of febrile neutropenia or sepsis. Hemorrhagic cystitis can result from the exposure of urothelium to acrolein, a metabolic degradation product of the CTX. Fassas et al [42] reported that 50% of patients developed febrile neutropenia after chemotherapy for stem cell mobilization. Four of these 12 patients had documented infections, including one patient who had serious polymicrobial sepsis. Eight of 11 patients described by Kozak et al [46,47] developed febrile neutropenia but other investigators report a lower incidence of toxicity [43,44].

Hematopoietic stem cell graft source

HSC may be obtained by direct aspiration from the bone marrow or by their removal from the circulation after mobilization. Marrow harvest is performed in the operating room under general or spinal anesthesia and causes short-lived postoperative pain. HSC are collected from the peripheral blood by leukopheresis using peripheral venous access; occasionally, a central venous catheter is required. Peripheral blood stem cell collections contain more HSC, resulting in a shorter period of post-transplant neutropenia. They contain approximately 10 times more lymphocytes than bone marrow harvests and this influences the post-transplant immune status of the recipient [67]. Peripheral blood stem cell collections technically are a more suitable product for ex vivo graft modifications, such as HSC selection or T-cell depletion.

Most investigators collected peripheral blood stem cells as the source of HSC. Generally, one to three leukopheresis procedures are required to collect sufficient stem cells for a transplant [43,44,46]. In the authors' experience, using large volume leukopheresis, 90% of patients have sufficient stem cells collected in one procedure. Occasionally, patients fail to mobilize stem cells into the circulation and these patients become ineligible for treatment with high-dose cytotoxic therapy. Inadequate stem cell mobilization occurred in 1 of 15 patients reported by Carreras [44]. Two of 11 of the patients reported by Kozak et al failed to mobilize stem cells [46]. Six of the 85 patients who had MS reported to the EBMTR used bone marrow harvest as the source of stem cells [62]. It is impossible to discern an effect between these different sources of stem cells on the outcome of MS after transplantation.

Ex vivo manipulation of the stem cell graft

Peripheral blood stem cell grafts contain significant numbers of immune cells. Adoptive transfer of autoimmune diseases after transplantation is well documented in animal models of autoimmunity and by transplanted lymphocytes in a number of clinical situations [68–70]. The most relevant example is the development of thyroiditis and vitiligo in transplant recipients of bone marrow from donors who have these autoimmune diseases [71–73]. Adoptive transfer of active autoimmunity does not occur in all instances, however. The recipient of an HSC graft from a donor who has rheumatoid arthritis [74] did not developed this disease in the first 4 years after transplantation. The authors have a patient who has not developed MS 5 years after receiving an allogeneic bone marrow transplant from a sibling who developed MS 1 year after the marrow donation. Autologous stem cell grafts, containing autoreactive lymphocytes, presumably could reinitiate the autoimmune disease after transplantation back into the patient, but this remains controversial.

Immune-mediated reactivity can be removed from a stem cell graft by lymphocyte depletion of the graft product using one of two ex vivo depletion strategies. Removing a population of cells that expresses a specific cell surface antigen, for example CD4-bearing lymphocytes, is a depletion or negative selection. The stem cell graft contains HSC and non–CD4-bearing lymphocytes. An alternate strategy purifies HSC, thus depleting the graft of all other contaminating cells. Older technology used a biotin-avidin interaction to enrich stem cells that express the CD34 surface antigen. Newer positive selection devices use immunomagnetic technology. Stem cell grafts are incubated with an anti-CD34 monoclonal antibody that is immobilized on a paramagnetic particle. The labeled HSC are retained in the magnetic field of a stem cell selector device while the remaining cells are washed away. The stem cells are washed and collected by releasing the magnetic field. Generally, a 10,000- to 100,000-fold depletion of lymphocytes can be obtained using the positive selection procedures. The purity and recovery of HSC vary with the processing technique.

The use of ex vivo selection technology to remove unwanted immune cells in the stem cell graft has not been consistent because of the controversy over its importance. Only 52 cases (61%) reported to the autoimmune disease working party registry of the EBMT used graft processing [62]. One study used unmanipulated stem cell grafts [65], whereas another used graft processing in 9 of their 24 patients [42]. Five studies used CD34 selection of the stem cell grafts [43–46,50]. Unprocessed stem cell grafts contained upwards of 50×10^6 T lymphocytes/kg [42], whereas the residual number of immune cells in processed grafts was dependent on the device used.

Processing with the Ceprate (Cellpro) reduced the T-cell burden to 7 × 10^4/kg [42]. The T-cell burden after selection with an Isolex 300i (Baxter) was variable across a range of 4–120 × 10^4/kg [43–45]. The T-cell burden was extremely low, less than 1 × 10^4/kg, after graft processing with a CliniMACS (Miltenyi Biotech) [44] (Atkins HA, Freedman MS, for the Canadian MS BMT study group, unpublished data, 2004).

It is difficult to relate the outcomes of the transplants back to whether or not the graft was processed, because of differences in the conditioning regimens and the stringency of lymphocyte depletion. Fassas et al did not detect a difference in the incidence of post-transplant MS progression in the 15 patients who received an unmanipulated graft compared with the 9 patients who received a CD34 selected graft [42]. The interpretation of this result is difficult because the processing procedure used in this study was only partially effective in removing contaminating T cells. Furthermore, the intensity of the conditioning regimen used was unlikely to completely ablate the immune system; the residual immunity masks any potential treatment benefit of removing immune cells from a stem cell graft. Thus, one must be cognizant of the intensity and effectiveness of the immune ablation and the rigor of the lymphocyte depletion of the stem cell graft when evaluating the role of graft processing.

Whether or not T-cell depletion increases the risk of opportunistic infections in the post-transplant period is ambiguous. Nash et al [43] report the death of one patient from Epstein-Barr Virus (EBV) lymphoproliferative disease after transplant in a patient who received a T-cell depleted HSC (TCD) graft and rabbit antithymocyte globulin (ATG), a recognized complication of severe T-cell immunodepletion. Reactivation of viral pathogens, however, such as CMV, has been reported in some [43,44], but not all, series [46,75] where T-cell depletion has been used, and CMV reactivation was seen in trials using unmanipulated grafts [65]. Similarly, the incidence of varicella zoster virus reactivation does not correspond to whether or not graft processing was used and ranges from 7% to 20% [43,44,46,50].

The role of biologic agents

Peritransplant administration of rabbit or equine ATG contributes to the immune ablation of the conditioning regimen. It also results in in vivo purging of reinfused lymphocytes. Most studies use ATG in the conditioning regimen for these purposes. Fully 80% of patients who had MS and were reported to the EBMTR received ATG [62]. The effectiveness of newer biologic agents, such as rituximab [75], daclizumab [76], and campath-1H [77], currently are being tested in clinical trials. A trial at Northwestern University proposes to study the effects of campath-1H, CTX, and stem cell transplantation in patients who have MS and who have failed interferon.

Transplant regimens

The conditioning regimen, used before the transplant, is composed of high-dose chemotherapy, radiotherapy, and other immune-suppressing agents. A variety of conditioning regimens have been used with the goal of depleting or ablating the autoreactive immune system. Several of these regimens have been adapted from the treatment of lymphoproliferative diseases. Another aim of the conditioning regimen is to eliminate the immune process in the CNS. This goal has been approached with the use of TBI or a systemically administered chemotherapeutic agent, such as busulphan or cytarabine, that cross the blood-brain barrier. Details of the conditioning regimens used are listed in Table 2.

Most investigators have used G-CSF after transplantation to aid neutrophil recovery after myeloablation. Neutrophil and platelet engraftment occurs within 1 to 2 weeks of HSC infusion; graft failure has not been reported to date. The median length of hospital stay for the transplant is approximately 25 days, although some patients require stays of up to 2 months for treatment of transplant-related complications [42,46,65]. There are no consistent differences in the rate or severity of treatment-related morbidity among the different conditioning regimens. This may reflect the small patient cohorts or the importance of patient selection and comorbidities.

The common short-term toxicity of conditioning regimens includes fatigue; decreased concentration; anorexia; a 10% to 15% loss in body weight; gastrointestinal mucosal breakdown, resulting in pain, ulceration, nausea, and diarrhea; fluid and electrolyte disturbances; alopecia; pancytopenia; the requirement for blood and platelet transfusions; febrile neutropenia; sepsis; and liver, renal, and lung toxicity. The frequency and severity of these side effects vary, depending on the intensity of the conditioning regimen. There also is marked interpatient variability in the severity of symptoms. These can be life threatening in some patients, yet others experience mild side effects. Survival and morbidity after transplantation are related to the patient's performance status, but it is difficult to discern any effect of MS disability on morbidity and mortality. Fortunately, the number of serious complications and deaths in published studies has been low. The noninfectious complications of the transplants in patients who have MS have been of moderate severity. Generally, the frequency of febrile neutropenia and the spectrum of infections during the period of neutropenia are typical of other autologous transplant populations receiving similar conditioning regimens.

A frequent "engraftment syndrome" is reported by some investigators [78]. Between 20% and 75% of patients who have MS, in some reports, present with noninfectious fevers, fatigue, and an erythematous maculopapular, or follicular, rash predominantly on the upper trunk [43,44]. Pruritis, minor pulmonary symptoms, and mild eosinophilia also may occur.

For most, symptoms last from 1 to 2 weeks and resolve spontaneously, whereas some patients may require a short pulse of steroids. Investigators using a TBI conditioning regimen report the syndrome most frequently, but it also is seen with non-TBI regimens. Patients undergoing autologous transplantation for malignancies also have developed this syndrome [79].

Because patients who have MS have abnormal bladder emptying, there is a concern about transplant complications related to the urinary tract. Exposure to acrolein, the toxic metabolite of CTX, may be prolonged, increasing the potential for hemorrhagic cystitis. This toxicity is minimized by forced diuresis, urinary catherization to maintain bladder drainage and the infusion of MESNA, which inactivates acrolein through a thiol-mediated chemical reaction. Only one patient has been reported with mild hemorrhagic cystitis [50], illustrating the effectiveness of these supportive measures. Catheterization results in a higher incidence of urinary tract infections than that seen in other transplant populations, however [43].

Possible late effects of chemotherapy include premature gonadal failure, shingles, and increased risk of secondary malignancies. There is a 10% to 20% incidence of late post-transplant disseminated or localized herpes varicella-zoster syndromes, consistent with other transplant populations. Somewhat more unusual are reports of CMV reactivation after autologous transplantation for MS. Although reactivation of CMV typically is a rare event after autologous HSCT for malignancies, in one series, reactivation of CMV occurred in 3 of 10 patients who had MS [65], and in 4 of 9 in another series [43]. This likely reflects the degree of immune ablation achieved by the conditioning regimens.

Mortality after autologous transplantation for malignancy is 2% to 10% and is dependent on the strength of the conditioning regimen and patient factors, including age, comorbidities, and performance status. Mortality has been reduced in recent years because of improved supportive care. The mortality of registry collections of patients who have and MS are undergoing transplantation does not seem excessive. The EBMTR reports a 4.7% mortality rate from treatment-related complications. Of the four patients who died within 60 days of their transplant, one succumbed to cardiac toxicity and three to infection [62]. Other fatal side effects include one instance each of veno-occlusive disease of the liver [75] and EBV lymphoproliferative disease [43]. The regimens containing busulphan or TBI generally are more intense with higher transplant-related mortality.

Outcome—clinical

An array of endpoints, including progression of disabilities, subjective and objective relapses, MRI lesions, and changes in cerebrospinal fluid (CSF) oligoclonal bands have been used to assess residual disease activity after transplantation. Up to 40% of patients who had MS progressed in different studies, with median post-transplant follow-ups of between 9 and 40 months.

The variability in outcome is multifactoral. Patient and disease-related factors may explain the difference in freedom from disease progression among the studies that used a BEAM conditioning regimen [42,46,65].

Differences in outcome also may reflect varied durations of follow-up, with some studies documenting increasing treatment failures with longer observation [42,43,50]. The distribution of time-to-progression events across the entire follow-up period and the lack of a plateau on the progression-free survival curves suggest that the underlying MS process may have been delayed but not eliminated. Some studies show a plateau in the time-to-progression curve after the early post-transplant period [80]. An optimist might suggest that the transplant controlled disease activity. Although studies to date enrolled patients who failed other therapies and tended to have advanced disease or a poor prognosis, caution is required when interpreting data on disease activity until there is sufficient long-term follow-up.

Using the first progression as the endpoint for a time-to-treatment failure analysis can underestimate the success of treatment. A more robust endpoint is continued progression over a prolonged period of observation. Early failure of treatment resulting from progression is seen in several patients. These patients accumulate disabilities in the early post-transplant period and then stabilize; this could reflect CNS damage occurring before immune ablation or as a result of the conditioning regimen. It is important to ascertain if these patients follow a course of progressive accumulation of disabilities or if their disabilities plateau.

More intense conditioning regimens provide better disease control. Studies using myelotoxic but not myeloablative regimens, such as BEAM or Carmustine (BCNU)/CTX, tend toward a higher failure rate than the stronger myeloablative regimens using Busulphan (Bu)/CTX or CTX/TBI. Incomplete disease control may occur after even the highest dose conditioning regimens if autoreactive lymphocytes are reintroduced into the patient in the stem cell graft. The ongoing Canadian MS-BMT study examines the effect of the most intense conditioning regimen combined with stringent lymphocyte depletion of the stem cell graft to test the hypothesis that complete ablation of the autoreactive immune system is necessary to provide complete and long-lasting disease control.

Fassas et al compared progression, defined as a rise in EDSS of 1.0 point (0.5 point if the baseline EDSS was greater than 5.0) persisting for more than 6 months with events, defined as any progression or relapse [42]. Progression-free survival was 76% at 3.7 years post transplant, but the event-free survival was markedly lower. In a similar analysis, Saiz et al [80] found only 5 of their 14 patients were free from relapses and deterioration on the Ambulation Index, yet 4 years after transplant nearly 85% of their patients were progression free. The relative stability of neurologic function in view of ongoing relapses suggests that these transplants may have "reset" the disease to an earlier phase. It has widely been believed that stopping the relentless deterioration of the patient's neurologic performance was essential for patients and their physicians to accept the risks of the transplant procedure, but less intense transplant conditioning regimens may provide significant disease control. Which strategy results in the best outcome for the patient, resetting the autoimmunity to an earlier stage in the disease course or eliminating the autoreactive process? Future studies must be directed at balancing the degree of disease control with treatment intensity and its attendant side effects.

Outcome—imaging

MRI metrics examined include the number of Gd-enhanced lesions, T2 lesion number, total T2 lesion volume, and atrophy. Gd-enhanced lesions either are absent or markedly reduced after cytotoxic therapy, reflecting control of the inflammatory process. Post-transplant Gd-enhanced activity generally was seen only in patients who had clinical evidence of progressive disease [43,50]. The appearance of new T2 lesions was reduced or absent in most patients after transplantation [65]. A 6% to 20% mean reduction in total T2 lesion volume was reported after transplantation [43]. Most of the reduction occurs in the first year after transplant with a slower resolution thereafter [80]. There is a broad range of changes, however, in total T2 lesion volume and unspecified numbers of patients had increased lesions. Four of the five patients in one series who had an increase in post-transplant total T2 lesion volume had clinically evident progression [50].

Despite the profound effect on inflammatory activity, there was ongoing evidence of atrophy, measured either as change in total brain volume [81], change in third ventricle diameter [50], or corpus callosum area [80]. Inglese et al noted an annual brain volume loss of nearly 2% during the first 2 years after transplant [81]. There was no correlation with baseline EDSS or T2 lesions appearing after transplantation. Third ventricle diameter increased by 10% to 50% in 8 of 21 patients after transplantation [50]. Most reduction in corpus callosal area occurred in the first year after transplantation. The investigators speculated that the apparent tissue loss might reflect changes in tissue water as a result of suppression of inflammation. There was ongoing loss of volume, however, in the second and third years [80]. The degree of ongoing corpus callosal atrophy was similar in magnitude to the loss of total brain volume. Interestingly, atrophy is progressive despite a reduction in the total T2 lesion volume and the absence of inflammatory changes. The MRI studies illustrate the impact of transplantation on reducing the inflammatory but not the neurodegenerative component of MS.

Outcome—pathology and immunology

A reduction or disappearance in oligoclonal bands in the CSF has been seen in approximately one quarter of patients when examined after transplantation. This occurred after treatment with busulphan, a drug with good CNS penetration, and TBI [43,45,75,82]. A reduction in oligoclonal bands has not been seen after treatment with drugs that do not cross the blood-brain barrier [83]. Serial CSF examination during the 2 years after transplantation shows a progressive reduction in CSF oligoclonal immunoglobulins in the initial three patients in the authors' series. These data suggest that aggressive transplant conditioning regimens can alter the immune system in the CNS.

Neuropathologic examination has been performed in two patients who died of transplant-related complications. Multiple small, demyelinated plaques with decreased axonal density were found 22 days after transplant [45]. Macrophages and round cells, presumably oligodendrocytes, were present at the edges of the lesions; only rare T and B cells were seen. Similarly, multiple demyelinating lesions with reduced axon density were seen in the second patient 63 days after transplantation [84]. There were focal perivascular infiltrates of macrophages and CD8 cells but no CD4 cells, plasma cells, or B cells. Some macrophages contained antimyelin peptides as evidence of recent demyelination. Most of the lesions were partly remyelinated [85]. Although the neuropathology was similar to that seen in other autopsy series of patients who had MS, it is unclear what the inflammatory change found these cases represents. It might reflect a response to damage in the CNS initiated before transplant, a response to the agents administered before transplantation, or the start of a clean-up process before the start of repair.

All patients become transiently lymphopenic after transplantation. Recovery of natural killer cells and B-cell subpopulations occurs in the first 3 to 6 months after transplantation. Thymopoiesis recovers within the first year of transplantation [82], but patients continue to have a persistent CD4 lymphopenia for 2 years or more. After transplantation, a diverse polyclonal T-cell receptor repertoire redevelops, but peripheral blood mononuclear cell proliferative responses to a panel of myelin peptides are reported to decrease. Alterations in the cytokine production by mononuclear cells and matrix protein production are reported. Further study of the changes induced in the immune system by transplantation ultimately may allow more selective methods of immune manipulation in MS.

Future considerations—patient selection

Which patients who have MS should be considered for immune ablation and autologous HSCT? Experience to date, and evidence that immune ablation is effective in reducing or eliminating inflammation in the CNS, suggests benefits from earlier intervention in this disease. Still, patients should have had a reasonable (at least 6 months, but ideally 1 year) chance to respond to the current disease modifying drugs, such as interferon or glatiramer acetate. There is ongoing debate as to whether or not mitoxantrone should be tried before considering a transplant, but in the population that has aggressive disease, that drug has not completely selected for transplantation arrested disease activity or progression [86–88].

Given the risks of the procedure, ethicists might advocate that individuals should be highly likely to develop significant life-altering disabilities over a short period despite all current therapies. There are no concrete prognostic indices of MS today, but natural history studies tells us that patients who have repeated attacks early in their disease course, incomplete recovery between attacks, and early involvement of pyramidal or cerebellar functional systems are most likely to progress. Untreated patients who have reached EDSS 3.0 with 5 attacks or more in the first 2 years after diagnosis have a nearly 95% chance of deterioration to an EDSS greater than or equal to 6.0 over the next decade [89]. Clearly, such patients warrant a more aggressive therapeutic approach.

Candidates should retain reasonable residual neurologic function, thereby ensuring a selection of patients who are more likely to be in the inflammatory stage of their illness and, provided there is elimination of ongoing progression, should retain high functionality. Patients who have advanced disabilities have been less responsive to transplantation. For similar reasons, patients who have PPMS are not optimal candidates, as only modest reported benefits were seen in those few that have undergone the procedure. This situation may change if regenerative strategies based on cellular therapeutics become feasible. The authors [90] and other investigators [91] consider the best candidates to be otherwise healthy, still mobile with an EDSS less than or equal to 6.0, and have ongoing inflammation despite currently accepted modalities of treatment.

Future considerations—allogeneic transplantation

Studies to date have used cytotoxic therapy to destroy the autoreactive immune system. Another strategy is to use allogeneic stem cell grafts to induce a graft-versus-host immune system reaction. Allogeneic stem cell grafts collected from a related or unrelated healthy donor typically are matched with the recipient at the major histocompatibility loci, but differences between the donor and recipient at minor histocompatibility gene loci allow donor lymphocytes to attack and destroy recipient lymphocytes. This immunologically mediated treatment effect, or graft-versus-autoimmunity phenomenon, can occur in the context of HSCT after immune suppressing but nonmyeloablative doses of therapy [92,93]. This strategy was tested extensively for low-grade lymphoproliferative diseases [94]. Although the risk of regimen-related toxicity is low, allogeneic immune attack of recipient organs leading to acute or chronic GVHD can occur [95]. Because of its higher mortality, workers in this field are cautious. Trials of nonmyeloablative transplantation in autoimmune diseases are being proposed [96].

Future considerations—beyond repair of the immune system

Stem cells exist in many organs in the body and are responsible for development and regeneration. Totipotent embryonal stem cells may be harnessed into new therapies, but their use is controversial. Primitive stem cells from one organ may be able to repair other damaged organs, and bone marrow stem cells exhibit such plasticity. Recipient-derived circulating blood cells are able to form endothelium and cardiomyocytes in heart transplant recipients [97]. Donor-derived cells are found in the liver [98], gastrointestinal tract [99], and brain [100,101] of allogeneic bone marrow transplant recipients. Bone marrow–derived cells are capable of differentiating into many specialized cell types, including oligodendrocytes and neurons. The progeny of grafted bone marrow cells are capable of differentiating into neurons in the brains of allogeneic transplant recipients who died [100,101], but the functionality of these cells has not been demonstrated. Reparative signals from damaged organ systems, in particular the brain, can drive the fate of stem cells, either nascent, injected, or implanted into the body [102]. This has spurred the testing of their ability to repair hearts damaged by coronary artery syndromes [103]. Similar repair mechanisms may operate in the CNS. Stem cell transplantation in rats aid functional recovery after stroke [104]. With improved understanding of the signals required to manipulate stem cell plasticity and repair, stem cell transplantation may be helpful in reconstructing the damage caused by MS.

Mesenchymal stem cells (MSC) are bone marrow–derived cells that repopulate the stromal elements of the marrow [105]. Neuronal precursors derived from MSC could be implanted directly into the brain to see if these are capable of initiating reparative processes. Such cells have been shown to migrate to sites of myelin damage, differentiate into functional oligodendrocytes, and aid functional recovery in rodent models. Similar studies using peripherally derived Schwann cells implanted into MS lesions, however, were not capable of anything more than survival [106]. MSC possesses the ability to modulate immune reactions and control life-threatening GVHD [107,108]. This immunosuppressive effect one day could be harnessed to treat autoimmunity. MSC are expanded ex vivo easily and can be directed by biochemical signals to differentiate into a number of different tissues in tissue culture, including neurons. Ongoing insights in this field open a number of new therapeutic avenues.

Summary

If the premise that MS is an acquired autoimmune process that produces chronic CNS inflammation is correct, it is reasonable to consider that a complete ablation of the immune system would remove the cells responsible and stop future damage. Careful monitoring of autologous transplant recipients can provide insights into the roles of genetic susceptibility, environmental elements, and inflammatory and neurodegenerative processes that contribute to the pathogenesis of this disease. The rationale for investigating this treatment becomes more robust given the potential that infused bone marrow–derived stem cells may be able to respond to CNS signals, guiding their differentiation into neurons or glia that are capable of promoting functional recovery.

Significant advances in the use of immune ablative therapy in the treatment of MS have occurred over the past several years. This promising therapy is one of the first to demonstrate that the natural history of aggressive MS, which causes progressive disability and incapacity through the relentless accumulation of immune-mediated brain damage, can be changed. The experience of centers investigating this treatment provides important lessons. The benefits of transplants are more likely to occur in patients treated early in the course of their disease. Patients who have MS experience predictable regimen-related toxicity, similar to other patient populations. Dose intensification seems to be associated with better disease control, but lesser degrees of immune ablation still provide important benefits to selected patients who have aggressive MS, resetting their illness to a more responsive stage. As the cohort of patients undergoing autologous stem cell transplantation grows, a better understanding of patient variables and treatment outcomes will allow tailoring of the intensity of immune ablation to optimize disease control and minimize toxicity. Future developments in this field include examining alternate methods of immune ablation, for instance using allogeneic stem cell grafts or newer biologic agents, and addressing the problems of improving preexisting disabilities, using cytokines and cellular therapies to guide CNS repair. Despite promising results, the potential side effects of the cytotoxic therapy and unanswered questions about long-term disease control warrant that this treatment remain investigational.

References

[1] Gonen O, Catalaa I, Babb JS, et al. Total brain N-acetylaspartate: a new measure of disease load in MS. Neurology 2000;11;54:15–9.

[2] Fu L, Matthews PM, De Stefano N, et al. Imaging axonal damage of normal-appearing white matter in multiple sclerosis. Brain 1998;121:103–13.

[3] Trapp BD, Peterson J, Ransohoff RM, et al. Axonal transection in the lesions of multiple sclerosis. N Engl J Med 1998;338:278–85.

[4] Kuhlmann T, Lingfeld G, Bitsch A, et al. Acute axonal damage in multiple sclerosis is most extensive in early disease stages and decreases over time. Brain 2002;125(Pt 10):2202–12.

[5] Filippi M, Bozzali M, Rovaris M, et al. Evidence for widespread axonal damage at the earliest clinical stage of multiple sclerosis. Brain(Pt 2):433–7.

[6] Markovic-Plese S, Pinilla C, Martin R. The initiation of the autoimmune response in multiple sclerosis. Clin Neurol Neurosurg 2004;106:218–22.

[7] Qin Y, Duquette P. B-cell immunity in MS. Int MS J 2003;10:110–20.

[8] Vanderlugt CL, Miller SD. Epitope spreading in immune-mediated diseases: implications for immunotherapy. Nat Rev Immunol 2002;2:85–95.

[9] Confavreux C, Vukusic S. Non-specific immunosuppressants in the treatment of multiple sclerosis. Clin Neurol Neurosurg 2004;106:263–9.
[10] Goodkin DE, Rudick RA, VanderBrug MS, et al. Low-dose oral methotrexate in chronic progressive multiple sclerosis: analyses of serial MRIs. Neurology 1996;47:1153–7.
[11] Cook SD, Devereux C, Troiano R, et al. Total lymphoid irradiation in multiple sclerosis: blood lymphocytes and clinical course. Ann Neurol 1987;22:634–8.
[12] Hohol MJ, Olek MJ, Orav EJ, et al. Treatment of progressive multiple sclerosis with pulse cyclophosphamide/methylprednisolone: response to therapy is linked to the duration of progressive disease. Mult Scler 1999;5:403–9.
[13] Sipe JC, Romine JS, Koziol JA, et al. Cladribine in treatment of chronic progressive multiple sclerosis. Lancet 1994;344:9–13.
[14] Rice GP, Filippi M, Comi G. Cladribine and progressive MS: clinical and MRI outcomes of a multicenter controlled trial. Cladribine MRI Study Group. Neurology 2000;54:1145–55.
[15] Moreau T, Coles A, Wing M, et al. CAMPATH-IH in multiple sclerosis. Mult Scler 1996;1: 357–65.
[16] Coles AJ, Wing M, Smith S, et al. Pulsed monoclonal antibody treatment and autoimmune thyroid disease in multiple sclerosis. Lancet 1999;354:1691–5.
[17] Khatri BO, McQuillen MP, Hoffmann RG, et al. Plasma exchange in chronic progressive multiple sclerosis: a long-term study. Neurology 1991;41:409–14.
[18] Weiner HL, Dau PC, Khatri BO, et al. Double-blind study of true vs. sham plasma exchange in patients treated with immunosuppression for acute attacks of multiple sclerosis. Neurology 1989;39:1143–9.
[19] Hartung HP, Gonsette R, Konig N, et al. Mitoxantrone in progressive multiple sclerosis: a placebo-controlled, double-blind, randomised, multicentre trial. Lancet 2002;28: 2018–25.
[20] Tabbara IA, Zimmerman K, Morgan C, et al. Allogeneic hematopoietic stem cell transplantation: complications and results. Arch Intern Med 2002;162:1558–66.
[21] IBMTR. 2004 Summary slide set. Available at: http://www.ibmtr.org/newsletter/sums_update.html. Accessed August 2004.
[22] Atkinson K, Nivison-Smith I, Hawkins T. Haemopoietic stem cell transplantation in Australia, 1992–95: a report from the Australian Bone Marrow Transplant Recipient Registry. Aust N Z J Med 1997;27:408–19.
[23] Dix SP, Geller RB. High-dose chemotherapy with autologous stem cell rescue in the outpatient setting. Oncology (Huntingt) 2000;14:171–85.
[24] Karussis D, Vourka-Karussis U, Mizrachi-Koll R, et al. Acute/relapsing experimental autoimmune encephalomyelitis: induction of long lasting, antigen-specific tolerance by syngeneic bone marrow transplantation. Mult Scler 1999;5:17–21.
[25] van Gelder M, Kinwel-Bohre EP, van Bekkum DW. Treatment of experimental allergic encephalomyelitis in rats with total body irradiation and syngeneic BMT. Bone Marrow Transplant 1993;11:233–41.
[26] Burt RK, Traynor AE, Pope R, et al. Treatment of autoimmune disease by intense immunosuppressive conditioning and autologous hematopoietic stem cell transplantation. Blood 1998;92:3505–14.
[27] van Gelder M, van Bekkum DW. Effective treatment of relapsing experimental autoimmune encephalomyelitis with pseudoautologous bone marrow transplantation. Bone Marrow Transplant 1996;18:1029–34.
[28] Nagata S, Suda T. Fas and Fas ligand: lpr and gld mutations. Immunol Today 1995;16: 39–43.
[29] Nose M, Nishihara M, Kamogawa J, et al. Genetic basis of autoimmune disease in MRL/lpr mice: dissection of the complex pathological manifestations and their susceptibility loci. Rev Immunogenet 2000;2:154–64.
[30] Pestronk A, Drachman DB, Teoh R, et al. Combined short-term immunotherapy for experimental autoimmune myasthenia gravis. Ann Neurol 1983;14:235–41.

[31] Kawahito Y, Cannon GW, Gulko PS, et al. Localization of quantitative trait loci regulating adjuvant-induced arthritis in rats: evidence for genetic factors common to multiple autoimmune diseases. J Immunol 1998;161:4411–9.

[32] Ikehara S, Inaba M, Yasumizu R, et al. Autoimmune diseases as stem cell disorders. Tohoku J Exp Med 1994;173:141–55.

[33] Georges GE, Storb R. Stem cell transplantation for aplastic anemia. Int J Hematol 2002;75:141–6.

[34] Nelson JL, Torrez R, Louie FM, et al. Pre-existing autoimmune disease in patients with long-term survival after allogeneic bone marrow transplantation. J Rheumatol Suppl 1997;48:23–9.

[35] McAllister LD, Beatty PG, Rose J. Allogeneic bone marrow transplant for chronic myelogenous leukemia in a patient with multiple sclerosis. Bone Marrow Transplant 1997;19:395–7.

[36] La Nasa G, Littera R, Cocco E, et al. Allogeneic hematopoietic stem cell transplantation in a patient affected by large granular lymphocyte leukemia and multiple sclerosis. Ann. Hematol 2004;83:403–5.

[37] Mandalfino P, Rice G, Smith A, et al. Bone marrow transplantation in multiple sclerosis. J Neurol 2000;247:691–5.

[38] McKendry RJ, Huebsch L, Leclair B. Progression of rheumatoid arthritis following bone marrow transplantation. A case report with a 13-year followup. Arthritis Rheum 1996;39:1246–53.

[39] Jacobs P, Vincent MD, Martell RW. Prolonged remission of severe refractory rheumatoid arthritis following allogeneic bone marrow transplantation for drug-induced aplastic anaemia. Bone Marrow Transplant 1986;1:237–9.

[40] Snowden JA, Kearney P, Kearney A, et al. Long-term outcome of autoimmune disease following allogeneic bone marrow transplantation. Arthritis Rheum 1998;41:453–9.

[41] Tyndall A, Gratwohl A. Cutting edge report—use of high-dose immunoablative therapy with hematopoietic stem cell support therapy in the treatment of severe autoimmune diseases. 2004. Available at: www.rheuma21st.com/archives/cutting_edge_tyndall_immuno_therapy.html. Accessed August 2004.

[42] Fassas A, Anagnostopoulos A, Kazis A, et al. Autologous stem cell transplantation in progressive multiple sclerosis–an interim analysis of efficacy. J Clin Immunol 2000;20:24–30.

[43] Nash RA, Bowen JD, McSweeney PA, et al. High-dose immunosuppressive therapy and autologous peripheral blood stem cell transplantation for severe multiple sclerosis. Blood 2003;102:2364–72.

[44] Carreras E, Saiz A, Marin P, et al. CD34 + selected autologous peripheral blood stem cell transplantation for multiple sclerosis: report of toxicity and treatment results at one year of follow-up in 15 patients. Haematologica 2003;88:306–14.

[45] Openshaw H, Lund BT, Kashyap A, et al. Peripheral blood stem cell transplantation in multiple sclerosis with busulfan and cyclophosphamide conditioning: report of toxicity and immunological monitoring. Biol Blood Marrow Transplant 2000;6(5A):563–75.

[46] Kozak T, Havrdova E, Pit'ha J, et al. High-dose immunosuppressive therapy with PBPC support in the treatment of poor risk multiple sclerosis. Bone Marrow Transplant 2000;25:525–31.

[47] Kozak T, Havrdova E, Pit'ha J, et al. Immunoablative therapy with autologous stem cell transplantation in the treatment of poor risk multiple sclerosis. Transplant Proc 2001;33:2179–81.

[48] Ekestern E, Lebhart G. Mortality from multiple sclerosis in Austria 1970–2001: dynamics, trends, and prospects. Eur J Neurol 2004;1:511–20.

[49] Warren S, Warren KG, Svenson LW, et al. Geographic and temporal distribution of mortality rates for multiple sclerosis in Canada, 1965–1994. Neuroepidemiology 2003;22:75–81.

[50] Burt RK, Cohen BA, Russell E, et al. Hematopoietic stem cell transplantation for progressive multiple sclerosis: failure of a total body irradiation-based conditioning regimen to prevent disease progression in patients with high disability scores. Blood 2003; 102:2373–8.

[51] Arbona C, Prosper F, Benet I, et al. Comparison between once a day vs twice a day G-CSF for mobilization of peripheral blood progenitor cells (PBPC) in normal donors for allogeneic PBPC transplantation. Bone Marrow Transplant 1998;22:39–45.

[52] Kroger N, Zander AR. Dose and schedule effect of G-GSF for stem cell mobilization in healthy donors for allogeneic transplantation. LeukLymphoma 2002;43:1391–4.

[53] Picardi M, De Rosa G, Selleri C, et al. Spleen enlargement following recombinant human granulocyte colony-stimulating factor administration for peripheral blood stem cell mobilization. Haematologica 2003;88:794–800.

[54] Kroger N, Renges H, Sonnenberg S, et al. Stem cell mobilisation with 16 microg/kg vs 10 microg/kg of G-CSF for allogeneic transplantation in healthy donors. Bone Marrow Transplantation 2002;29:727–30.

[55] Falzetti F, Aversa F, Minelli O, et al. Spontaneous rupture of spleen during peripheral blood stem-cell mobilisation in a healthy donor. Lancet 1999;353:555.

[56] Brown SL, Dale DC. Spontaneous splenic rupture following administration of granulocyte colony-stimulating factor (G-CSF): occurrence in an allogeneic donor of peripheral blood stem cells. Biol Blood Marrow Transplant 1997;3:341–3.

[57] Becker PS, Wagle M, Matous S, et al. Spontaneous splenic rupture following administration of granulocyte colony-stimulating factor (G-CSF): occurrence in an allogeneic donor of peripheral blood stem cells. Biol Blood Marrow Transplant 1997;3: 45–9.

[58] Canales MA, Arrieta R, Gomez-Rioja R, et al. Induction of a hypercoagulability state and endothelial cell activation by granulocyte colony-stimulating factor in peripheral blood stem cell donors. J Hematother Stem Cell Res 2002;11:675–81.

[59] Kuroiwa M, Okamura T, Kanaji T, et al. Effects of granulocyte colony-stimulating factor on the hemostatic system in healthy volunteers. Int J Hematol 1996;63:311–6.

[60] Snowden JA, Biggs JC, Milliken ST, et al. A randomised, blinded, placebo-controlled, dose escalation study of the tolerability and efficacy of filgrastim for haemopoietic stem cell mobilisation in patients with severe active rheumatoid arthritis. Bone Marrow Transplant 1998;22:1035–41.

[61] Openshaw H, Stuve O, Antel JP, et al. Multiple sclerosis flares associated with recombinant granulocyte colony-stimulating factor. Neurology 2000;54:2147–50.

[62] Fassas A, Passweg JR, Anagnostopoulos A, et al. Hematopoietic stem cell transplantation for multiple sclerosis. A retrospective multicenter study. J Neurol 2002;249:1088–97.

[63] Kastan MB, Schlaffer E, Russo JE, et al. Direct demonstration of elevated aldehyde dehydrogenase in human hematopoietic progenitor cells. Blood 1990;75:1947–50.

[64] Breban M, Dougados M, Picard F, et al. Intensified-dose (4 gm/m^2) cyclophosphamide and granulocyte colony-stimulating factor administration for hematopoietic stem cell mobilization in refractory rheumatoid arthritis. Arthritis Rheumatol 1999;42:2275–80.

[65] Mancardi GL, Saccardi R, Filippi M, et al. Autologous hematopoietic stem cell transplantation suppresses Gd-enhanced MRI activity in MS. Neurology 2001;57:62–8.

[66] Freedman MS, Bowman MJ, Atkins HA. Canadian BMT study group: reduction in gadolinium enhancing lesions and clinical stability in Multiple Sclerosis patients receiving a combination of cyclophosphamide and filgrastim (G-SCF) in preparation for stem cell mobilization. Neurology 2004;58.

[67] Couban S, Simpson DR, Barnett MJ, et al. A randomized multicenter comparison of bone marrow and peripheral blood in recipients of matched sibling allogeneic transplants for myeloid malignancies. Blood 2002;100:1525–31.

[68] Legendre C, Caillat-Zucman S, Samuel D, et al. Transfer of symptomatic peanut allergy to the recipient of a combined liver-and-kidney transplant. N Engl J Med 1997;337:822–4.

[69] Walter EA, Greenberg PD, Gilbert MJ, et al. Reconstitution of cellular immunity against cytomegalovirus in recipients of allogeneic bone marrow by transfer of T-cell clones from the donor. N Engl J Med 1995;333:1038–44.

[70] Bollard CM, Savoldo B, Rooney CM, et al. Adoptive T-cell therapy for EBV-associated post-transplant lymphoproliferative disease. Acta Haematol 2003;110:139–48.

[71] Alajlan A, Alfadley A, Pedersen KT. Transfer of vitiligo after allogeneic bone marrow transplantation. J Am Acad Dermatol 2002;46:606–10.

[72] Neumeister P, Strunk D, Apfelbeck U, et al. Adoptive transfer of vitiligo after allogeneic bone marrow transplantation for non-Hodgkin's lymphoma. Lancet 2000;15: 1334–5.

[73] Kishimoto Y, Yamamoto Y, Ito T, et al. Transfer of autoimmune thyroiditis and resolution of palmoplantar pustular psoriasis following allogeneic bone marrow transplantation. Bone Marrow Transplant 1997;19:1041–3.

[74] Snowden JA, Atkinson K, Kearney P, et al. Allogeneic bone marrow transplantation from a donor with severe active rheumatoid arthritis not resulting in adoptive transfer of disease to recipient. Bone Marrow Transplant 1997;20:71–3.

[75] Rastetter W, Molina A, White CA. Rituximab: expanding role in therapy for lymphomas and autoimmune diseases. Annu Rev Med 2004;55:477–503.

[76] Bielekova B, Richert N, Howard T, et al. Humanized anti-CD25 (daclizumab) inhibits disease activity in multiple sclerosis patients failing to respond to interferon beta. Proc Natl Acad Sci U S A 2004;101:8705–8.

[77] Coles A, Deans J, Compston A. Campath-1H treatment of multiple sclerosis: lessons from the bedside for the bench. Clin Neurol Neurosurg 2004;106:270–4.

[78] Oyama Y, Cohen B, Traynor A, et al. Engraftment syndrome: a common cause for rash and fever following autologous hematopoietic stem cell transplantation for multiple sclerosis. Bone Marrow Transplant 2002;29:81–5.

[79] Spitzer TR. Engraftment syndrome following hematopoietic stem cell transplantation. Bone Marrow Transplant 2001;27:893–8.

[80] Saiz A, Blanco Y, Carreras E, et al. Clinical and MRI outcome after autologous hematopoietic stem cell transplantation in MS. Neurology 2004;62:282–4.

[81] Inglese M, Mancardi GL, Pagani E, et al. Brain tissue loss occurs after suppression of enhancement in patients with multiple sclerosis treated with autologous haematopoietic stem cell transplantation. J Neurol Neurosurg Psychiatry 2004;75:643–4.

[82] Sun W, Popat U, Hutton G, et al. Characteristics of T-cell receptor repertoire and myelin-reactive T cells reconstituted from autologous haematopoietic stem-cell grafts in multiple sclerosis. Brain 2004;12:996–1008.

[83] Saiz A, Carreras E, Berenguer J, et al. MRI and CSF oligoclonal bands after autologous hematopoietic stem cell transplantation in MS. Neurology 2001;56:1084–9.

[84] Kuhlmann T, Metz I, Jansen G, et al. Histopathology of MS lesions after high-dose chemotherapy and haematopoietic stem cell rescue. American Academy of Neurology 2004. Abstract P02.120. Neurology 2004;62(suppl 5):A154.

[85] Bruck W, Porada P, Poser S, et al. Monocyte/macrophage differentiation in early multiple sclerosis lesions. Ann Neurol 1995;38:788–96.

[86] Hartung HP, Gonsette R, Konig N, et al. Mitoxantrone in progressive multiple sclerosis: a placebo-controlled, double-blind, randomised, multicentre trial. Lancet 2002;28: 2018–25.

[87] Millefiorini E, Gasperini C, Pozzilli C, et al. Randomized placebo-controlled trial of mitoxantrone in relapsing-remitting multiple sclerosis: 24-month clinical and MRI outcome. J Neurol 1997;244:153–9.

[88] Edan G, Miller D, Clanet M, et al. Therapeutic effect of mitoxantrone combined with methylprednisolone in multiple sclerosis: a randomised multicentre study of active disease using MRI and clinical criteria. J Neurol Neurosurg Psychiatry 1997; 62:112–8.

[89] Weinshenker BG, Bass B, Rice GP, et al. The natural history of multiple sclerosis: a geographically based study. 2. Predictive value of the early clinical course. Brain 1989;112: 1419–28.
[90] Freedman MS, Atkins HL. Suppressing immunity in advancing MS: too much too late, or too late for much? Neurology 2004;62:168–9.
[91] Fassas A, Kimiskidis VK. Autologous hemopoietic stem cell transplantation in the treatment of multiple sclerosis: rationale and clinical experience. J Neurol Sci 2004;15;223: 53–8.
[92] Kojima R, Kami M, Kim SW, et al. Induction of graft-versus-autoimmune (GVA) disease effect against refractory psoriasis by complete donor-type chimerism and graft-versus-host disease after allogeneic hematopoietic stem cell transplantation. Bone Marrow Transplant 2003;32:439–42.
[93] Slavin S, Nagler A, Varadi G, et al. Graft vs autoimmunity following allogeneic non-myeloablative blood stem cell transplantation in a patient with chronic myelogenous leukemia and severe systemic psoriasis and psoriatic polyarthritis. Exp Hematol 2000;28: 853–7.
[94] Seftel MD, Lavoie J, Barnett MJ, et al. Treatment of lymphoid malignancies with non-myeloablative stem cell transplantation. Hematology 2002;7:151–5.
[95] Maloney DG, Sandmaier BM, Mackinnon S, et al. Non-myeloablative transplantation. Hematology. Am Soc Hematol Educ Program 2002;392–421.
[96] Oyama Y, Traynor AE, Barr W, et al. Allogeneic stem cell transplantation for autoimmune diseases: nonmyeloablative conditioning regimens. Bone Marrow Transplant 2003; 32(Suppl 1):S81–3.
[97] Quaini F, Urbanek K, Beltrami AP, et al. Chimerism of the transplanted heart. N Engl J Med 2002;346:5–15.
[98] Korbling M, Katz RL, Khanna A, et al. Hepatocytes and epithelial cells of donor origin in recipients of peripheral-blood stem cells. N Engl J Med 2002;346:738–46.
[99] Okamoto R, Yajima T, Yamazaki M, et al. Damaged epithelia regenerated by bone marrow-derived cells in the human gastrointestinal tract. Nat Med 2002;8:1011–7.
[100] Cogle CR, Yachnis AT, Laywell ED, et al. Bone marrow transdifferentiation in brain after transplantation: a retrospective study. Lancet 2004;363:143–7.
[101] Mezey E, Key S, Vogelsang G, et al. Transplanted bone marrow generates new neurons in human brains. Proc Natl Acad Sci U S A 2003;100:1364–9.
[102] Martino G. How the brain repairs itself: new therapeutic strategies in inflammatory and degenerative CNS disorders. Lancet Neurol 2004;3:372–8.
[103] Yau TM, Tomita S, Weisel RD, et al. Beneficial effect of autologous cell transplantation on infarcted heart function: comparison between bone marrow stromal cells and heart cells. Ann Thorac Surg 2003;75:169–76 [discussion 176–7].
[104] Li Y, Chen J, Wang L, et al. Treatment of stroke in rat with intracarotid administration of marrow stromal cells. Neurology 2001;56:1666–72.
[105] Horwitz EM, Keating A. Nonhematopoietic mesenchymal stem cells: what are they? Cytotherapy 2000;2:387–8.
[106] Kohama I, Lankford KL, Preiningerova J, et al. Transplantation of cryopreserved adult human Schwann cells enhances axonal conduction in demyelinated spinal cord. J Neurosci 2001;21:944–50.
[107] Le Blanc K, Rasmusson I, Sundberg B, et al. Treatment of severe acute graft-versus-host disease with third party haploidentical mesenchymal stem cells. Lancet 2004;363:1439–41.
[108] Rossiev VA, Makarov SV, Aleksandrova II, et al. Experience with high-dose immunosuppressive therapy followed by transplantation of autologous stem hematopoietic cells in patients with multiple sclerosis. Ter Arkh 2002;74:35–8.

NEUROLOGIC CLINICS

Neurol Clin 23 (2005) 301–306

Index

Note: Page numbers of article titles are in **boldface** type.

0733-8619/05/$ - see front matter
doi:10.1016/S0733-8619(04)00124-0 ***neurologic.theclinics.com***

Changing Your Address?

Make sure your subscription changes too! When you notify us of your new address, you can help make our job easier by including an exact copy of your Clinics label number with your old address (see illustration below.) This number identifies you to our computer system and will speed the processing of your address change. Please be sure this label number accompanies your old address and your corrected address—you can send an old Clinics label with your number on it or just copy it exactly and send it to the address listed below.

We appreciate your help in our attempt to give you continuous coverage. Thank you.

W. B. Saunders Company
SHIPPING AND RECEIVING DEPTS.
151 BENIGNO BLVD.
BELLMAWR, N.J. 08031

SECOND CLASS POSTAGE
PAID AT BELLMAWR, N.J.

This is your copy of the
__________ CLINICS OF NORTH AMERICA

00503570 DOE—J32400 101 NH 8102

JOHN C DOE MD
324 SAMSON ST
BERLIN NH 03570

XP-D11494

JAN ISSUE

Your Clinics Label Number

Copy it exactly or send your label along with your address to:
W.B. Saunders Company, Customer Service
Orlando, FL 32887-4800
Call Toll Free 1-800-654-2452

Please allow four to six weeks for delivery of new subscriptions and for processing address changes.

Order your subscription today. Simply complete and detach this card and drop it in the mail to receive the best clinical information in your field.

YES! Please start my subscription to the **CLINICS** checked below with the ❑ first issue of the calendar year or ❑ current issues. If not completely satisfied with my first issue, I may write "cancel" on the invoice and return it within 30 days at no further obligation.

Please Print:

Name ______________________________

Address ______________________________

City ______________ State ______________ ZIP ______________

Method of Payment

❑ Check (payable to **Elsevier**; add the applicable sales tax for your area)

❑ VISA ❑ MasterCard ❑ AmEx ❑ Bill me

Card number ______________________ Exp. date ______________

Signature ______________________________

Staple this to your purchase order to expedite delivery

❑ **Adolescent Medicine Clinics**
- ❑ Individual $95
- ❑ Institutions $133
- ❑ *In-training $48

❑ **Anesthesiology**
- ❑ Individual $175
- ❑ Institutions $270
- ❑ *In-training $88

❑ **Cardiology**
- ❑ Individual $170
- ❑ Institutions $266
- ❑ *In-training $85

❑ **Chest Medicine**
- ❑ Individual $185
- ❑ Institutions $285

❑ **Child and Adolescent Psychiatry**
- ❑ Individual $175
- ❑ Institutions $265
- ❑ *In-training $88

❑ **Critical Care**
- ❑ Individual $165
- ❑ Institutions $266
- ❑ *In-training $83

❑ **Dental**
- ❑ Individual $150
- ❑ Institutions $242

❑ **Emergency Medicine**
- ❑ Individual $170
- ❑ Institutions $263
- ❑ *In-training $85
- ❑ Send CME info

❑ **Facial Plastic Surgery**
- ❑ Individual $199
- ❑ Institutions $300

❑ **Foot and Ankle**
- Individual $160
- Institutions $232

❑ **Gastroenterology**
- ❑ Individual $190
- ❑ Institutions $276

❑ **Gastrointestinal Endoscopy**
- ❑ Individual $190
- ❑ Institutions $276

❑ **Hand**
- ❑ Individual $205
- ❑ Institutions $319

❑ **Heart Failure (NEW in 2005!)**
- ❑ Individual $99
- ❑ Institutions $149
- ❑ *In-training $49

❑ **Hematology/ Oncology**
- ❑ Individual $210
- ❑ Institutions $315

❑ **Immunology & Allergy**
- ❑ Individual $165
- ❑ Institutions $266

❑ **Infectious Disease**
- ❑ Individual $165
- ❑ Institutions $272

❑ **Clinics in Liver Disease**
- ❑ Individual $165
- ❑ Institutions $234

❑ **Medical**
- ❑ Individual $140
- ❑ Institutions $244
- ❑ *In-training $70
- ❑ Send CME info

❑ **MRI**
- ❑ Individual $190
- ❑ Institutions $290
- ❑ *In-training $95
- ❑ Send CME info

❑ **Neuroimaging**
- ❑ Individual $190
- ❑ Institutions $290
- ❑ *In-training $95
- ❑ Send CME info

❑ **Neurologic**
- ❑ Individual $175
- ❑ Institutions $275

❑ **Obstetrics & Gynecology**
- ❑ Individual $175
- ❑ Institutions $288

❑ **Occupational and Environmental Medicine**
- ❑ Individual $120
- ❑ Institutions $166
- ❑ *In-training $60

❑ **Ophthalmology**
- ❑ Individual $190
- ❑ Institutions $325

❑ **Oral & Maxillofacial Surgery**
- ❑ Individual $180
- ❑ Institutions $280
- ❑ *In-training $90

❑ **Orthopedic**
- ❑ Individual $180
- ❑ Institutions $295
- ❑ *In-training $90

❑ **Otolaryngologic**
- ❑ Individual $199
- ❑ Institutions $350

❑ **Pediatric**
- ❑ Individual $135
- ❑ Institutions $246
- ❑ *In-training $68
- ❑ Send CME info

❑ **Perinatology**
- ❑ Individual $155
- ❑ Institutions $237
- ❑ *In-training $78
- ❑ Send CME info

❑ **Plastic Surgery**
- ❑ Individual $245
- ❑ Institutions $370

❑ **Podiatric Medicine & Surgery**
- ❑ Individual $170
- ❑ Institutions $266

❑ **Primary Care**
- ❑ Individual $135
- ❑ Institutions $223

❑ **Psychiatric**
- ❑ Individual $170
- ❑ Institutions $288

❑ **Radiologic**
- ❑ Individual $220
- ❑ Institutions $331
- ❑ *In-training $110
- ❑ Send CME info

❑ **Sports Medicine**
- ❑ Individual $180
- ❑ Institutions $277

❑ **Surgical**
- ❑ Individual $190
- ❑ Institutions $299
- ❑ *In-training $95

❑ **Thoracic Surgery (formerly Chest Surgery)**
- ❑ Individual $175
- ❑ Institutions $255
- ❑ *In-training $88

❑ **Urologic**
- ❑ Individual $195
- ❑ Institutions $307
- ❑ *In-training $98
- ❑ Send CME info

*To receive in-training rate, orders must be accompanied by the name of affiliated institution, dates of residency and signature of coordinator on institution letterhead. Orders will be billed at the individual rate until proof of resident status is received.